# Disaster Mental Health Counseling

**Mark A. Stebnicki, PhD, LPC, DCMHS, CRC, CCM, CCMC,** is a professor and coordinator of the Military and Trauma Counseling Certificate Program he developed in the Department of Addictions and Rehabilitation Services at East Carolina University. He holds a doctoral (PhD) and master's degree in rehabilitation counseling. Dr. Stebnicki is a licensed professional counselor (LPC) in North Carolina and holds three national certifications: Diplomate in Clinical Mental Health Specialist (DCMHS) in Trauma Counseling through the American Mental Health Counselors Association (AMHCA); Certified Rehabilitation Counselor (CRC); and Certified Case Manager (CCM). He is also certified by the Washington, DC-based crisis response team, the National Organization for Victim Assistance (NOVA), and North Carolina's American Red Cross Disaster Mental Health crisis team. Dr. Stebnicki is an active teacher, researcher, and practitioner with over 30 years of experience working with the mental health and psychosocial rehabilitation needs of persons who have traumatic stress, chronic illnesses, and disabilities. In 2016, Dr. Stebnicki developed a military counseling training program for the state of North Carolina. The credential, The Certified Clinical Military Counselor (CCMC), is for those who train professional counselors to work with the medical, psychosocial, vocational, and mental health needs of active duty personnel, veterans, and family members.

Dr. Stebnicki has written seven books (four edited books with Dr. Irmo Marini), most recently *The Psychological and Social Impact of Illness and Disability* (7th ed.; forthcoming, Springer Publishing Company) and *The Professional Counselors' Desk Reference* (2016, Springer Publishing Company); and four single-author books, most recently *Empathy Fatigue: Healing the Mind, Body, and Spirit of Professional Counselors* (2008, Springer Publishing Company). He has over 28 articles in peer-reviewed journals, and has presented at over 100 regional, state, and national conferences, seminars, and workshops, on topics such as youth violence, traumatic stress, empathy fatigue, and the psychosocial aspects of adults with chronic illnesses and disabilities. Dr. Stebnicki has served on multiple professional counseling and accreditation boards. He served on the crisis response team for the Westside Middle School shootings in Jonesboro, Arkansas (March 24, 1998) and has done many stress debriefings with private companies, schools, and government employees after incidents of workplace violence, hurricanes, tornadoes, and floods. His youth violence program, the Identification, Early Intervention, Prevention, and Preparation (IEPP) Program, was awarded national recognition by the American Counseling Association (ACA) Foundation for its vision and excellence in the area of youth violence prevention. Other accolades include consulting with former President Bill Clinton's staff on addressing the students of Columbine High School after their critical incident (April 20, 1999).

# Disaster Mental Health Counseling

## Responding to Trauma in a Multicultural Context

Mark A. Stebnicki, PhD, LPC, DCMHS, CRC, CCM, CCMC

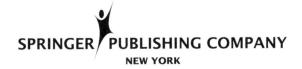

SPRINGER PUBLISHING COMPANY
NEW YORK

Springer Publishing Company, LLC
11 West 42nd Street
New York, NY 10036
www.springerpub.com

*Acquisitions Editor*: Nancy Hale
*Compositor*: Westchester Publishing Services

*ISBN*: 978-0-8261-3288-8
*e-book ISBN*: 978-0-8261-3289-5

**Instructor's Materials: Qualified instructors may request supplements by e-mailing textbook@springerpub.com:**
*Instructor's Manual*: 978-0-8261-3324-3
*Instructor's PowerPoints*: 978-0-8261-3325-0

16 17 18 19 20 / 5 4 3 2 1

**Library of Congress Cataloging-in-Publication Data**

Names: Stebnicki, Mark A., author.
Title: Disaster mental health counseling : responding to trauma in a multicultural context / Mark A. Stebnicki.
Description: New York : Springer Publishing Company, LLC, [2017] | Includes bibliographical references.
Identifiers: LCCN 2016035332 (print) | LCCN 2016037356 (ebook) | ISBN 9780826132888 (hard copy : alk. paper) | ISBN 9780826132895 (ebook)
Subjects: | MESH: Stress Disorders, Traumatic—therapy | Counseling—methods | Disaster Victims—psychology | Emigrants and Immigrants—psychology
Classification: LCC RC552.P67 (print) | LCC RC552.P67 (ebook) | NLM WM 172.5 | DDC 616.85/210651—dc23
LC record available at https://lccn.loc.gov/2016035332

Printed in the United States of America by McNaughton & Gunn.

*This book is dedicated to all those who have served in the military who have been deployed to war-torn countries and mobilized for humanitarian missions, civilian personnel who have served as first responders in homeland disasters, and disaster mental health and all counseling-related professions. You have served our homeland with honor and distinction. Your compassion, empathy, and professionalism for humanitarian causes during times of disaster are unparalleled. You have all assisted the minds, bodies, and spirits of many survivors on their transformational journey to healing trauma.*

# CONTENTS

# PREFACE

In the predawn hours of April 18, 1906, one of the largest natural disasters in the United States took place, killing over 3,000 persons. It was the San Francisco earthquake, estimated to be about a 7.8 magnitude by today's Richter scale rating. As a result of this earthquake, commercial buildings toppled, houses collapsed and shifted from their foundations, and water mains and gas lines were twisted and ruptured. This earthquake in California was felt along the fault-line from about 300 miles north to south. Within a 5-mile radius of the epicenter, more than 28,000 structures were totally decimated by explosions, blasts, and fires. In the aftermath, about 80% of San Francisco was destroyed. Over half of the city's population (400,000) was displaced. Persons were left homeless and thousands were listed as missing. Some moviegoers may have noted some similarities between the April 1906 earthquake and the May 2015 Hollywood movie release of *San Andreas*. Yet, Hollywood's depiction of major natural disasters and zombie apocalypses does not quite grasp the significant loss and grief or emotional and psychological trauma associated with person-made and natural disasters.

How easily we have forgotten this event among all the other disasters that have occurred before and after September 11, 2001.

Today, we are in the midst of a paradigm shift in the counseling and psychology profession when it comes to providing disaster mental health response to individuals and groups that have been affected. Extraordinary stressful and traumatic events, both person-made and natural disasters, have accelerated worldwide within the past 16 years. In the United States, the horrific terrorist attacks of Tuesday, September 11, 2001, as well as Hurricane Katrina, which took place on August 29, 2005, left emotional, physical, spiritual, and environmental scars on our minds, bodies, and spirits. In some ways, these 21st-century events mirrored the 20th-century San Francisco earthquake. However, comparisons are never therapeutic because all disasters and traumas have their own unique set of populations affected, natural and person-made characteristics, and other attributes that harm our minds, bodies, and spirits.

As we prepare for the next disaster, how easily we have forgotten the cataclysmic event that took place on December 26, 2004, where a tsunami and earthquake, registering 9.0 off the west coast of northern Sumatra, which claimed the lives of approximately 300,000 and injured over half-a-million people. To date, thousands of individuals have not been found in 14 countries that were affected, such as Sri Lanka, India, Indonesia, Malaysia, and Thailand. Where did all the disaster mental health counselors, international volunteers, angels, and earthly saints go who descended on these countries? Did they have to retreat back home for the sake of their own emotional, physical, and spiritual well-being? Who has taken their place? The desolation left in the aftermath of these particular critical events creates a sort of historical trauma among world cultures.

The foundation for this book was inspired by my own experiences in disaster and trauma response. During March 1998, I worked and lived in Jonesboro, Arkansas, where I served on the crisis response team for the Westside Middle School shootings. It was here where four students and one teacher were killed and 15 others were injured by 11- and 13-year-old shooters. Since that time, I have been trained in various crisis response models and have provided stress debriefings and group crisis response to persons employed in state and county government, private companies, day-care centers and schools, persons in the media, and survivors of brutal crimes, as well as individuals who have been at the epicenter of hurricanes, floods, and tornadoes.

Disasters occur in many different forms such as fires, floods, hurricanes, tornadoes, drought, earthquakes, school shootings, bombings at sporting events, biological epidemics and pandemics such as viruses, sociopolitical unrest, and war. These critical incidents require our complete and full attention. It necessitates a high level of empathy and compassion toward survivors of such traumatic events. As mental health professionals, we are constantly in a state of disaster preparedness. As a consequence, we have the potential to be emotionally, socially, physically, spiritually, and vocationally exhausted. I would propose that many of us are experiencing empathy fatigue as a direct consequence of providing services at the most intense levels of human suffering. The ensuing wars in Afghanistan, Iraq, the Middle East, and the fight against the terror group ISIS are also constant reminders of how fragile our physical safety, mental health, and overall well-being can be. For many, planet Earth does not appear to be a safe place to live because of the multitude of natural and person-made disasters.

Even though many Americans may be far from the epicenter of such critical incidents, many are affected at some level of consciousness by these critical incidents in the homeland and globally. Disaster scenarios are replayed on the nightly news, by quick-release television and Hollywood-style movies, and in the print and electronic media. We can watch tragedies and catastrophic events unfold in real time as they occur globally on a weekly basis. Despite the enormous loss of human life, psychological grief, physical pain, and spiritual suffering seen on the nightly news, first responders and disaster mental health professionals cannot watch from the sidelines. Failure to respond is not an option.

The consequence of extraordinary stressful and traumatic events affects the planet as a whole. So how do we come out of the darkness and into the light to be able to bring new meaning to such traumatic and critical events? As mental health counseling professionals, how can we facilitate good emotional, social, physical, psychological, spiritual, and occupational healing? Do we really understand other cultures' experiences of disaster and trauma? Are all disasters and the traumatic experiences treated the same or are they different in terms of the mental health response? And how can we actually help? These are just some questions that will be answered in *Disaster Mental Health*

*Counseling*. Thus, it is my intention that mental health professionals and others in the helping professions acquire the insight, knowledge, and skills to work optimally with individuals and groups that may be culturally different.

*Disaster Mental Health Counseling: Responding to Trauma in a Multicultural Context* provides a unique resource guide with practical application for graduate students, counselor educators and supervisors, and mental health practitioners to prepare to meet the intense challenges of disaster response in the 21st century. Each section of the book defines, describes, and applies the knowledge, awareness, and skills to work in a variety of disaster mental health counseling scenarios. Considerations are given to working with a variety of different cultures and special populations.

This book honors particularly the collective wisdom of indigenous cultural practices and philosophical beliefs of various world cultures and how they heal from traumatic experiences. Special consideration is given to understanding how disaster mental health counselors can provide culturally relevant approaches that recognize personal perspectives from disaster survivors, case study scenarios, guidelines for interventions, and best-practice strategies.

*Disaster Mental Health Counseling* is unique because of its cutting-edge research in areas related to the neurosciences of stress and trauma; interventions with the emerging populations of immigrants, refugees, and asylum seekers exposed to trauma from war-torn countries; its understanding of military versus civilian trauma interventions; the impact that global terrorism has on Americans; and how the search for personal meaning and cultivating resiliency and coping resources can be facilitated with disaster and trauma survivors.

Other topics that set apart *Disaster Mental Health Counseling* from other traditional books on trauma counseling and crisis response offer holistic perspectives in a range of important life areas. Chapters pertaining to the medical, psychosocial, vocational, and career transition suggest that co-occurring mental and physical health conditions can hinder the trauma survivors' abilities to get back to normal daily routines.

*Disaster Mental Health Counseling* goes beyond the traditional counseling theories and interventions text in that it offers real-world functional assessments, explains culturally relevant interventions, and provides readers with a structured approach for healing trauma: the Personal Growth Program to Heal Trauma (PGP-HT). Overall, mental health professionals should find *Disaster Mental Health Counseling* a practical guide for cultivating coping resources and resiliency approaches that are mindful of working with individuals, families, groups, communities, and cultures as they heal from experiences of disaster and trauma.

Indeed, disaster mental health counseling is intense work. These experiences can result in the counselors' own wounds that are continually revisited by their clients' life stories of chronic illness, disability, trauma, grief, loss, and extraordinary stressful events. Thus, guidelines are offered for the assessment and prevention of empathy fatigue and other professional fatigue syndromes. The intent is to recognize how to decrease the acute and cumulative long-term stressors associated with disaster and trauma response. Mostly, it is of paramount importance that mental health professionals develop a regular practice of self-care. I hope that you enjoy reading *Disaster Mental Health Counseling* as much as I enjoyed writing this work.

As an aid to using this book in the classroom, supplementary PowerPoints and an Instructor's Manual are available. To access these materials, qualified instructors should e-mail textbook@springerpub.com to receive a code to be used to download.

# CHAPTER 1

# Defining the Role and Function of Disaster Response

Extraordinary stressful and traumatic events, whether naturally occurring (e.g., hurricanes, earthquakes, floods), person made (e.g., school shootings, war, terrorism), or catastrophic injury and illness (e.g., brain injury, spinal cord injury, AIDS), are common experiences in the lives of many Americans (Elliott, 1997; Marini & Stebnicki, 2012). It is estimated that the typical American spends nearly 12 years of his or her life in a state of limited functioning because of chronic illness and disability acquired through disease or injury (Eisenberg, Glueckauf, & Zaretsky, 1999; Livneh & Antonak, 2012). Today cybercrimes, sordid acts of violence posted as social media, and digital terrorism have added another dimension of victim–survivorhood in the personal lives. In fact, worldwide, millions have fallen victim to computer fraud and hacking, costing the public personal loss of their hard-earned income. A minimum $500,000 loss per incident is reported among corporate institutions (Richardson, 2008). Overall, the loss of revenue in the private and public sectors is calculated in billions of dollars. It would appear that our lives are not safe engaging in our daily routines of social media, online banking, and the online purchase of goods and services.

Today, we are in the midst of a paradigm shift in coordinating efforts to deal with person-made, natural, technological, and biological disasters. These critical incidents have accelerated worldwide over the past 16 years. A humanitarian effort is required. It may have been the 1906 San Francisco earthquake that killed well over 3,000 persons that awakened Americans to the fact that we require a well-coordinated central command structure to assist immediately with the medical, physical, and mental health rescue of the survivors.

As the United States prepares for disasters in the 21st century, it is crucial not to forget the lessons learned from past tragedies like the horrific terrorist attacks of September 11, 2001, or Hurricane Katrina of August 2005. The next disaster is waiting for us on the five o'clock news. Globally, we may have already forgotten the cataclysmic event that took place on December 26, 2004, when a tsunami following an earthquake registering 9.0 off the west coast of northern Sumatra injured and claimed the lives of millions of people; to date, thousands have not been found in countries that were affected, such as Sri Lanka, India, Indonesia, Malaysia, and Thailand. The desolation left in the aftermath of this naturally occurring event creates a sort of historical trauma among world cultures closest to the epicenter. This chapter addresses the role and function of disaster response and the need for critical incident response teams that can assist with the immediate medical and mental health care needs of those affected by such incidents.

## WHAT IS A DISASTER?

*Disaster* is derived from the Latin words *dis* (against, away, or without) and *astrum* (star or planet), which some interpret as "the stars are against you" (Farber, 1967; Miller, 1998) or "without a star" (Solnit, 2009). One can measure disaster from a statistical perspective in terms of the degree, type, intensity, amount of loss to human life, injury and acquired disability, damage to the structural architectural environment, and the major devastation to the Earth itself. Disaster at the epicenter looks much different than calculating human causalities or architectural-infrastructural and financial-economic loss. To fully understand the mental health conditions related to disaster from ground zero (as opposed to flying over a disaster site in a helicopter), a definition must include the impact it has on the medical, physical, psychological, vocational, social, emotional, cognitive, cultural, spiritual, and psychosocial well-being of humankind. A good definition of disaster must also comprehensively delineate how to intervene in a variety of critical events: natural, person made, and/or technological.

The literature poses multiple definitions of the term *disaster* and is typically classified by categories, types, and etiologies of such critical events. Table 1.1 provides the primary categories of natural, person-made, and technological disasters, most of which are experienced in the global community. In regard to the typology of disasters, I prefer the term *person made* to other terms frequently seen in the literature, such as *man made* or *human made*. Despite the fact that males, rather than females, are perpetrators of most violent acts in society, the use of *man made* is not gender neutral and leaves out the reality that females do in fact perpetrate some acts of violence in society (e.g., bombings, terrorism). Additionally, it is my opinion that the use of *human made* does not reflect well on the positive attributes of human beings on the planet. The term *person made* implies individual personal responsibility for acts of violence (e.g., school shooting, bombings, rape, torture, terrorism). Although the person may not act alone during person-generated critical incidents, it is this collection of pathological attributes and traits expressed by each person, or perpetrator, which contributes toward acts of person-made disaster and trauma.

Although you may not be a survivor of a major earthquake (natural), war and ethnic genocide (person made), or a nuclear power plant contamination (technological), this book emphasizes the unique psychological, psychosocial, and sociocultural considerations for mental health professionals who deal with individuals and groups that have experienced natural, person-made, and technological disasters. Just as all chronic and persistent health conditions (e.g., diabetes, chronic obstructive pulmonary disease, cancers) are not medically defined, diagnosed, or treated the same, the chronic and

## TABLE 1.1 Categories, Types, and Etiology of Disasters

| Natural | Person Made | Technological |
|---|---|---|
| Avalanche/landslide | Bombing | Biological |
| Climate change | Building—structural collapse | Building—structural collapse |
| Disease and virus epidemic and pandemic | Cyber, computer, Internet, satellite technology issues | Cyber, computer, Internet, satellite technology issues |
| Drought | Economic recession and depression | Electrical and power plant outage and failure |
| Earthquake | Ethnic conflict | Environmental pollution, toxic spills, contamination, nuclear and other industrial incidents |
| Environmental pollution | Environmental pollution, toxic spills, contamination, nuclear, and other industrial incidents | Transportation incidents (i.e., plane, train, bus, auto crash, shipwreck) |
| Extreme heat and cold | Famine | |
| Flood | Force or voluntary displacement of ethnic populations | |
| Hurricane | Financial collapse | |
| Ice and snow storm | Genocide | |
| Insect, plant, and animal plague | Mass rioting | |
| Meteor | Overpopulation | |
| Thunderstorm, lightning, and high wind | Political violence | |
| Tornado | Public violence (i.e., theaters, shopping malls, sporting events) | |
| Tsunami | School violence | |

*(continued)*

| TABLE 1.1 Categories, Types, and Etiology of Disasters *(continued)* | | |
|---|---|---|
| **Natural** | **Person Made** | **Technological** |
| Wildfire | Transportation incidents (i.e., plane, train, bus, auto crash, shipwreck) | |
| | Terrorist acts | |
| | Torture | |
| | War | |

persistent mental health costs of natural, person-made, and technological disasters should not be defined, diagnosed, or treated the same by mental health counselors. Accordingly, any definition of disaster and disaster mental health counseling must consider the unique psychosocial and sociocultural attributes of the individuals, groups, and cultures that have been exposed to extraordinary stressful and traumatic events.

Solnit (2009) suggests that disasters, at their root meaning, are tragic, horrific, grievous, and have no redeeming value or positive effects to a culture, although disasters have the potential to provide an extraordinary window into how a culture can survive and heal from traumatic events. Attributing the meaning and purpose of a disaster to one's life or culture can be a path toward healing from traumatic experiences. Also within the definition of disaster, it may be judicious to include the interconnectedness of the concepts of being "the survivor," based on empowering individuals with coping and resiliency skills, versus being "the victim," usually a seriously injured individual or casualty of a disaster incident. Overall, in studying the epidemiology of disaster, the literature is clear that disaster knows no color, race, ethnicity, gender, socioeconomic group, and has no geographic preference.

The defining characteristics of almost all disasters are the individual's perception of the potential threat on the person's survival and positive coping abilities and the perception that critical events are uncontrollable and unpredictable (Friedman & Marsella, 1996). The following section helps functionally describe and define *disaster*. Regardless of how close one is from the epicenter, disaster is generally part of the human experience. With crisis comes opportunities for rebuilding and getting back to balance and learning how to live life again, only with a new meaning and purpose. Disaster organizations and volunteers play a significant role in helping cultures rise up from the ashes. The humanitarian effort in disaster response requires organized groups of like-minded individuals who have compassion, cultural sensitivity, and core principles dedicated to assisting others in healing from traumatic experiences.

## DISASTER ORGANIZATIONS

The section that follows discusses the role and function of four major organizations and agencies that have significant responsibilities, federal support, and influence at many levels during times of natural, person-made, and/or technological disasters. These organizations perform a critical operation in the humanitarian response to natural, person-made, and technological disasters. These organizations and agencies help define *disaster*. They are the American Red Cross (ARC), International Federation of Red Cross and Red Crescent Societies (IFRC), Federal Emergency Management Agency (FEMA), and Centers for Disease Control and Prevention (CDC). There are, of course, other disaster agencies that facilitate similar services from a state, regional, and local level in both the United States and worldwide. The intent is to describe disaster response emphasizing the importance of first responders and how mental health professionals can partner with other disaster response agencies that serve those affected by natural, person-made, and/or technological disasters. It is through partnering, capacity building, and coordinating efforts that best outcomes result when dealing with survivors at the epicenter of disaster. Without such organizations that have the ability to plan, organize, lead, and communicate with different operational networks, there is potential for chaos, civil unrest, and exacerbation of the traumatic experiences. Governments and organizations that believe in a compassionate response to provide humanitarian aid to human pain and suffering have found that partnering with others provides additional support systems in disaster planning, preparation, response, and recovery. Clearly, serving the humanitarian needs in large-scale disasters requires a central command structure that has a multidisciplinary close support system: one that can deploy a unified effort in the planning, preparation, and aftercare of mental and physical health care needs in a dynamic forward operations environment.

### American Red Cross

The ARC (n.d.-a) organization was founded in 1881 in Washington, DC, by Clara Barton. Barton and her colleagues created a model for organizing public health, education, safety, and a humanitarian response to disaster. Historically, disaster organizations such as the ARC began their mission with a public health and safety agenda, providing first aid, water safety, and public health nursing programs. The ARC early in its history also served America's veterans, providing public health, in-home care for veterans with disabilities, and health education for the veteran and family members. Disaster organizations as a whole were not designed to serve in the capacity of providing disaster mental health response. Rather, their mission was to serve in matters of public health, education, and safety with civilian populations. It was not until later that disaster organizations expanded their roles and functions serving the psychological and humanitarian needs in times of critical incidents, bringing balance back to communities, regions, and the nation.

The ARC model was based on Europe's international Red Cross model. The ARC was ratified in the United States in 1882 and received its first congressional charter in 1900 to serve as the primary organization in America to form a national leadership that initially served in the capacity of public health, education, and public safety. Later in its history, the

ARC expanded its humanitarian efforts for organizing, planning, and implementation of disaster response in a variety of critical incidents in all 50 states. The ARC also coordinates disaster response with Homeland Security and State Police agencies. Also, at the request of the various American military branches, the ARC mobilizes a volunteer force of medical support, food, shelter, and clothing needs to civilian survivors in war-torn countries across the globe. It also coordinates and deploys in disaster incidents with other international Red Cross organizations to provide an international presence of support.

ARC's mission perhaps serves as a model to help define disaster. The constructs within ARC's mission statement may provide a glimpse into a working definition of disaster and disaster mental health response. Its mission is stated as: "The American Red Cross prevents and alleviates human suffering in the face of emergencies by mobilizing the power of volunteers and generosity of donors" (ARC, n.d.-b, p.1).* The emphasis in this definition is on serving the humanistic needs of individuals and groups in crisis. This organization may assist in expanding the role and function of mental health providers within disaster mental health response. The ARC coordinates with national, state, and regional professional psychological, counseling, and mental health organizations with the intent to integrate the mental health triage and screening component of services during critical incidents. Some states provide training and certification for mental health counselors, psychologists, and social workers to be available for brief assessment, triage, and brief solution-focused interventions. Practitioners must be certified through ARC disaster mental health training programs so as to be allowed onsite during a critical incident. These approaches and interventions are discussed throughout this book. Given ARC's lengthy history in disaster preparation, critical incident management, and postdisaster support, mental health professionals have much to gain by translating ARC's mission and objectives into models of disaster mental health counseling.

## International Federation of Red Cross and Red Crescent Societies

One particular organization that has been a mainstay internationally in disaster response is the IFRC (2015). The IFRC was founded in 1919, in Paris, in the aftermath of World War I. The IFRC defines *disaster* as "a sudden, calamitous event that seriously disrupts the functioning of a community or society and causes human, material, and economic losses that exceed the community's or society's ability to cope using its own resources" (p. 1). IFRC's definition appears to imply a sense of powerlessness, vulnerability, and inescapable hazard that individuals and groups experience during and after a disaster. Undoubtedly, within this definition are the substantial negative impacts that disaster and traumatic experiences have on one's mind, body, and spirit.

Although the IFRC appears to place less emphasis on the mental health aspects of disaster response (e.g., assessment, triage, intervention), compared with the ARC and professional counseling associations in the United States, the IFRC appears to be a

*Reprinted from http://www.redcross.org/about-us/who-we-are/mission-and-values by the American Red Cross by permission of: American Red Cross.

leader in organizing, planning, and implementing the humanistic effort of compassion relief worldwide. Given the international presence during natural, person-made, and technological disasters, there appears to be a significant emphasis for IFRC volunteers to have an increased cultural understanding and sensitivity to work within specific populations or geographic areas where they are mobilized.

It would appear that disaster mental health counselors have much to learn from the IFRC from a sociocultural perspective, given their deployments to various geographic regions globally. Truly, the nature of disaster response is a multicultural experience. Disaster mental health counselors, pending few or no language barriers, have unused opportunities to develop the requisite knowledge and skills needed when working with critical incidents cross-culturally.

## Mercy Corps

Mercy Corps (2016), founded in 1979, is a global organization of over 4,000 staff members and volunteers who assist indigenous groups in over 40 countries to assist in the humanitarian response in natural disasters and those civilians affected by war. More than 93% of Mercy Corps's field staff members are indigenous to the countries they serve. Mercy Corps's website indicates that they have no political or religious agenda. They have served over 190 million individuals and have partnered with local cultural community leaders to facilitate, coordinate, and organize resources that are culturally relevant in times of emergency response.

Mercy Corps focuses on efforts of sustainable and innovative change to assist culturally indigenous groups to thrive and not just survive. There are multiple projects that focus on such global initiatives of sustainable agriculture, education, health care, women's rights, disaster preparedness, mental health care, special populations at risk, urban planning, and many other life areas of concern. It appears to have a strong commitment to research, development, and implementation of evidence-based practices. It has published multiple case studies, evaluations, reports, and other technical documents to share with the world community of its innovative achievements.

The board of directors of Mercy Corps is composed primarily of many prestigious well-to-do, high-achieving Americans who identify as college professors and university administrators; corporate chief executive officers (CEOs) in the fields of business, education, energy, and technology; entrepreneurs in a variety of professions; best-selling authors; and many other innovators. Mercy Corps is a 501c (3) tax-exempt organization that relies on large and small donations to serve the needs of the most disadvantaged populations at home and abroad.

## Federal Emergency Management Agency

FEMA (2015) is another example of a disaster organization that is similar yet different from State Police agencies and National Guard organizations that serve to protect citizens in the aftermath of disasters. FEMA, now under the Department of Homeland Security, is responsible for coordinating efforts and partnering with local authorities to cultivate unified efforts in the protection of U.S. citizens.

FEMA was signed into law under President Carter's administration in April 1979. Its mission ". . . is to support our citizens and first responders to ensure that as a nation we work together to build, sustain and improve our capability to prepare for, protect against, respond to, recover from and mitigate all hazards" (p. 1). FEMA's organizational chart shows multiple departments, divisions, offices, and regional authorities organized under the Department of Homeland Security. FEMA is a substantial U.S. government agency that appears military-like at least organizationally, with its chain of command, partnerships with other emergency management regional authorities, and the extensive personnel at many different levels of operation. It has a considerable budget that helps coordinate emergency management systems through local, state, regional, and tribal emergency management systems. Given the size, influence, and status of FEMA within the disaster response community, it is in a unique position to act as a catalyst to create dynamic partnerships with public security, public health, and other public safety agencies.

In response to looking at disaster scenarios over the next 15 years, which FEMA calls "the age of uncertainty," it has launched a Strategic Foresight Initiative (SFI; FEMA, 2012) that addresses a range of critical incidents. The SFI report identifies challenges within the emergency management community in dealing with such issues as the shift in demographics, unauthorized immigrants coming into the United States, older aging adult populations, persons with chronic illnesses and disabilities, technology, terrorism in the homeland, pandemics, drought, and multiple other critical incidents. Throughout the SFI report is the underlying theme that "the emergency management community faces increasing complexity and decreasing predictability in its operating environment . . ." (p. 2). Hence, it appears to be predicting critical events in multiple areas with comprehensive plans to handle everything from natural, person-made, and technological disasters and nothing short of a zombie apocalypse. Overall, the SFI report details the emergency and disaster response communities' limitations, vulnerabilities, and challenges in negotiating multiple resources by the year 2030.

One gets the sense after reading the SFI report that much like the military, public safety, and public health surveillance systems, there are no days off. Thus, FEMA must maintain a status of active duty at all times, fulfilling its obligation to the homeland by standing ready to react and respond to any critical incident that may arise at any given moment. The point is that emergency management and being in a constant state of disaster preparedness, at whatever level of contribution, can be an exhausting existence. Many seasoned mental health professionals know early in their career what it is like being on-call 24/7/365. It is extremely difficult to plan time for health and wellness activities, family events, and social activities. Such a lifestyle creates the physical, psychological, emotional, social, spiritual, and occupational exhaustion of what I have called empathy fatigue. Chapter 19 presents in detail how to cultivate resiliency and self-care activities to reduce the effects of empathy fatigue and other professional fatigue syndromes.

The affirming outcome of FEMA's SFI document is the contribution of over 800 experts from various disciplines, which was garnered over a 4-day workshop. The contributors report good information and statistical facts by which decisions can be made within the emergency management community. FEMA has undertaken a complexity of different responsibilities to plan, organize, lead, and support essential capabilities, innovative models and tools, and dynamic partnerships with businesses, nonprofits, public works, and other local, state, regional, and tribal government authorities. Clearly, FEMA has defined and delineated the role and function of *emergency management* through its organizational structure, action plan, and strategic initiatives.

Absent from the SFI report, as noted in the statement of "15 strategic needs," are the psychological, emotional, social, cultural, spiritual, and psychosocial costs relating to how we may respond to everything from an Ebola epidemic in the United States to another meteor falling somewhere in New Mexico, or a San Francisco earthquake like the one that occurred 100 years ago. As mental health professionals, there are therapeutic advantages to "talking about the elephant in the room" and what the future of disaster response holds in 2030. Being proactive is critical in the prediction, planning, and creation of options and alternatives in disaster scenarios. The wisdom we can gain from a unified effort is how to cope, adapt, and be more resilient during unpredictable natural, person-made, and/or technological critical events that occur on the planet by 2030.

## Centers for Disease Control and Prevention

In the 21st century, the CDC (2015b) is considered the first responder in the mobilization of resources to protect the medical and physical health concerns of U.S. citizens. The CDC monitors and responds to deadly life-threatening viruses and biological toxins that may cause severe health risks to Americans. It acts in the role of the first responder, much like law enforcement agencies, firefighters, and paramedics who provide physical and medical rescue in times of disaster. The CDC is another federal government agency that stands ready to guard and protect Americans from health, safety, and security threats, both foreign and domestic. They have an emergency operations center that functions much like a hospital emergency department that has continuous operations 24/7 and 365 days a year, with state-of-the-art technology for receiving, reporting, and communicating health-related threats to the proper authorities. They have a critical incident management system that handles the health, safety, and well-being of all Americans across all 50 states. Overall, the CDC fields more than 1,500 calls per month from health care facilities, public health agencies and organizations, military bases, and other state and federal entities.

Although the CDC has a much different threat to contend with than person-made critical incidents, it has an enormous task of protecting both our physical and mental health from a variety of chronic illnesses, diseases, and disabilities. The CDC (2015b) indicates in its mission statement, "CDC works 24/7 to protect America from health, safety, and security threats, both foreign and domestic. Whether diseases start at home or abroad, are acute or chronic, curable or preventable, human error or deliberate attack, CDC fights disease and supports communities and citizens to do the same" (p. 1). To accomplish this mission, the CDC requires a significant budget for research and development using the scientific and medical models to conduct clinical trials, monitor diseases and illnesses, and cultivate and support cutting-edge research that could save millions of lives worldwide.

There appears to be a significant interest in chronic illnesses and diseases that occur around the globe. The primary intent is to be proactive in monitoring the health and welfare, exposure to viruses, and life-threatening illnesses of individuals and groups from other countries. Epidemics and pandemics are a stark reminder of how porous the borders are in the United States. The transmission of illnesses and diseases finds many ways to terrorize the human blood and immune system. This can happen through insects, birds, and rats, or by water and air. Global disease threats never sleep or take a day off. Once exposed to an epidemic or pandemic virus, the human body has the potential to proliferate unhealthy bacteria, abnormal cells, pathogens, and microorganisms that are toxic, life threatening, and deadly. It is much like the chain reaction in the emotional brain, sympathetic–parasympathetic nervous system, and stress hormones that launch a panic or anxiety attack.

The Ebola outbreak in West Africa has taken center stage in the war of lethal diseases. For many readers, West Africa may not seem close to where you live in the world, so Ebola may not be viewed as a concern. However, there are 27,000 Ebola cases reported worldwide in at least nine countries. In 2015, there were four confirmed cases of Ebola in the United States (CDC, 2015c). Overall, in 2015 there were 11,000 deaths due to confirmed cases of the deadly Ebola virus. Contact tracing is critical in the Ebola outbreak because the natural host has not yet been identified. Thus, scientists are not quite sure how it spreads. Much like a California wild fire, there is little that can be done at this time to contain the virus and keep it from spreading. Unfortunately, education, information, preparation, and planning for disaster may be all we can do for this year. It is perplexing to humanity and may prompt an existential crisis for some to think of deadly viruses as a natural disaster, at least in terms of its classification. Indeed, any virus is biological in nature. However, the Ebola virus is a mutation that the human DNA has manufactured. It is not generated synthetically in some clinical laboratory setting.

It is clear that in defining disaster, we must consider the biopsychosocial aspects of what the human body is capable of producing. Aside from other human-generated critical events (e.g., war, torture, weapons, and chemicals of mass destruction), the CDC has an enormous task to serve and protect the overall health and wellness of Americans. The CDC has extensive information on its website (CDC, 2015a) relating to the psychological, emotional, and mental health aspects of disaster. It partners with other government agencies such as the Substance Abuse and Mental Health Services Association (SAMHSA, 2015). There is a wealth of information for both consumers and medical and mental health care practitioners treating patients who may have been at the epicenter of a natural, person-made, and/or technological disaster.

## CONCLUDING REMARKS

It is imperative that the disaster response community be organized to ensure that mental health practitioners can build, sustain, and improve our capability to prepare for, protect against, and respond to a variety of natural, person-made, and technological disasters. Currently, there is a movement for recognizing the psychological, psychosocial, and emotional impacts of posttrauma experiences, as well as complex and prolonged grief, when disaster strikes. The psychological effects and the need for mental health interventions are well documented in the literature. In the next chapter, some professional counseling associations and organizations are drawn together, which have cultivated relationships with federal, state, and international critical incident management organizations and agencies that help lead the humanitarian effort in healing from disaster.

## REFERENCES

American Red Cross. (n.d.-a). Our history. Retrieved from http://www.redcross.org/about-us/history

American Red Cross. (n.d.-b). Mission & values: Red Cross mission, vision, and fundamental values. Reprinted from http://www.redcross.org/about-us/who-we-are/mission-and-values by permission of: American Red Cross.

Barton, C. (1898). *The Red Cross*. Washington, DC: American National Red Cross.

Centers for Disease Control and Prevention. (2015a). Coping with a disaster or traumatic event. Retrieved from http://emergency.cdc.gov/mentalhealth

Centers for Disease Control and Prevention. (2015b). Emergency preparedness and response. Retrieved from http://emergency.cdc.gov/cerc/index.asp

Centers for Disease Control and Prevention. (2015c). 2014 Ebola outbreak in West Africa: Case counts. Retrieved from http://www.cdc.gov/vhf/ebola/outbreaks/2014-west-africa/case-counts.html

Eisenberg, M. G., Glueckauf, R. L., & Zaretsky, H. H. (1999). *Medical aspects of disability: A handbook for the rehabilitation professionals*. New York, NY: Springer Publishing.

Elliott, D. (1997). Traumatic events: Prevalence and delayed recall in the general population. *Journal of Consulting and Clinical Psychology, 65*, 811–820.

Farber, I. J. (1967). Psychological aspects of mass disasters. *Journal of the National Medical Association, 59*, 340–345.

Federal Emergency Management Agency. (2012). Crisis response and disaster resilience 2030: Forging strategic action in an age of uncertainty. Progress report highlighting the 2010–2011 insights of the Strategic Foresight Initiative. Retrieved from http://www.fema.gov/media-library-data/20130726 -1816-25045-5167/sfi_report_13.jan.2012_final.docx.pdf

Federal Emergency Management Agency. (2015). About FEMA. Retrieved from http://www.fema.gov/ about-agency

Friedman, M. J., & Marsella, A. J. (1996). Posttraumatic stress disorder: An overview of the concept. In A. J. Marsella, M. J. Friedman, E. T. Gerrity, & R. M. Scurfield (Eds.), *Ethnocultural aspects of posttraumatic stress disorder: Issues, research, and clinical applications* (pp. 11–32). Washington, DC: American Psychological Association.

The International Federation of Red Cross and Red Crescent Societies. (2015). What is a disaster? Retrieved from https://www.ifrc.org/en/what-we-do/disaster-management/about-disasters/what-is-a -disaster

Livneh, H., & Antonak, R. F. (2012). Psychological adaptation to chronic illness and disability: A primer for counselors. In I. Marini & M. A. Stebnicki (Eds.), *The psychological and social impact of illness and disability* (6th ed., pp. 95–107). New York, NY: Springer Publishing.

Marini, I., & Stebnicki, M. A. (2012). *The psychological and social impact of illness and disability* (6th ed.). New York, NY: Springer Publishing.

Mercy Corps. (2016). About us. Retrieved from https://www.mercycorps.org/about-us

Miller, L. (1998). *Shocks to the system: Psychotherapy of traumatic disability syndromes.* New York, NY: W. W. Norton.

Richardson, R. (2008). CSI computer crime and security survey. Retrieved from http://www.sis.pitt .edu/jjoshi/courses/IS2150/Fall11/CSIsurvey2008.pdf

Solnit, R. (2009). *A paradise built in hell: The extraordinary communities that arise in disaster.* New York, NY: Penguin Books.

Substance Abuse and Mental Health Services Association. (2015). Disaster preparedness and recovery. Retrieved from http://store.samhsa.gov/term/Disaster-Preparedness-Recovery

# CHAPTER 2

# What Is Disaster Mental Health Counseling?

In my clinical practice as a licensed professional counselor (LPC) in Arkansas and North Carolina, I have provided stress debriefings, group crisis response, and disaster mental health (DMH) counseling to individuals and groups in middle schools, high schools, and colleges/universities; communities and neighborhoods; private companies; not-for-profit organizations; journalists in print and electronic media; military veterans; and employees working for state and county governments. I have been at the epicenter of hurricanes and floods while living on the North Carolina coast and in the Midwest and mid-South where tornadoes occur frequently in the spring and summer months. I have also provided crisis response to survivors of brutal crimes and sexual assaults, as well as witnesses to homicides, fatal motor vehicle accidents, child accidental swimming pool drownings, bank robberies, and incidents of workplace accidents and violence. My most intense experience was when I served on the crisis response team (CRT) for the Westside Middle School shootings, Jonesboro, Arkansas. I lived in Jonesboro and worked in the department of psychology and counseling at Arkansas State University. I was in Jonesboro on March 24, 1998, where four students and one teacher were killed and 15 others were injured by 11- and 13-year-old shooters who would be tried as juvenile offenders and released as adults at 21 years of age.

During most of these critical incidents (CIs), where I intervened within 24 to 48 hours, I primarily facilitated DMH response based on the 40-hour training I received by the Washington, DC-based National Organization for Victims Assistance (NOVA, 2015). Since Westside, I have been trained in various other models of crisis, trauma, stress debriefing, and DMH response. Each model has its own theory base, interventions, and means for assessing, triaging, and providing mental health interventions for individuals and groups.

When mental health practitioners are mobilized for disaster response, most seasoned professionals use a wide range of eclectic counseling approaches. These are typically interventions that have been learned through a variety of experiences. At times, professionals facilitate DMH counseling in ways that match their style of therapy and/or what works best for them when serving individuals and groups while at ground zero.

*DMH counseling* helps clarify some of the confusion related to definitions, concepts, and models of intervention through an extensive use of research-based literature and resources for best practices. It is of paramount importance that mental health professionals be open to the idea that each CI has its own unique psychological, social, emotional, cultural, and psychosocial response. Not all natural, person-made, or technological/biological disasters should be treated the same.

The various definitions and models of DMH response may appear the same, similar, but yet different. Competent and ethical mental health counselors are aware of the appropriate application for diagnosing, triaging, and intervening across different settings, cultures, and types of traumatic experiences. In other words, competent mental health professionals understand the cultural and clinical differences between a tornado in rural Arkansas, a wildfire in California or Canada, and a Chicago neighborhood exploding in gun violence. Overall, as most seasoned counselors and psychotherapists might agree that establishing a person-centered and culturally appropriate rapport is essential in developing an optimal working alliance with individuals and groups, empathy and compassion for a survivor's sense of loss, grief, and suffering can go a long way in healing trauma.

## DEFINING DMH COUNSELING

Disaster response is not a new phenomenon in the field of mental health counseling. In the early 1970s, the psychology and counseling literature was replete with brief and immediate interventions for clients who were in crisis (Aguilera & Messick, 1974; Lester & Brockopp, 1973; Specter & Claiborn, 1973). Perhaps the defining characteristics of almost all mental health disasters are the individual's perception of potential threat on the person's survival and his or her perception of how he or she can or cannot control and predict the critical event (Friedman & Marsella, 1996). Some practitioners and researchers across a variety of disciplines describe the role and function of DMH based on their particular occupation (i.e., psychiatry, psychology, mental health), as a "first responder" (i.e., paraprofessional crisis worker, firefighters, paramedics, law enforcement), or within a cultural content (i.e., impact of tsunami on Asian countries, psychological impact of Hurricane Katrina on African Americans). Included within the various definitions and constructs of DMH is the survivor's experience of *vulnerability* and being a *victim* or *survivor* of a CI. This construct is most often contained within the definition of DMH counseling because of the inescapable sense of unexpectedness, unpredictability, shock, and powerlessness associated with being at the epicenter of such traumatic experiences.

Other constructs related to the general definition of disaster are delineated in McFarlane and Norris's (2006) research. These authors suggest disasters have an acute onset, are collectively experienced by groups, and have a beginning and ending point. Because disasters are experienced by large and small groups of people, then by their nature they involve a community of individuals that make attempts to get back to their daily normal routines. Thus, the concept of "community resilience" has been used in the literature (Norris, Stevens, Pfefferbaum, Wyche, & Pfefferbauam, 2008), which studies groups' and cultures' capacities to bounce back from adversity. This concept also takes into account how resilient communities and cultures are collectively and how effective disaster readiness and response become of particular importance, especially when dealing with chronic, reoccurring conditions that may be natural (e.g., hurricanes, tornadoes, floods), technological/biological (e.g., cyber bullying, environmental hazards), or person made (e.g., war, ethnic cleansings, forced geographic relocation). Indeed, the concept of resiliency has been studied quite extensively in multiple contexts, but it becomes particularly critical when defining variables that assist individuals and groups to bounce back from adversity while reducing acute and posttraumatic stress symptoms.

## Trauma Versus Crisis

Trauma, as experienced by individuals, groups, and cultures, has existed since the beginning of time. Defining trauma has been a challenge for persons in the social and behavioral sciences, as well as in humanistic theories of counseling. Accordingly, there continues to be a lack of consensus related to terms, concepts, definitions, and models that relate to the field of traumatology and crisis intervention theory. This chapter helps elucidate some of these distinctions in definitions, constructs, and theories related to disaster, trauma, and crisis. Otherwise, some professionals may confuse traditional counseling and psychotherapy theories and interventions with brief interventions related to critical incident stress debriefing (CISD), crisis interventions, or trauma response.

*Trauma counseling* is a broad term used to describe a type of counseling approach that is aimed at reducing the emotional and psychological effects of trauma and the prevention of posttraumatic stress disorder (PTSD; Raphael & Dobson, 2001). Wilson, Friedman, and Lindy (2001) suggest that Sigmund Freud grappled extensively with the concept of PTSD from 1895 to 1920 in several written works and lectures. Freud understood the anxiety and stress associated with violence and one's traumatic reaction. He concluded that if a traumatic event was at the magnitude and intensity that were overwhelmingly beyond one's coping resources, then the trauma experience could breach the stimulus barrier of the ego defenses, producing a psychic reaction that could influence one's behaviors and personality. It is not the intent of this chapter to review the historical theoretical debate surrounding PTSD but rather point out the complexity of the phenomena of PTSD and constructs related to trauma and crisis.

The terms *crisis* and *trauma* are often used interchangeably in the trauma and disaster mental health literature. Yet, there are distinct differences because of the theories and constructs that underlie these terms (Echterling, Presbury, & Edson McKee, 2005). The term *crisis intervention* was an approach that was first developed from Caplan's (1964) original model of preventive intervention that followed a stressful life event. *Crisis* was derived from the early Greek word *krinein* that translates into "to decide." The Chinese character or symbol of *crisis* has the meaning generally of the potential benefits that one can learn from the opportunity of a crisis or the detrimental effects that could potentially occur in the aftermath of a critical event.

Early crisis intervention models applied brief crisis interventions with incidents of bereavement, motor vehicle accidents, and acute illness and injury, and have been shown to be effective when used with high-risk populations to reduce suicide (Raphael & Dobson, 2001). The concept of crisis suggests that the individual is confronted by an enormous life-changing event (e.g., divorce, loss of a loved one, job lay-off, diagnosis of an illness or disease, culture shock), whereas trauma typically refers to a serious physical and/or psychological injury sustained as a result of a life-threatening or horrific experience. There are obvious mental health consequences, symptoms, and conditions associated with both crisis and trauma (e.g., PTSD, anxiety, and major depressive disorders).

It is my contention from a person-centered perspective that the trauma survivor defines his or her experience of crisis or trauma. In other words, the individual chooses the language and depiction of his or her traumatic or crisis experience, not the mental health counselor. The competent and skilled mental health practitioner listens to the client's core communication of how he or she describes his or her experience and then focuses on the client's story within a person-centered and cultural context.

Mental health counselors can help clarify the client's experiences of crisis or trauma. However, definitions, theoretical models, and psychological debate are of little importance to the pain and suffering felt by trauma survivors. Life is somewhat different, however, for researchers and theorists in the fields of traumatology and DMH counseling. It is in this context where terms are defined, conceptualized, theorized, and summarized with the intent to offer guidelines for evidence-based treatment protocols. Foundationally, DMH counseling approaches need to be effective and functional in order for persons to develop enough coping resources and resiliency to heal from trauma.

Overall, crisis and trauma theory in evidence-based practice can complement the therapeutic process. However, it is important that the survivor validate and confirm his or her perceptions of mental health counseling interventions and level of "helpfulness" in terms of getting back to balance and achieving optimal levels of mental and emotional well-being. Thus, it is essential that DMH counseling theories and approaches integrate well with clients' experiences of trauma or crisis.

## In Search of a Holistic Definition of DMH

It is beyond the scope and intention of this chapter to describe, delineate, compare, and contrast the theoretical and conceptual models in trauma, crisis, and disaster response. This work would be more appropriate for a doctoral dissertation. The interested readers should consult the References at the end of this chapter. The literature itself uses the terms *trauma*, *crisis*, and *disaster* the same, differently, and interchangeably, which does not assist in building theoretical constructs, developing screening instruments, or offering guidelines of symptom checklists.

Many contributors to theory, research, and practice in DMH counseling have provided models and theories for effective integrative therapies to assist persons in crisis or trauma. Levers, Ventura, and Bledsoe (2012) provide salient features of trauma-informed and trauma-specific models that are systematic approaches for treating individuals in crisis who have sustained a variety of traumatic experiences. Trauma-informed and trauma-specific models reflect interventions, therapies, and treatment programs designed to intervene in specific CIs and traumatic events. In order to achieve the effectiveness of trauma interventions, protocols, or therapies, these programs must be measured and validated alongside current evidence-based practices. These are difficult tasks for researchers because the authors who endorse specific models of trauma interventions (e.g., dialectical behavior therapy [DBT], mindfulness stress reduction, cognitive behavioral therapy [CBT], exposure therapy, eye movement desensitization and reprocessing [EMDR]) imply some level of significance or improvement in emotional regulation, reduction in stress and posttraumatic stress, interpersonal effectiveness, or other self-reported affirmations as they relate to use with specific populations and critical events.

## Proposed Definition for DMH Counseling

There are a variety of psychological and emotional symptoms exhibited by shared trauma experiences and by individuals and groups closest to the epicenter of disaster. Thus, any definition related to disaster and DMH counseling must be holistic and person-centered in nature. It should also include the cost to one's social, emotional, physical, and psychological health and well-being. Thus, I propose the following definition for *DMH counseling* as it relates to material discussed in this text. DMH counseling *involves immediate and short- and long-term counseling interventions that result from natural, person-made, technological, and/or biological catastrophic events where such critical events impact the medical, physical, psychological, social, emotional, cognitive, cultural, spiritual, occupational, and psychosocial well-being of individuals, groups, and world cultures.*

Implied in this definition offered for *DMH counseling* is that counseling interventions must be intentional and achieve some level of effectiveness as measured by the individual, family, and/or cultures' perception of improving one's physical, emotional, psychological, mental, and spiritual well-being. Also implicit in this definition is that (a) DMH response utilizes the knowledge and skills of the counseling profession to facilitate interventions during disaster and trauma response, (b) all interventions should be holistic in nature where professional counselors choose specific interventions based on the specific CI and population they are serving, and (c) all interventions are culturally based and may require attunement to a specific culture.

Essentially, the therapeutic alliance and person-centered relationship is the foundation of connection and rapport with persons traumatized by disasters. From the client perspective, mere use of the terms *trauma*, *crisis*, or *disaster* may or may not resonate with the client's physical, psychological, emotional, cognitive, or sociocultural experiences. For many survivors who have been at the epicenter of a life-threatening CI, the need for survival, getting back to balance, and achieving optimal health and well-being are of critical importance. No words can describe the horrific, life-threatening, or catastrophic experiences that some individuals have endured. Thus, from the humanistic point of view, the persons themselves define their experiences of trauma, crisis, or disaster.

## The Impact of Trauma and Disaster on Culture

Trauma and disaster impact both the individual and how he or she interacts with the culture and environment. All indigenous cultural groups have healing practices. There is an observable form, structure, organization, theory, ritual practice, philosophical belief, and system for healing the mind, body, and spirit. Individuals and groups that have shared trauma stories and experiences of vulnerability have much to share with the mental health profession. Thus, mental health counselors have an obligation to be aware of how disasters impact the traumatic experiences of different individuals within a cultural context and with vulnerable or special populations. Otherwise, DMH interventions may not be facilitated in a culturally appropriate or sensitive manner. There is much to learn from the plethora of trauma stories and stories of resiliency and healing as told by individuals and groups from a variety of different cultures and populations.

In fact, mental health professionals in the United States have much to learn from the disaster response experiences of the International Federation of Red Cross and Red Crescent Societies (IFRC, 2015) group of volunteers who are deployed to different regions of the globe. Facilitating mental health counseling interventions cross-culturally is challenging primarily because Western models of DMH response, psychological first aid, or trauma counseling may not fit neatly into a disaster survivor's cultural worldview.

Herein lies the confusion and problems with developing a usable definition of DMH counseling and the accompanying mental health models that are the foundation of disaster response. The primary issue here is that models of crisis, trauma, or DMH response are built primarily on definitions, constructs, and perceptions related to Western models of counseling theory and technique. The term *DMH counseling* is an oxymoron in a sense. This is primarily because mental health counseling has a predisposition and bias that relates to Western models of psychological first aid, crisis response, mental health assessment, triage, and trauma interventions. The expectation and anticipation with such models imply that disaster survivors must verbalize or talk about their traumatic experiences. The underlying thesis is that "verbally sharing your story" is psychologically healthy. For instance, in the American Red Cross (ARC) model of DMH services there are components that specifically relate to (a) mental health or psychological first aid, psychological triage, and mental health surveillance; (b) promoting resiliency and coping skills that are enhanced by psychological first aid and psychoeducation; and (c) providing targeted DMH crisis interventions, assessment and referral, and support and advocacy (ARC, 2012). This may not be culturally appropriate for some individuals and groups, which is discussed in detail in chapters related to multicultural counseling. Consequently, an operational definition of DMH counseling must include culturally relevant concepts, approaches, and interventions. Definitions and constructs in DMH counseling must bridge the gap between Western mental health counseling and intervening in disaster scenarios with culturally different groups in the United States and global populations.

Most world cultures heal from trauma through their tribal rituals, village, communicating with family elders, and seeking wisdom from shaman and other spiritual leaders (Moodley & West, 2005). Many cultural groups inside and outside the United States do not have therapeutic engagements with licensed mental health practitioners. Thus, I contend that our current models of DMH response may not fit neatly with a variety of cultural and subcultural groups. For example, Syrian refugees, immigrants, and asylum seekers may not adapt well to Western mental health diagnosis and treatment models during trauma and disaster response (Stebnicki, 2015). Accordingly, *DMH counseling*, with an emphasis on *responding to trauma in a multicultural perspective*, helps elucidate the impact that culture has on the traumatic experiences of disaster survivors cross-culturally. This book offers culturally centered approaches that have some universal value during a disaster response (i.e., empathy, screenings for mood and affect disorders). However, the cultural application of such interventions (i.e., cultural empathy) is described for real-world application.

## COMMONLY USED TERMS AND DEFINITIONS IN THE FIELD OF DMH COUNSELING

Pursuant to my research for *DMH counseling* and my professional experiences in DMH response, the focus on disaster response has changed somewhat, primarily because of the (a) nature and severity of the CIs (e.g., increase in mass shootings such as school and workplace violence resulting in multiple deaths), (b) types of interventions and services provided (e.g., debriefings, defusing, critical incident response [CIR] with public and private entities), (c) shift toward serving different groups of primary and secondary survivors (e.g., paramedics, police, nurses, counselors), and (d) research suggesting that immediate and brief interventions decrease the negative long-term symptoms associated with posttraumatic stress symptoms (e.g., depression, suicide, nightmares). The following (listed alphabetically) are commonly used terms, definitions, and constructs in the field of DMH response. These terms are used interchangeably throughout this text, depending on the context of the subject matter.

> *Critical incident (CI):* Events that are disruptive and stressful, with the origin being in multiple life environments (i.e., workplace, school, neighborhood) and multiple life areas (i.e., workplace violence, school shootings, civil unrest). CIs range on a continuum of minor to catastrophic. As in most other definitions, the person's or trauma survivor's perception of the CI helps define his or her experience that may be somewhat stressful (e.g., having an argument with your spouse or supervisor at work) to extremely stressful and disabling (e.g., motor vehicle accident, brain or spinal cord injury).

> *Critical incident response (CIR):* A well-coordinated and planned effort that has a defined organizational structure of roles, tasks, and responsibilities, typically performed in teams of specialists (i.e., law enforcement, paramedics, rescue workers, mental health specialists). Typically, CIR remains onsite in terms of disaster relief, triages mental and physical conditions, and provides after-care supports and resources to survivors.

> *Critical incident stress debriefing (CISD):* CISD refers to a formal, structured protocol originally developed by Mitchell (1983) as a direct, action-oriented crisis intervention

process designed to prevent traumatic stress symptoms for both primary and secondary survivors. CISD is recognized as the most widely utilized among disaster response teams, military, and emergency service personnel (Meichenbaum, 1994). CISD can further be defined as a team-oriented approach, a group process, and should not be a substitute for psychotherapy.

*Critical incident stress management (CISM):* CISM utilizes a comprehensive approach of stress management education, programs, interventions, and strategies designed to prevent posttraumatic stress symptoms and secondary traumatic stress in primary and secondary survivors.

*Crisis response team (CRT):* The NOVA (2016) uses a group debriefing model as the primary intervention. The CRT is a group of well-trained and certified individuals who provide trauma mitigation and psychoeducation after a CI. CRT members are deployed in both small- and large-scale disasters. The CRT is a well-coordinated and planned effort that has specific roles, tasks, and responsibilities managed by team leaders to provide onsite disaster relief, offer triage of mental and physical conditions, and provide supports and resources to survivors in the aftermath of disaster.

*Debriefing:* Debriefing is a common term (originally used by military personnel) to describe an approach that involves forming small and large groups of primary and secondary survivors to educate and discuss one specific CI. Debriefings typically last 60 to 90 minutes and are facilitated by trained and qualified personnel. Sessions focus primarily on the ventilation and validation of the individual's and group's emotional and psychological impacts associated with the traumatic event. Debriefings also use prediction and preparation interventions to help facilitate resources and coping skills among the group of survivors.

*Defusing:* Defusing is basically a shortened version of the CISD model. It is designed to either eliminate the need for a formal debriefing or enhance the CISD. Defusing takes place immediately or relatively soon after a CI and includes three parts: (a) introduction, (b) exploration, and (c) information.

*Extraordinary stressful and traumatic event (ESTE):* ESTE is a sudden stressful or traumatic event that is typically outside the normal range of ordinary human experience and is so overwhelmingly stressful to an individual or group that initially it has little or no coping skills to deal with the event. ESTEs are events that range from moderate to severe based on the individual survivor's perception of the ESTE.

It is important to note that there are similar terms used in nonmental health crisis response organizations, government entities, and the military. For instance, the Federal Bureau of Investigation (FBI, 2016) uses the term *critical incident response group* that was established in 1994 to integrate tactical negotiations, behavioral analysis, and crisis management resources as a coordinated effort for rapid response in CIs. The other government agencies as described in Chapter 1 (e.g., Federal Emergency Management Agency [FEMA], Centers for Disease Control and Prevention [CDC], ARC) all have their own definitions, models, and protocols for handling CIs. Primarily, CRTs focus on the health and safety of U.S. citizens in times of natural (e.g., floods, hurricanes), biological (e.g., hazardous material containment), and person-made disasters (e.g., mass shootings). The mission is clearly focused on first-responder activities. In the aftermath, there may be mental health professionals called upon to provide screenings, triage, or brief crisis interventions.

## ASSUMPTIONS IN DMH RESPONSE

DMH counselors should consider the following assumptions when providing interventions (Stebnicki, 2001, 2016a).

1. *Recognize the person as a survivor.* Viewing persons as "victims" of traumatic events discounts their survival skills and negatively reinforces the stereotype of being helpless, hopeless, dependent, and defenseless. Although the person may be a victim of a crime or motor vehicle accident, perceiving and intervening with an individual in this role will hinder his or her abilities to cope and adapt.

2. *Accept that the stressors accompanying traumatic events are real and legitimate for primary survivors.* Persons involved with extraordinary stressful and traumatic events are typically physiologically and psychologically affected and require some short-term therapeutic interventions. This does not mean that the person is "going crazy" or is "emotionally weak." Rather, the physiological and psychological effects the person is experiencing are a normal response to an extraordinary stressful event. Research indicates that approximately 20% to 30% of those individuals most directly affected by the event require long-term mental health services. Additionally, persons with disabilities and other vulnerable populations, such as persons with life-threatening illnesses and older individuals, may be at risk of increased psychological and emotional trauma, complicating their preexisting issues; in particular, hindering their ability for healthy coping and adjustment. Regardless of preexisting traits or conditions, survivors of the previous traumatic events are at risk for revictimization by recent CIs.

3. *There is a high incidence of secondary posttraumatic symptoms that affects family members, friends, and communities as a whole.* The phenomenon of "vicarious victimization" (Young, 1998) and empathy fatigue (Stebnicki, 2016b) suggest that persons can be emotionally, physically, vocationally, and spiritually exhausted as secondary survivors of an exposure to disaster. Depending on how close the family members, friends, communities, or mental health professional are to the "epicenter" of a CI, they may also be at risk of experiencing the full range of posttraumatic stress symptoms expressed as grief and loss.

4. *Interventions should be person centered as opposed to treating a diagnostic category.* The *Diagnostic and Statistical Manual of Mental Disorders* (5th ed.; DSM-5; American Psychiatric Association, 2013) does not allow PTSD to be diagnosed for 30 days following exposure to traumatic events. Regardless, primary and secondary survivors are affected by traumatic events and each individual responds differently. Persons who report a history of trauma are not members of

a homogenous population. Thus, treatment efforts must consider the unique individual, cultural, and environmental characteristics by focusing on symptom relief of the person's acute stress and coping strategies. Regardless of the results of the person's clinical assessment (i.e., PTSD), the individual's response to prior traumatic events and coping mechanisms may offer more of an insight for brief or solution-focused interventions.

5. *Posttraumatic stress symptoms must be viewed in terms of the person's cultural and institutional environment.* Individuals and groups have their own unique identities that merit using different approaches. Mental health professionals must view survivors in relationship to their cultural, sociopolitical, and institutional environments and assess which factors may hinder the persons' or groups' abilities to cope and adjust. Mental health conditions associated with the traumatic event may not reside solely within the individual. Rather, there may be outside variables that do not integrate coping and adjustment with groups and individuals.

6. *Empowering survivors with multiple resources and support systems facilitates better coping abilities and recovery.* Family, friends, churches, and other support groups can be a major source for coping and psychosocial adaptation.

7. *Individuals heal at different rates.* Individuals' coping abilities and their adjustment to the grief and loss associated with traumatic events vary and do not fit neatly into a theoretical stage model of adaptation or adjustment. Viktor Frankl (1963) sums up this point by suggesting that it is not necessarily the nature of the trauma itself that most affects one's ability to cope psychologically with its consequences, but rather the person's own attitude toward the trauma.

8. *Preexisting physical, emotional, cognitive, or financial limitations may intensify a crisis event and produce more complex reactions of grief and loss.* It is important to recognize that when traumatic events occur with persons who have existing mental or physical disabilities, the crisis event may combine with the preexisting underlying chronic illness or disability and produce a synergistic effect, which may intensify the person's response to the extraordinary stressful and traumatic event. Primarily, exposure to CIs for vulnerable populations may be "trigger events," which can exacerbate current medical conditions and may cause some persons to relapse.

## THE PROFESSION OF DMH COUNSELING

The new Council for Accreditation of Counseling and Related Educational Programs' (CACREP, 2015) 2016 standards now incorporate content areas related to "crisis intervention, trauma-informed, and community-based strategies, such as Psychological First Aid" (p. 11). Thus, the new standards require all CACREP-accredited programs to include content across the curriculum under the domains of Professional Counseling Orientation and Ethical Practice, Human Growth and Development, and Counseling and Helping Relationships. The Standards Revision Committee for the 2016 CACREP standards (Beckett, 2009), which included members of the American Counseling Association

(ACA), had a strong commitment to redefining the role and function of the professional counselor for the 21st century. Many professional counselors are called upon to serve as DMH responders in a variety of CIs. Professional counseling associations are integral to deploying volunteers in mass natural and person-made disasters. Thus, preprofessionals training in crisis, trauma, and disaster response is essential. Current practicing LPCs also have a number of specialty certifications and trainings they can attend through continuing educational activities to fulfill the role and function of DMH responders. Accordingly, this section describes professional counseling and related associations and organizations that have taken the lead in cultivating volunteer efforts and the workforce for DMH response.

## American Counseling Association

The ACA (2016a), the largest international association for LPCs, has created a new counseling specialty focus with training opportunities for LPCs in the emerging area of DMH counseling. ACA's definition suggests that disaster results in a social disruption in which the social function and structure of the community is threatened. Although this definition is not as comprehensive as the IFRC (2015) and others, the ACA does advocate for LPCs to possess the knowledge and skills to work effectively with the emotional, cognitive, behavioral, physiological, and religious/spiritual aspects of individuals and groups healing from trauma.

The ACA, in collaboration with ACA's Traumatology Interest Network and the ARC (ACA, 2016b), have taken the lead nationally to develop a coordinated list of active volunteers who are independent practitioners and currently provide training materials online and workshops that deal with the natural and person-made disasters.

## American Mental Health Counselors Association

The American Mental Health Counselors Association (AMHCA, 2016) endorses the philosophy that mental health counseling is a distinct profession that requires specialized education, training, and clinical practice; it combines traditional mental health counseling and psychotherapy approaches to assist individuals and groups in problem-solving and problem resolution of mental health, substance abuse, and crisis issues. Mental health counselors engage in therapeutic relationships and use the clinical approaches of assessment and diagnosis, psychotherapy, and treatment planning, as well as a variety of counseling theories and techniques to facilitate therapy, psychoeducational, and prevention programs, and to intervene in a variety of crises affecting one's mental health.

Exposure to traumatic events such as natural disasters, mass violence, terrorism, or other unanticipated events that affect the individual's and group's mental health and well-being requires well-coordinated efforts partnering with a variety of professional counseling associations, such as the ACA (2016b), and governmental agencies such as the Substance Abuse and Mental Health Services Administration's (SAMHSA's) Disaster Distress Helpline (DDH; SAMHSA, 2016). SAMHSA's DDH is charged with offering a national mental health crisis hotline that is open 24 hours per day year-round to support individuals who have experienced emotional distress related to natural (i.e., tornadoes, floods, hurricanes, wildfires, earthquakes) and person-made disasters (i.e., mass violence, civil unrest). The crisis lines are staffed by qualified mental health professionals who are trained in addressing short-term crisis and coordinating immediate services such as evacuations, shelters, food and clothing distribution centers, and other crisis referral and information resources.

## American Psychological Association

The American Psychological Association (APA, 2016) understands the psychological impact that disasters have on individuals, families, and communities. As a result, the APA partnered with the ARC in 1992 to launch the Disaster Response Network (DRN). APA's DRN began with a group of approximately 2,500 trained psychologists from the United States and Canada to coordinate, collaborate, and provide mental health interventions with the ARC during times of disaster. APA's DRN works in the various aspects of disaster response, including disaster preparation, response, and recovery. APA's DRN connects with other local, regional, and state ARC teams to recruit and train volunteers of mental health professionals (i.e., LPCs, licensed clinical social workers [LCSWs]) who are ready to mobilize and respond to the mental health needs on ARC disaster sites. The brief interventions include stress debriefing, offering mental health screening and triage, providing emotional supports, and cultivating resources to build coping and resiliency skills.

## National Association of Social Workers

The National Association of Social Workers (NASW, 2016) has long been involved in disaster relief and has provided trauma interventions to trauma survivors in civilian and military CIs. The NASW advocates that social workers are uniquely suited to provide disaster relief services to disaster survivors during the disaster predation, response, and recovery phases. Social workers have had a long history in the coordination of disaster relief and social justice interventions with other disaster relief organizations such as Charity Organization Societies (COS; Zakour, 1996). In the 19th century, social workers intervened in rural and urban environments to improve the physical and mental health of disparate populations living in substandard housing, poor working conditions, and other areas of society that decreased one's social, emotional, and psychological functioning. The NASW coordinates with state chapters and other counseling-related professional organizations to train and recruit DMH volunteers who are ready to be mobilized to ARC disaster sites.

## CONCLUDING REMARKS

Even though there is not a homeland DMH agency responsible to prepare, plan, prevent, coordinate, organize, and direct a national plan of disaster response, there are multiple professional counseling associations and a few governmental agencies that have taken the lead in DMH response. It has been my experience that DMH counseling at present appears to be cobbled together by local community mental health providers, churches, and paraprofessionals with occasional backup support from national counseling associations. Part of the reason this does not exist in disaster scenarios is that, understandably, people need medical care first, along with food, shelter, and clothing. However, from a mental health perspective, individuals and groups in crisis need compassionate and empathetic interventions. This can be shown by actions at first, but listening to the traumatic experiences and stories of survivors is psychological or what I would call *empathy first aid* (EFA), which is also a critical intervention that can help heal trauma. Perhaps it is time to embrace the holistic view of interventions of the mind, body, and spirit within the emergency management community. It is imperative that the DMH community be organized to ensure that we can build, sustain, and improve our capability to prepare for, protect against, and respond to CIs for the intent of reducing psychological, social, and emotional costs to traumatic experiences at the epicenter of a natural, person-made, and/or technological disaster.

## REFERENCES

Aguilera, D. C., & Messick, J. M. (1974). *Crisis intervention: Theory and methodology* (2nd ed.). St. Louis: C. V. Mosby.

American Counseling Association. (2016a). About ACA. Retrieved from http://www.counseling.org/about-us/about-aca

American Counseling Association. (2016b). Disaster mental health: Terms to know. Retrieved from http://www.counseling.org/knowledge-center/trauma-disaster

American Mental Health Counselors Association. (2016). Home page. Retrieved from http://www.amhca.org

American Mental Health Counselors Association. (2016). Facts about clinical mental health counselors. Retrieved from http://www.amhca.org/?page=facts

American Psychiatric Association. (2013). *Diagnostic and statistical manual of mental disorders* (5th ed.). Arlington, VA: American Psychiatric Publishing.

American Psychological Association. (2016). Disaster resource network. Retrieved from http://www.apa.org/practice/programs/drn

American Red Cross. (2012). Disaster mental health handbook of disaster services. Retrieved from http://www.cdms.uci.edu/PDF/Disaster-Mental-Health-Handbook-Oct-2012.pdf

Beckett, C. (2009). New CACREP standards frame counselors' skills in disaster response. Retrieved from http://www.cacrep.org/wp-content/uploads/2012/07/New-CACREP-Standards-frame-counselors-skills-in-disaster-response-February-2009.pdf

Caplan, G. (1964). *Principles of preventative psychiatry.* New York, NY: Basic Books.

Council for Accreditation of Counseling and Related Educational Programs. (2015). 2016 CACREP standards. Retrieved from http://www.cacrep.org/wp-content/uploads/2012/10/2016-CACREP-Standards.pdf

Echterling, L. G., Presbury, J. H., & Edson McKee, J. (2005). *Crisis intervention: Promoting resilience and resolution in troubled times.* Upper Saddle River, NJ: Pearson Prentice Hall.

Federal Bureau of Investigation. (2016). Critical incident response group. Retrieved from https://www.fbi.gov/services/cirg

Frankl, V. E. (1963). *Man's search for meaning.* New York, NY: Pocket Books.

Friedman, M. J., & Marsella, A. J. (1996). Posttraumatic stress disorder: An overview of the concept. In A. J. Marsella, M. J. Friedman, E. T. Gerrity, & R. M. Scurfield (Eds.), *Ethnocultural aspects of posttraumatic stress disorder: Issues, research, and clinical applications* (pp. 11–32). Washington, DC: American Psychological Association.

The International Federation of Red Cross and Red Crescent Societies. (2015). What is a disaster? Retrieved from https://www.ifrc.org/en/what-we-do/disaster-management/about-disasters/what-is-a -disaster

Lester, D., & Brockopp, G. W. (1973). *Crisis intervention and counseling by telephone.* Springfield, IL: Charles C. Thomas.

Levers, L. L., Ventura, E. M., & Bledsoe, D. E. (2012). Models for trauma intervention: Integrative approaches to therapy. In L. L. Levers (Ed.), *Trauma counseling: Theories and interventions* (pp. 493–503). New York, NY: Springer Publishing.

McFarlane, A. C., & Norris, F. (2006). Definitions and concepts in disaster research. In F. Norris, S. Galea, M. Friedman, & P. Watson (Eds.), *Methods for disaster mental health research* (pp. 3–19). New York, NY: Guilford Press.

Meichenbaum, D. (1994). *A clinical handbook/practical therapist manual for assessing and treating adults with post-traumatic stress disorder (PTSD).* Waterloo, ON, Canada: Institute Press.

Mitchell, J. T. (1983). When disaster strikes: The critical incident stress debriefing process. *Journal of Emergency Medical Services, 8*(1), 36–39.

Moodley, R., & West, W. (2005). *Integrating traditional healing practices into counseling and psychotherapy.* Thousand Oaks, CA: Sage Publications.

National Association of Social Workers. (2016). Social workers and disaster relief services. Retrieved from http://www.socialworkers.org/ldf/legal_issue/200509.asp?back=yes

National Organization for Victims Assistance. (2015). Home page. Retrieved from http://www. trynova.org

National Organization for Victims Assistance. (2016). Help crisis victims. Retrieved from http:// www.trynova.org/help-crisis-victims/overview

Norris, F. H., Stevens, S. P., Pfefferbaum, B., Wyche, K. F., & Pfefferbaum, R. L. (2008). Community resilience as a metaphor, theory, set of capacities, and strategy for disaster readiness. *American Journal of Psychology, 41*, 127–150.

Raphael, B., & Dobson, M. (2001). Acute posttraumatic interventions. In J. P. Wilson, M. J. Friedman, & J. D. Lindy (Eds.), *Treating psychological trauma & PTSD* (pp. 139–158). New York, NY: Guilford Press.

Specter, G. A., & Claiborn, W. L. (1973). *Crisis intervention: A topical series in community-clinical psychology.* New York, NY: Behavioral Publications.

Stebnicki, M. A. (2001). The psychosocial impact on survivors of extraordinary stressful and traumatic events: Principles and practices in critical incident response for rehabilitation counselors. *New Directions in Rehabilitation, 12*(6), 57–72.

Stebnicki, M. A. (2015, October). *The psychosocial cost of war on non-military civilian populations: A global perspective.* Presentation made at the Annual Conference of the Licensed Professional Counseling Association of North Carolina, Raleigh, NC.

Stebnicki, M. A. (2016a). Disaster mental health response and stress debriefing. In I. Marini & M. A. Stebnicki (Eds.), *The professional counselors' desk reference.* New York, NY: Springer Publishing.

Stebnicki, M. A. (2016b). From empathy fatigue to empathy resiliency. In I. Marini & M. A. Stebnicki (Eds.), *The professional counselor's desk reference* (2nd ed., pp. 533–545). New York, NY: Springer Publishing.

Substance Abuse and Mental Health Services Administration. (2016). Disaster distress helpline. Retrieved from http://www.samhsa.gov/find-help/disaster-distress-helpline

Wilson, J. P., Friedman, M. J., & Lindy, J. D. (2001). Treatment goals for PTSD. In J. P. Wilson, M. J. Friedman, & J. D. Lindy (Eds.), *Treating psychological trauma & PTSD* (pp. 3–27). New York, NY: Guilford Press.

Young, M. A. (1998). *The community crisis response team manual* (2nd ed.). Washington, DC: National Organization for Victim Assistance.

Zakour, M. J. (1996). Disaster research in social work. In C. L. Streeter & S. A. Murty (Eds.), *Research in social work and disasters* (pp. 7–26). New York, NY: Haworth.

# CHAPTER 3

# The Search for Meaning in Trauma and Disaster

Today's practitioners of the healing arts have the challenge of restoring faith and hope in communities and cultures that have been ravaged by naturally occurring and person-made events. There is a psychological and emotional cost to those at the epicenter of trauma and disaster; it is a wounded soul. Professional helpers at all levels of service (e.g., first responders, disaster mental health professionals, Red Cross volunteers) have the task of bringing balance back to the mind, body, and spirit of individuals, groups, and communities affected by trauma and disaster. The therapeutic value of empathy, compassion, good intention, and commitment from mental health professionals should not be underestimated in the search for meaning in person-made and natural disasters.

Clearly, the search for personal meaning in one's traumatic experience is an existential and spiritual pursuit (Stebnicki, 2006). Questions such as *What kind of God could allow such suffering or horrific acts to take place (to me) or in my world? Why do bad things happen to good people?* or *Why do good things happen to bad people?* cannot be addressed with psychological first aid, stress debriefing, or providing food, shelter, and clothing. These are important questions on the way to one's healing journey that require someone to help guide the process in the search for meaning of trauma and disaster.

In many cultures, the most significant and meaningful questions in life are related to where we came from before birth and where we will transcend at the time of our death (Pedersen, 2000). Pearlman and Saakvitne (1995) suggest that the loss of meaning, connection, and hope after a traumatic event can be overwhelmingly destructive in a spiritual sense to both clients and counselors. The counselor's vicarious traumatization and empathy fatigue has a profound effect on his or her spiritual health. To give our whole emotional attention to another person who metaphorically questions "What happens if I say damn you God?" (Arokiasamy, 1994) or "Why do bad things happen to good people?" (Kushner, 1980) requires a compassionate and empathic response that is both existential and spiritual in nature. Thus, taking care of the soul or being conscious of our spiritual health is critical to personal survival, especially in the search for meaning in trauma and disaster.

## THE ROLE OF SPIRITUALITY IN THE SEARCH FOR MEANING

Spirituality plays a prominent role in the lives of individuals from many different cultural and ethnic backgrounds (Stebnicki, 2016b). Some authors (Pargament & Zinnbauer, 2000; Shafranske & Malony, 1996) have suggested that counselors have an ethical obligation to explore the spiritual aspects of their clients' lives. It is consistent with multicultural interactions and facilitating culturally sensitive counseling approaches. Thus, to work effectively with the individual's spiritual identity and worldview and to assist in the search for meaning, the literature suggests that counselor educators and clinical supervisors need to intentionally inquire about how supervisors are addressing their clients' spiritual needs and spiritual health (Bishop, Avila-Juarbe, & Thumme, 2003; Cashwell & Young, 2004; Polanski, 2003; Stebnicki, 2007). Accordingly, skilled and competent counselor educators and clinical supervisors prepare preprofessional counselors for addressing the spiritual needs of their clients in the search for meaning of their traumatic or disaster experiences.

Miller (2003) suggests that mental health professionals must first be comfortable with exploring their own spirituality before delving into their clients' existential and spiritual experiences of loss, grief, life-threatening illness, and trauma. It also necessitates that we do not feel obligated to provide all the answers to know everything that God, our higher power, spirit guides, or the universe has to teach us. For some mental health professionals, this ambiguity and parallel experience of spiritual confusion exist within our own existential angst. Horrific experiences of genocide, torture, human trafficking, and other trauma reach beyond the range of ordinary human experience that words cannot express. It permeates our levels of consciousness. The client's existential and/or spiritual crisis may become the counselor's crisis, resulting in an empathy fatigue reaction (Stebnicki, 2016a). Thus, it becomes the ethical obligation of professional counselors to sustain empathic wellness, seek meaning and purpose of the work we do with trauma survivors, and function optimally so that professional fatigue syndromes do not overwhelm our ability to assist others.

Too often we think about mental health counseling as a one-way street in which the professional or "expert" is all knowing and is the only person empowered to possess all healing resources. By the very nature of this relationship, there is both an ethical obligation and assumption that mental health professionals reach out in compassion and empathy to heal the client's trauma experience or wounded soul. Consequently, the compassionate and empathic mental health professional, at the end of the day, will know that the healing journey has begun for his or her client, with one small step toward finding meaning in his or her traumatic experience.

### Viktor Frankl

Dr. Viktor Frankl (1963), a psychiatrist who spent World War II in a Nazi concentration camp, was one of the first psychotherapists to discuss those extraordinary experiences of people who survived the death camps of Nazi Germany despite hunger, humiliation, fear, deep injustice, and torture. Frankl, an existential theorist who introduced the most significant Western psychological movement of its time through *Man's Search for Meaning*, provided a dramatic narrative of humankind's capacity for coping and resiliency despite the most horrific treatment imaginable. Logotherapy, an original psychotherapeutic approach Frankl developed, provides a foundation for treating survivors of extraordinary stressful and traumatic events.

The key proposition in logotherapy is to find meaning in one's existential pain and suffering. For Frankl, it was all about perception of one's circumstances in life and then changing this attitude toward an unalterable fate (e.g., life-threatening disease, chronic illness, loss of a loved one). As Frankl states: "Suffering ceases to be suffering in some way at the moment it finds a meaning, such as the meaning of sacrifice" (p. 179). He further suggests that one of the basic tenets of logotherapy is not to gain pleasure or avoid pain, but rather to seek meaning in life. It was through these death camp experiences where he explains that it is critical to find meaning in one's physical, emotional, and spiritual pain and suffering. In Frankl's final analysis, he wrote:

> It becomes clear that the sort of person the prisoner became was the result of an inner decision, and not the result of camp influences alone. Fundamentally, therefore, any man can, even under such circumstances, decide what shall become of him—mentally and spiritually. (p. 105)

Frankl concludes that it is this type of spiritual freedom and the freedom to make choices that cannot be taken away from an individual even under the most brutal of circumstances. Changing our attitude and perception toward a critical life event is empowering for many individuals. Attitudinal change does not mean forgetting traumatic experiences. Rather, Frankl suggests that we can make a choice in the present moment to change the way we perceive our past. Accordingly, past critical life events do not define who we are in the present moment. Finding new meaning and purpose for our life is how we can heal trauma and cultivate resiliency.

## THE WOUNDED HEALER EXPERIENCE

The "wounded healer" is an archetypal representation that psychologist Carl Jung used to describe the phenomenon and dynamic that take place between the client and the therapist when the therapist constantly revisits his or her own emotional and psychological wounds (Campbell, 1976). The basis of this phenomenon has been explained as negative countertransference experienced by the therapist. Jung felt that a wounded healer experience could harm the therapeutic alliance within the client–counselor relationship because it leaves the therapist vulnerable to not only his or her own issues but also those of his or her clients. The term itself is actually derived from an ancient Greek legend of a physician named Asclepius who had mystical powers to heal his own wounds and created a sanctuary to treat others (National Library of Medicine [NLM], 2016). In fact, modern medicine has symbolically adopted part of this ancient philosophy as recognized by the *caduceus* (two intertwined snakes grasping a staff) that is the familiar physician symbol of the medical profession.

Truly, multiple client stories of extraordinary stressful and traumatic events, as well as exposure to the client's chronic physical and mental health conditions, place mental health professionals at risk for their own feelings of helplessness and hopelessness (Stebnicki, 2008). So, the question becomes who pays attention to and takes care of the wounded healer. Nouwen (1972) speaks to this type of counselor experience from his concept of the "wounded healer," stating:

> When our souls are restless, when we are driven by thousands of different and often conflicting stimuli, when we are always "over there" between people, ideas and the worries of this world, how can we possibly create the room and space where someone else can enter freely without feeling himself an unlawful intruder? Paradoxically, by withdrawing into ourselves, not out of self-pity but out of humility, we create the space for another to be himself and to come to us on his own terms. (p. 91)

Miller (2003) proposes that from the "wounded healer" framework counselors bring a compassionate spirit to the client–counselor relationship. Further, the client's expectations of his or her counselor are that he or she does not possess any psychological, emotional, or spiritual vulnerability. Thus, the counselor is seen as a role model for emotional and spiritual wellness by the client who feels wounded. However, the counselor who attempts to act as a "role model" may not be dealing honestly and openly with his or her client. Showing vulnerability as a therapist and facilitating empathic understanding suggest to our clients that we responsibly share or disclose our wounds alongside of them (Miller & Baldwin, 1987). Client stories that have such themes as addictions, physical or sexual abuse, and psychological trauma adversely affect the mind, body, and spirit of both the client and the mental health professional. Remembering emotions related to such painful events creates an emotional scrapbook that can be extremely painful and difficult.

An integral part of Navajo medicine is the use of storytelling and remembering painful and traumatic memories (Tafoya & Kouris, 2003). The purpose of storytelling is to help make sense of a traumatic event and to bring harmony to the mind, body, and spirit. In the Navajo culture, the person who requires healing takes part in a ceremony that includes family and friends who gather for various rituals. Interestingly, the responsibility for healing is shared by most of the community, not just the person and the healer. Storytelling is done through ceremonial chants, dances, prayers, and stories about the creation of the Navajo people. In the Navajo tradition, it is particularly meaningful to communicate how all things in the universe are interconnected. Storytelling in the Navajo culture is said to be healing medicine because stories have the power to clarify one's identity, purpose, meaning, connection, and harmony with the spirit world. Although some stories are healing, others have the potential to carry multiple layers of meaning that may be interpreted and perceived by others as a myth or poison that weakens the spirit of the individual and the culture (Coulehan, 1980). In drawing on Nouwen's (1972) concept of the "wounded healer," he states:

Many people suffer because of the false supposition on which they have based their lives. That supposition is that there should be no fear or loneliness, no confusion or doubt. But these sufferings can only be dealt with creatively when they are understood as wounds integral to our human condition. (p. 93)

Facilitating empathic approaches in the counseling relationship requires that we help our clients unfold the layers of their stress, grief, loss, or traumatic experiences by searching through their emotional scrapbook. The search for personal meaning and purpose of our client's pain and suffering may contribute to the counselor's empathy fatigue experience. If counselors are mindful of this experience and view this as an opportunity for nurturing personal growth and development, they will then learn resiliency strategies that can help replenish their wounded spirit.

## EMPATHY AS THE SOUL OF THE COUNSELOR: AN INDIGENOUS WORLDVIEW

In many cultures, the soul is regarded as the seat of the individual's emotions, feelings, and spiritual experiences. In Jungian symbolism, the center of the person's psyche is referred to as the "self" or "soul." Many mental health professionals spend a tremendous amount of psychic energy in being empathic and looking for the emotional parts of their clients' souls that have been lost to incest, physical abuse, addictions, loss of a loved one, chronic illness, or psychological and physical trauma. Empathy as the soul of the counselor figures prominently in the subjective experiences of understanding the experience of the "fatigued" professional. This is a significant point because there is a parallel experience between the mental health professional and fatigue syndromes (i.e., burnout, compassion, empathy fatigue) that ultimately end up affecting the mind, body, spirit, and soul (Stebnicki, 2008).

The transition from being a mental health counselor trained in the West to a culturally competent healer requires openness to indigenous health and healing practices. West (2005) suggests that if we truly want to experience the richness of each client's cultural healing system, then we need to honor his or her belief system. Thus, integrating traditional approaches in therapy (e.g., stress management, cognitive behavioral therapy [CBT], relaxation, visualization) with more indigenous practices with culturally different clients may offer mental health professionals another dimension to facilitate therapeutic approaches. Developing an understanding and appreciation of this has profound implications for practice. It should be emphasized that many indigenous healing practices may also benefit the mental health professional program of self-care.

From an indigenous worldview, illness within the mind, body, and spirit means there is a blocking of the flow of "good" energy. In Central African cultures, the belief exists that there is a "sleeping sickness of the soul," which is exhibited by one's indifference to the pain and suffering of others (Graham, 2005). Addictions are just one example of how the flow of energy can be blocked and prevents us from engaging in our daily routines (e.g., job, family, relationships, recreation).

Regardless of your belief system, any form of energy that is blocked can distort our perceptions and attitudes about life. This ultimately affects our minds, bodies, and spirits. It can decrease our feelings and compassion for the good work that we do for others. We can easily acquire unhealthy habits and grow into an out-of-balance life. Thus, being open to our spirit helpers and letting the universal life-energy flow can decrease the possibilities of empathy fatigue. This is an ongoing challenge for anyone who has had the opportunity to provide service to another human being.

Beginning-level or seasoned mental health therapists should be open to the idea of embracing cultural differences by paying attention to indigenous health and healing approaches. This may be used as therapeutic leverage for culturally different clients. The journey to become a mental health professional requires personal and professional growth experiences that may not be provided by traditional counselor education programs or continuing education credits through workshops and conferences. Thus, developing one's mind, body, and spirit requires openness to the idea that as we challenge our clients to grow, we too must grow.

## Use of Empathy in Facilitating Meaning

Empathy as a trait or state of the mental health professional is not simply a counseling approach or strategy whereby the counselor grasps the meaning of the client's issues (e.g., transition from a loss), then associates this with a specific feeling (e.g., stress, depression, anxiety) and relates this to the person's overall experience (e.g., overall sense of loss and grief). Rather, it is suspected that more seasoned mental health counselors use an empathic-intuitive connection to experience their clients' verbal and nonverbal communication. In other words, the more established and seasoned therapist has developed a sixth sense or "third eye" for intuitiveness (Stebnicki, 2008). Mental health counselors who have engaged in multiple sessions over the years are much better than beginning-level counselors at sensing whether their clients' verbal reports of emotion are congruent with their nonverbal behaviors and cognitions, or whether their clients could potentially harm themselves or others. Accordingly, it is suspected that over the years more seasoned practitioners have learned how to integrate their clients' thoughts, feelings, and cognitions with spiritual and existential meaning and purpose. More specifically, the seasoned mental health counselor facilitates counseling approaches that integrate traditional Western psychotherapy approaches with his or her client's culturally specific belief system.

## One Spirit

Many cultures of the world believe that there is a divine spiritual energy or life force that has created order in the universe since the beginning of time. For example, in the African-centered worldview (Graham, 2005), spirituality is defined as (a) a creative life force, (b) the very essence of all things that connects human beings to others, and (c) the power that interconnects all elements of the universe: people, animals, and earthly things such as plants. Interestingly, on the other side of the world native or indigenous Indian tribes of North American ancestry have a very similar belief system about divine spiritual energy. The Great Spirit, as referred to by many Native peoples, is the creator of all things. Likewise, in this view, all things are related and interconnected to The Great Spirit, particularly the mind, body, and spirit. If one's mind is out-of-harmony with his or her spirit, then there is disharmony in all systems. Thus, One Spirit in a cultural sense suggests that the individual does not have to visit a physician to heal his or her body, see a mental health counselor to heal his or her mind, or attend a faith-based institution to heal his or her spirit. The One Spirit entity is loving, compassionate, humanistic, all knowing (noetic), and represents holistic healing at its best.

Many gifted healers and ancient sages have claimed to see the aura of this spiritual energy flowing through themselves and others as they perform their healing rituals. As Seaward (1997) explains, this spiritual energy binds us to the source of God at all times. This connection will never be broken because all living things emanate from this divine source. There is a sense that this universal spirit communicates and nourishes one's soul. Regardless of one's belief in a God, universal spirit, or higher power, this *chi* or *ki* continuously flows even in the wounded soul. This stress can be felt by many in the mental health profession, especially in the presence of clients who are suffering due to trauma and disaster in their lives. Even a wounded soul experience can provide the trauma survivor with the greatest opportunity for growth of soul and spirit. Understanding spiritual principles from a cultural perspective first and foremost requires the recognition that almost all cultures have some spiritual and religious beliefs, values, philosophical ideology, structure, and organization. Cultivating the client's spiritual beliefs and values resonates as a coping resource and can serve as therapeutic leverage with many clients.

## THE MYSTERY OF MAKING MEANING

The paradoxes of facilitating meaning of one's traumatic experiences are many. Those who want a parsimonious explanation are surely disappointed. It is the common experience, however, in client–counselor therapeutic engagements that a thought, feeling, cognition, or experience of sorts moves the trauma or disaster survivor forward in his or her healing. As alluded to in various chapters throughout this book, premental health wellness predicts posttrauma/disaster mental health and wellness or unwellness. Trauma and disaster survivors who have a tank half-full of resiliency and coping abilities predictably have better opportunities for making sense and meaning of adversity. Those with a tank half-empty may not fare so well. It is this group of individuals during disaster triage that exhibits a decreased ability to cope with trauma and disaster (e.g., smoking/drinking more than normal, isolation and detachment, severe physical ailments, severe depression, and panic).

The survivor's obedience to internal and external forces of wellness or unwellness is critical for disaster mental health counselors to reveal during therapeutic interactions. This can occur with some basic foundational questions: *Help me understand what you are feeling, thinking, or experiencing now. After you look back over the past several days of what you experienced, what are some resources and supports that could help pull you through this week?* As the mental health counselor puts aside the art and science of the mental health profession, we are mindful of how to slip into the role of the empathic and compassionate visitor. We can provide survivors with the hope of being with them at least throughout the first few hours and day so as to assist them in opening windows and doors. This process occurs best with natural environmental supports of family, friends, faith-based organizations, and the community. Thus, the mystery of making meaning begins with facilitating culturally attuned approaches that assist in bringing the survivor back to balance and feeling a sense of normalcy without fear of falling into the abyss.

There are many rich healing traditions indigenous to various cultures around the world that are integrated into many counseling and psychotherapy practices today (Mijares, 2003; Moodley & West, 2005). Mental health counselors who are particularly skilled in multicultural counseling interventions know that establishing rapport with a culturally different client is critical to achieving a good working alliance. It may mean careful attending to their clients' nonverbal or covert description of disharmony in their mind, body, and spirit. Mental health counselors who are skilled in multicultural counseling use their cultural intellect (i.e., knowledge and awareness of the client's cultural belief system) and their intuitive sense to understand their clients' meaning of life and worldview.

Mental health counselors must try and understand their clients holistically from a cultural perspective. This includes, but is not limited to, understanding cultural aspects of the client's: (a) beliefs about good mental health and wellness, (b) psychosocial and spiritual well-being, (c) style of expressed and unexpressed emotions, (d) verbalized feelings and specific meaning behind the emotions expressed, and (e) overall experience of acculturated values. Understanding cultural differences requires cultural identity work by both the counselor and the client.

Everyone has a cultural identity and is a collective member of an array of other cultural groups and subgroups that represent such things as gender (male/female), geographic regions of the United States (Southern rural/urban), age (younger/older), language (English/Spanish, or multilingual), religious/spiritual beliefs (Catholic/Protestant), and many other characteristics. An excellent starting point for the mental health professional is to begin a journey of understanding your own cultural beliefs and identity. The inability to understand one's own cultural beliefs and identity can create some disharmony during client sessions if the counselor has no anchor for his or her own mind, body, and spirit. Not having a good sense of interconnectedness or a well-developed sense of compassion for disaster or trauma survivors can have negative consequences. Some mental health professionals may view themselves in a "job" rather than in a "career" that fulfills one's requirement for meaning and purpose in life.

Culturally competent mental health professionals have learned to use the subjective experiences of culturally different individuals to skillfully build a rapport and establish a working alliance. Just as in the scientific paradigm, the counselor may make a hypothesis about his or her client; measure/assess his or her behaviors and weight this against others in the norm group; focus on critical incidents associated with specific behaviors, feelings, and beliefs; and then make some interpretation or hypothesis about the client. The mental health professional's clinical judgment may or may not support the theory he or she has created about his or her client's dysfunctional life patterns. However, culturally competent mental health professionals should be attuned to the subjective experiences of their clients' cultural worldview. Interpreting verbal and nonverbal behaviors or relying heavily on traditional helping strategies may not provide the mental health counselor with a richer opportunity for understanding and clarifying his or her own cultural identity. The point is that disaster mental health counselors often must develop a sixth sense to search the essence of survival of the client's mind, body, and spirit. This information, which is often hidden by self and others, can assist mental health counselors in developing appropriate treatment approaches that serve to bring meaning and purpose to extraordinary stressful and traumatic events.

## CONCLUDING REMARKS

Culturally competent mental health professionals have learned to use the subjective experiences of culturally different individuals to skillfully build a rapport and establish a working alliance. Making meaning of trauma and disaster happens over the range of the survivor's experiences, thoughts, and feelings. The timing of making sense and meaning of a critical incident is not a process with a beginning and ending point. Rather, for some, it is a lifelong process. Indeed, resiliency and coping skills help support psychosocial adjustment to adversity. Disaster mental health professionals can play a key role in this challenge of promoting faith and hope for trauma and disaster survivors.

## REFERENCES

Arokiasamy, C. R. (1994). *What happens if I say, "Damn you, God?"* Carbondale, IL: Avanti.

Bishop, D. R., Avila-Juarbe, E., & Thumme, B. (2003). Recognizing spirituality as an important factor in counselor supervision. *Counseling and Values, 48*(1), 34–46.

Campbell, J. (1976). *The portable Jung.* New York, NY: Penguin Books.

Cashwell, C. S., & Young, J. S. (2004). Spirituality in counselor training: A content analysis of syllabi from introductory spirituality courses. *Counseling and Values, 48*(2), 96–109.

Coulehan, J. (1980). Navajo Indian medicine: Implications for healing. *Journal of Family Practice, 10*, 55–61.

Frankl, V. E. (1963). *Man's search for meaning.* New York, NY: Pocket Books.

Graham, M. (2005). Maat: An African-centered paradigm for psychological and spiritual healing. In R. Moodly & W. West (Eds.), *Integrating traditional healing practices into counseling and psychotherapy* (pp. 210–220). Thousand Oaks, CA: Sage Publications.

Kushner, H. S. (1980). *When bad things happen to good people.* New York, NY: Avon Books.

Mijares, S. G. (2003). *Ancient wisdom: Psychological healing practices from the world's religious traditions.* New York, NY: Routledge.

Miller, G. (2003). *Incorporating spirituality in counseling and psychotherapy: Theory and technique.* Hoboken, NJ: Wiley.

Miller, G. D., & Baldwin, D. C. (1987). Implications of the wounded-healer paradigm for the use of the self in therapy. In M. Baldwin & V. Satir (Eds.), *The use of self in therapy* (pp. 130–151). New York, NY: Haworth.

Moodley, R., & West, W. (2005). *Integrating traditional healing practices into counseling and psychotherapy.* Thousand Oaks, CA: Sage Publications.

National Library of Medicine. (2016). Greek medicine. Retrieved from http://www.nlm.nih.gov/hmd/greek/greek_asclepius.html

Nouwen, H. J. M. (1972). *The wounded healer.* New York, NY: An Image Book/Doubleday.

Pargament, K. L., & Zinnbauer, B. J. (2000). Working with the sacred: Four approaches to religious and spiritual issues in counseling. *Journal of Counseling & Development, 78,* 162–171.

Pearlman, L. A., & Saakvitne, K. W. (1995). Treating therapists with vicarious traumatization and secondary traumatic stress disorders. In C. R. Figley (Ed.), *Compassion fatigue: Coping with secondary traumatic stress disorder in those who treat the traumatized* (pp. 150–177). Bristol, PA: Brunner/Mazel.

Pedersen, P. (2000). *A handbook for developing multicultural awareness* (3rd ed.). Alexandria, VA: American Counseling Association.

Polanski, P. J. (2003). Spirituality and supervision. *Counseling and Values, 47*(2), 131–141.

Seaward, B. L. (1997). *Stand like mountain, flow like water: Reflections on stress and human spirituality.* Deerfield Beach, FL: Health Communications.

Shafranske, E. P., & Malony, H. N. (1996). Religion and the clinical practice of psychology: The case for inclusion. In E. P. Shafranske (Ed.), *Religion and the clinical practice of psychology.* Washington, DC: American Psychological Association.

Stebnicki, M. A. (2006). Integrating spirituality in rehabilitation counselor supervision. *Rehabilitation Education, 20*(2), 137–159.

Stebnicki, M. A. (2007). Integrating spirituality in rehabilitation counseling. *Rehabilitation Education, 20*(2), 115–132.

Stebnicki, M. A. (2008). *Empathy fatigue: Healing the mind, body, and spirit of professional counselors.* New York, NY: Springer Publishing.

Stebnicki, M. A. (2016a). From empathy fatigue to empathy resiliency. In I. Marini & M. A. Stebnicki (Eds.), *The professional counselors' desk reference* (2nd ed., pp. 533–545). New York, NY: Springer Publishing.

Stebnicki, M. A. (2016b). Integrative approaches in counseling and psychotherapy. In I. Marini & M. A. Stebnicki (Eds.), *The professional counselors' desk reference* (2nd ed., pp. 593–604). New York, NY: Springer Publishing.

Tafoya, T., & Kouris, N. (2003). Dancing the circle: Native American concepts of healing. In S. G. Mijares (Ed.), *Modern psychology and ancient wisdom: Psychological healing practices from the world's religious traditions* (pp. 125–146). New York, NY: Haworth Integrative Healing.

West, W. S. (2005). Crossing the line between talking therapies and spiritual healing. In R. Moodley & W. West (Eds.), *Integrating traditional healing practices into counseling and psychotherapy* (pp. 38–49). Thousand Oaks, CA: Sage Publications.

# CHAPTER 4

# The Neuroscience of Stress and Trauma

Survivors of mass violence are at high risk for a wide range of psychiatric, neurobehavioral, and neurocognitive disorders as a result of experiencing extraordinary stressful and traumatic events. Compelling new research in neuroscience is at the forefront of understanding the physiological, emotional, psychological, and neurocognitive experiences of trauma survivors. Studying how the brain's complex neuropathways record, transpose, replicate, express, and persistently reproduce individuals' traumatic experiences requires new research paradigms in the biopsychosocial sciences.

The dynamic neural structure and function of the brain, as it relates to human emotions and acquired trauma, is a complex topic that goes beyond the scope and intention of this book. However, it is an important topic to discuss because of the mind–body connection and the impact that our culture has on the emotions we express as a result of extraordinary stressful and traumatic experiences. These topics are complex to discuss because of the current debate in neuroscience that demonstrates strong philosophical and theoretical differences between disciplines, experimental designs (e.g., populations selected for neuroexperimentation appear to be primarily White males with some animals used to generalize over to human emotions and behaviors), and, of particular importance, the cultural aspects related to human emotions, behaviors, and cognitions. Despite the healthy debate and open discussions in the neuroscience of trauma, the ultimate reward is to bridge the gap between science, medicine, and the development of evidence-based practices for pre- and posttrauma mental health interventions. Thus, a more comprehensive biopsychosocial understanding of stress, trauma, and its impact on the mind, body, and spirit has the potential to provide greater opportunities to decrease posttraumatic stress and other mental health symptoms as experienced by trauma survivors.

## NEUROBIOLOGICAL EXPRESSION OF TRAUMA AND CULTURAL IMPACT

A common core of human biology across all cultures is that 99.9% of our DNA is the same (Genome News Network, 2016; Weil, 1995). The widely accepted scientific theory of evolution (out-of-Africa) suggests that we can trace the roots of human existence back to Africa between 200,000 and 60,000 years ago (Cann, Stoneking, & Wilson, 1987). Biblically, it was thought that human life in the universe began somewhere at the end of the first Ice Age (10,000 BCE) or possibly 5,000 years BCE. Indeed, brain development has been evolving for quite a long time. Sankararaman et al. (2014) suggest that in current genomic studies, our human ancestors are a mix of Neanderthals that bred with modern humans from the European, East-Asian, and sub-Saharan Africa continents. Adding even more controversy to the evolutionary discussion, recent scientific debates suggest our DNA is now somewhere between 0.90% and 99.9% the same, or 0.01% to 0.09% different (The Tech Museum of Innovation, 2016).

From a Judeo–Christian theological point of view, (a) we are all created by God who created Adam and Eve; (b) we did not evolve through Neanderthals; (c) all life was designed by God, our creator; and (d) as humans, our DNA was created by the Divine Creator: God (Warren, 2002; Wilson, 2013). Regardless of your religious belief system(s), from a scientific empirical view, it has been discovered over the past several decades that DNA strands among all of the Earth's inhabitants are created almost equally despite a 0.01% to 0.09% difference. It is important to note, however, that even a 0.01% difference in our DNA creates variances in eye, hair, and skin color; physical shape and appearance; and the distinct genetic code that may predispose us to chronic illnesses or diseases, as well as other unique attributes and individual characteristics.

There is no one else on the planet exactly like you. It is equally important to note that, in considering the 0.01% to 0.09% individual difference in our DNA, our behavior, personality, cognitive interpretation, perception of our environment, verbal/nonverbal communication, mapping of all these states and traits, and way of turning on our stress mechanism are highly variable and individualized, yet very organized. Overall, considering this 0.01% to 0.09% difference and understanding how we think, feel, and behave appear to be developmental, cultural, and biopsychosocial in nature. Despite our highly evolved (or divinely designed) nature, we still view ourselves in relation to where we live in our environment and how we interact with others both intra- and interculturally.

From a neurobiological and neurocognitive perspective, emotions such as stress are mapped in our physiology, which has a relational meaning to each individual (Lazarus, 1999). Understanding the perceptual–cognitive–emotional meaning of stress for each individual is critical and has therapeutic value. Since the mid-1960s, scientists have conceived that certain "basic emotions" (i.e., anger, fear, sadness, happiness, disgust) are neurobiological in nature and that each emotion arises from an innate specific part of the brain, which can be measured from neurochemical and electrical impulses as seen using a variety of brain imaging technologies (e.g., rs-fcMRI, fMRI; Tracy & Randles, 2011). Counter to the "basic emotions" theory of the brain, Touroutoglou, Lindquist, Dickerson, and Barrett (2015) have shown in experimental studies that specific emotions, within the "salience network" of the brain, do not exist within the core structure of the human brain. Instead, they are associated with the perception and intensity of certain emotions that support the "conceptual act" theory of emotion. Thus, basic emotions do not arise from their own neural networks. Rather, they are constructed from the combination of activity in the core brain system that performs more basic functions such as memory, sensory perception, receptive language, and expressive language. Ultimately, the "conceptual act" theory of emotions predicts that the same intrinsic networks engage during a variety of emotions exhibited by individuals.

## The Conscious Expression of Emotions

Similar to Touroutoglou et al.'s (2015) perspective, Pessoa (2014) proposes that in the emotional architecture of the brain, neither emotions nor cognitions are mapped into compartmentalized parts of the right–left brain or in the amygdala. Rather, viewing emotions from a network perspective should supersede the hypothesis of looking at specific neural connections that surround basic emotions. There are complicating factors in mapping and measuring individual emotions that are expressed consciously versus those expressed nonconsciously. For example, LeDoux (2014) and others have extensively studied the emotions of fear and anxiety to see how the brain detects and responds to these emotions. From a neurobiological view, it is important to make the distinction between emotions that are expressed consciously and those that arise nonconsciously. There may be predisposing factors that precipitate the frequency and intensity of individual emotions such as fear and anxiety. Although conscious and nonconscious forms of emotional expression may be equally important to understand, LeDoux suggests that the conscious expression of emotions such as fear and anxiety has been overstudied. Thus, newer research designs must look at what aspects of the brain trigger the individual's threat detection and defense response from the nonconscious part of the brain.

From a humanistic and biopsychosocial perspective, individuals experience stress and trauma in relation to a particular event or situation. As suggested by newer research paradigms, these emotions are expressed both consciously and nonconsciously and cannot be mapped in one core structure of the brain such as the amygdala. Thus, the individual's perception and intensity of emotions associated with stressful and traumatic events should predict the expression of one's emotional response.

## Cultural Aspects of Neurobiology

Some researchers suggest there are important cultural differences in how emotions such as stress and trauma are expressed and experienced (Kitayama, Markus, & Matsumoto, 1995; Kohrt & Hruschka, 2010; Mauro, Sato, & Tucker, 1992). Lazarus (1999), for instance, views the psychobiological and cultural expressions of emotions as a result of person–environment interaction, not from a pure cultural base. He states "that a particular relational meaning leads to a particular emotion, and each emotion has its own relational meaning, or core relational theme" (p. 69). Thus, Lazarus is suggesting that the essence of human emotions may not be dependent on a particular culture because there are always within-group differences in how stress and trauma are experienced. Rather, it is how human emotions are appraised by others within the environment in which the person exists and interacts, as well as other moderating variables, that change the person's perception and expression of stress. From a neurobiology point of view, Lazarus's theory may be closely tied to Touroutoglou et al.'s (2015) hypothesis, suggesting that perception and intensity of emotions may predict the individual's response to certain experiences and emotions that may not be dependent on one's culture.

The neuroscience of emotions appears to be in its infancy. Multiple neurobiological researchers now suggest that extraordinary stressful and traumatic events create abnormalities such as atrophy of neural connections within the structures of the brain (Sapolsky, 1998; Vasterling & Brewin, 2005; Vasterling & Verfaellie, 2009). Several studies of animal and human populations using tissue samples revealed an increase in oxidative stress, chronic inflammation, and extracellular glutamate; this provided direct evidence of biochemical deficits in the brain (Prasad & Bondy, 2015). Exposure to chronic stress and trauma can also lead to neurocognitive abnormalities, as well as involving other body systems. This has been demonstrated by both brain imaging scans and neuropsychological test performance where persons having symptoms of posttraumatic stress exhibit neurocognitive limitations with such tasks as memory, concentration, focus, and activities of daily living.

The implications of neuroscience and the impact that trauma has on neurocognitive functioning within one's culture have far-reaching significance. From a historical and intergenerational trauma perspective, chronic exposure to stress and trauma has massive cultural implications, particularly for those who have been affected by continual horrific acts such as oppression, slavery, ethnic cleansing, and genocide. The psychosocial implications of historical and intergenerational trauma are discussed more extensively in other chapters. However, intriguing questions remain as to how traumatic events can change the neurobiological, neurocognitive, and mental health functioning of a culture on a long-term basis.

The point here is that there is a complex interplay between our biological, psychological, psychosocial, and cultural environment that may determine how we react to stress, traumatic stress, and other mental health symptoms. As Frankl (1963) proposes, it may not necessarily be the nature of trauma itself that predicts our response to trauma; rather, it is our perception and attitude toward the traumatic event. If in fact certain emotions can be mapped and integrated into our neurochemistry, then perhaps we can change our mind, body, and spirit through a change in our attitude, perception, and the way we activate and deactivate our specific stress mechanisms (e.g., use of bioneurocognitive feedback, mindfulness meditation, positive psychology, resiliency training). Accordingly, as mental health practitioners, we can use this knowledge to work more effectively with trauma survivors. The ultimate payoff is that if we look deeper into the biopsychosocial functioning and the neurobiological effects of trauma on the individual, then we might find important strategies that cultivate posttraumatic growth, resiliency, and hardiness.

## THE EMOTIONAL BRAIN

The field of psychoneuroimmunology (PNI), a word coined by Ader (1990) in 1981, has provided new insights into how our thoughts, emotions, and cognitions influence our total physiology. The task of PNI researchers is difficult because as Sapolsky (1998) asserts, our emotions, particularly during the stress response, have their own unique physiological arousal patterns of magnitude, frequency, and intensity. This is partly because people differ in how they turn on their stress mechanisms and respond to other emotions within the core structures of the brain. Additionally, it is hypothesized that our emotional experiences manifest in other complex ways neurologically, because we all possess different personality traits and states, behavioral response patterns, and motivational states (Mayne & Ramsey, 2001).

Sapolsky (1998) eloquently describes the emotional brain during an acute stress reaction. Initially, when we perceive an event to be highly stressful, our body goes into a fight-or-flight mode, which activates our sympathetic nervous system. This region of our autonomic nervous system begins in the brain and reaches out into every organ, blood vessel, hormone, and gland in our body. It is important to note that this same physiological reaction is turned on even when we anticipate or believe that something bad is going to happen.

Next, the hormones epinephrine and norepinephrine (the British refer to this as adrenaline and noradrenaline) are secreted into our body so that we can mobilize energy rapidly and react to a stressful or critical life event. The other half of the autonomic nervous system plays an opposing role and engages our parasympathetic system, which helps bring our nervous system into calm states of functioning. While the sympathetic system speeds up our heart rate, blood flow, and pulse rates, and releases adrenaline into the system, the parasympathetic system slows our body down so that we are not always in a state of fight-or-flight or hypervigilance.

Our immune system also plays a significant role in the impact that stress has on our body. The primary task of the immune system is to defend the body against infectious agents such as viruses, bacteria, fungi, and parasites. The system is quite complex because it has the task of remembering every cell in our body (i.e., brain cells, heart cells, muscle cells, lung cells, sensory nerve cells) and being able to sort these cells into the different organs and body systems. The immune system must also differentiate between normal and abnormal cell structures by recording and memorizing the distinctive cellular signature of each cell structure (referred to as immunologic memory). The core function of our immune system is to defend us when we come under attack by viruses, bacteria, or some other infectious anomalies.

Clinical studies have shown how some individuals who are in a constant state of hyperarousal due to high and intense levels of stress exposure have developed significant health problems (Goleman, 2003; Kabat-Zinn, 1990; Sapolsky, 1998; Wachen et al., 2013). For some, chronic stress and anxiety can become a persistent pattern involving one's physical, mental, emotional, and cognitive states of being. Once the biochemical reactions in the emotional brain are mapped due to intense and high levels of chronic stress exposure, this can increase oxidative stress, inflammation in tissue, and nitric oxide synthase, as well as the release of multiple stress hormones; this creates an enduring neurological pattern resulting in multiple mental health conditions (Prasad & Bondy, 2015). When physical injury occurs (e.g., traumatic brain injury [TBI], amputation, spinal cord injury), this places the individual in a whole other risk category for multiple mental health conditions (i.e., major depression, anxiety disorders, substance use disorders [SUDs], chronic pain conditions).

It should come as no surprise that untreated intense levels of emotional and psychological stress can become a risk factor for developing posttraumatic stress disorder. Many individuals internalize their physiological stress reaction and consequently never have an opportunity to store usable resources for healthy energy. Consequently, if we constantly mobilize energy, we never have the opportunity to store it so we can use these resources for calm and focused states of consciousness. Overall, there is a physical, emotional, cognitive, and biochemical cost to persistent sympathetic arousal and the heavy secretion of glucocorticoids and other toxins released in the nervous system. Primarily, high levels of glucocorticoids along with other processes that are toxic to the body are among the markers for depression and anxiety disorders (Sapolsky, 1998).

Applying the "basic emotions" theoretical perspective, Brother (1989) points to the amygdala–cortical pathway in the brain as part of the key neural circuitry that underlies emotions. The amygdala appears to be the specific structure of the brain that orchestrates the most intense electrical activation when reading, interpreting, or trying to understand the emotions of self and others. In fact, the amygdala is positively correlated with increases in negative affect and consistently shows robust activation during intense emotional experiences during brain imaging studies (Barrett, Moreau, Duncan, Rauch, & Wright, 2007). Thus, over time, those who are not able to express healthy emotions or those who suppress emotions such as stress, grief, or trauma appear to be affected biologically, physiologically, emotionally, psychologically, socially, and spiritually. Accordingly, chronic activation of the emotional brain and habitual repression of emotions can compromise our immune system, which increases our resistance to infections, chronic illness, and diseases (Pert, Dreher, & Ruff, 2005; Sapolsky, 1998; Weil, 1995).

## HEALING EMOTIONS IN THE BRAIN

The impact that our mind, body, and spirit has on our emotional and physical well-being has been well documented through time by archeological and historical record and ancient texts, communicated through religious and spiritual leaders, and displayed through ritual medicine practices by indigenous cultures across the planet (Eagle, 2003; Harner, 1990; Mehl-Madrona, 1997). Qualitatively, there is evidence for healing one's emotions related to stress and trauma. Empirical evidence for the mind–body connection or the brain's influence on human physiology dates back 100 years where some of the first studies designed appeared to convince scientists that there is a strong link between the nervous system and the immune system (Sapolsky, 1998). Accordingly, it is difficult to discuss the brain and emotions without pointing to the exceedingly intricate interplay of the various body systems involved in recording, transposing, replicating, expressing, and persistently reproducing the individual's stressful and traumatic experiences.

Building upon the shoulders of giants in the highly complex fields of physics, neurosciences, psychology, theology, and spirituality, Wilber (1996) comprehensively describes healing the mind, body, and spirit in his somewhat esoteric work *A Brief History of Everything*, in which he theoretically maps the biological, psychological, cognitive, and spiritual development of the individual. This philosophical rendering of the human condition offers a unique example of many issues that are cross-discipline, yet all relate to healing. Wilber's elegant model provides a clearer understanding of the complex interplay in healing the mind, body, and spirit, which may increase the mental health professional's capacity for understanding the experience of stress and trauma.

Indeed, humanists and neuroscientists have different perspectives on healing the emotional brain. For some, healing the emotional brain may actually begin outside the human physiology. How the person interacts with stress in his or her environment, the level and intensity with which the person experiences stress, and the type of critical incident he or she has been exposed to all seem to have predictive validity with how the person responds from a mind, body, and spiritual perspective. In the study of emotions and the brain, it has been hypothesized by some that there are discrete, basic, and universal emotions that individuals react to on a mind, body, and spiritual dimension (Bar-On & Parker, 2000; Mayne & Bonanno, 2001). Most persons have the capacity to express universal emotions (e.g., anger, love, happiness, sadness) with varying levels of degree and intensity. However, Mayne and Ramsey (2001) imply that expressing emotions (e.g., verbalizing, behaving, acting) can only be measured consciously by self-report measures and observations of the person's experience. We cannot fully understand the unconscious intention of individual emotions. Thus, it is critical that we understand different states of consciousness (self-awareness, thought, imagination) in healing emotions.

## The Expression of Empathy and the Brain

Newer studies on the verbal and nonverbal expression of emotions and the interpersonal communication experience shared between two individuals during therapeutic engagements create a physiological and emotional arousal between two individuals. Empathy has been well documented as a necessary human approach to facilitate during therapeutic interactions. This may contribute to an understanding of how empathic connections are made during counseling and psychotherapy versus those developed outside of session in the client's natural environment. For example, Marci, Ham, Moran, and Orr (2007) looked at 20 client–therapist pairs being treated for mood and anxiety disorders. They specifically focused on the therapeutic relationships that were formed during psychotherapy sessions. These researchers then took measures of the physiological reactions of both the client and the therapist and the client's perceived level of empathy as expressed by the therapist. They found that when high positive emotions and empathy were expressed by the therapist, similar physiological responses were experienced by the client and the therapist as measured by electrical skin conductance recordings, heart rate, voice dynamics, and body movement. Thus, it seems that a much stronger working alliance or social–emotional attachment is formed in therapy when clients perceive their therapists are communicating higher levels of empathy. This not only has implications for the therapeutic relationship, but also may bring promise to how the emotional brain can be developed in those critically affected by extraordinary stressful and traumatic events.

It is clear that neuroscientists, as well as clinical and experimental psychologists, all measure empathy and the emotional brain from different perspectives. From a purely dynamic physiological state, the expression of emotions has been shown to involve different body systems during therapeutic interactions. Integral studies in the mind, body, and spirit demonstrate how different emotions are experienced by the person. Indeed, there is a complex interplay of such mind–body neural connections within the structures of the brain. More experimental designs will be needed that measure the individual's perception of critical events (e.g., hurricanes, floods, fire, physically traumatic experiences) and how his or her autonomic nervous system (e.g., parasympathetic and sympathetic) is activated during times of an actual or anticipated stressful event. This is a critical area for study because many stress researchers believe that as much as 80% of all physical illnesses are caused by psychological and emotional stressors (Kabat-Zinn, 1990; Sapolsky, 1998; Selye, 1976; Weil, 1995).

The awareness of one's emotions is considered to be a prerequisite for empathy and is very closely associated with measuring the emotional intelligence of children, adolescents, and adults (Bar-On & Parker, 2000; Goleman, 2003). This may be an important area of research for healing emotions. Our ability to perceive and experience the emotions of others cannot exceed our ability to monitor our own emotional states (Lane, 2000). Even though we have no control over our autonomic nervous system, we do have some degree of control over our voluntary nervous system, such as is observed during biofeedback or mindfulness activities. Thus, becoming attuned to our thoughts, feelings, emotions, and behaviors is central to the mind–body connection of studying the emotional brain in healing through different states of consciousness.

## STATES OF CONSCIOUSNESS IN THE EMOTIONAL BRAIN

Consciousness is a process that involves awareness, thoughts, feelings, cognitions, perceptions, and sensations as they relate to how we experience ourselves and the world around us (Schlitz, Amorok, & Micozzi, 2005). It relates to how individuals think, feel, act, and behave, given a specific event, stimuli, environment, or energy that evokes the various sensory mechanisms of the brain. Of particular interest is the question: *How does the brain network and map this total sensory and extrasensory experience?* Consciousness is a highly complex construct and has a variety of meanings across the various specialty areas in neuroscience, psychology, and spirituality. Understanding the individual's particular state of consciousness requires conceptual frameworks and theoretical tools to make sense and meaning out of what the individual truly experiences (Tart, 2000). During the second half of the 20th century, Western psychology recognized only a few states of consciousness such as normal waking and sleeping states (Walsh & Vaughn, 1993). If the person did not exist in these ordinary states, then he or she was likely in an unconscious state lying in a hospital bed somewhere. However, many other states of consciousness exist than once thought given the complexities of how neuroscience has begun mapping the brain and emotions. For instance, shamanic cultures have been known to achieve nonordinary states of consciousness during healing rituals as they journey for spirits or power animals (Harner, 1990; Meadows, 1991). The way of the shaman requires a cultural understanding of indigenous peoples and how natural it is for the tribal leader or shaman to change into an "altered state," much like mediums, mystics, and empaths have done for centuries. From a Western cultural viewpoint, we might understand "altered states of consciousness" better as it relates to priests, ministers, monks, rabbis, or lay clergy who go into deep contemplative states of meditation and prayer. To fully understand the complexities of consciousness within the context of this chapter, readers are encouraged to consult the References section at the end of this chapter.

In the past decade, consciousness studies have particularly become an interest for neuroscientists and psychologists because of the impact that conscious and nonordinary states of consciousness has on the emotional brain (Hubbard, 2015; LeDoux, 2014, 1996; Tart, 2000). Tart proposes a newer term, *discrete states of consciousness,* which he suggests more accurately depicts this highly unique and dynamic pattern of psychological states and traits that operate in the core structures of the human brain. Consciousness plays a key role in understanding fear conditioning, anxiety, posttraumatic stress, and somatoform disorders. It also plays an important role in the overall perceptions of our mental and physical well-being and is critical regarding how we turn on/off our stress and trauma triggers.

## Empathetic and Transpersonal States of Consciousness

The construct of states of consciousness may be better understood using the emotion of empathy. Empathy, both considered a trait and state, requires a significant level of intuitiveness when perceiving, processing, and expressing any type of verbal and nonverbal expression of feeling, thought, or emotion (Huther, 2006). The capacity for empathy is primarily found in persons who possess this highly complex mechanism within the emotional brain. Interestingly, the idea that helping and human service professionals have a highly developed capacity for empathy is not necessarily accurate. Expressing empathy and possessing the capacity for warmth, compassion, genuineness, and understanding are positive attributes and good worker traits for professional counselors. However, there are other occupations and fields that require a high degree of empathy in order to be successful (e.g., salespersons, public relations, nurses, teachers). As described by career development theorists, persons must be motivated and have an expressed or manifested interest to work in certain occupations and careers. A key point here is that it is entirely possible that most individuals have the ability to cultivate an empathic state of consciousness to some degree. Just as humans are capable of warm greetings, good manners, and the expression of love, they can also choose empathy as a way of being. There are exceptions, of course (e.g., severe brain injury, neurocognitive impairments, and psychopathology).

Brennan (1987), a former research scientist with NASA and currently a therapist, healer, and author, has spent a lifetime researching the high sense perception (HSP) and the human energy field to try and affect the health and healing of individuals. It is evident in her writings that she and others like her who began careers outside the counseling and psychology field have a deep sense of compassion and empathy for others. Brennan (1987) explains that within the deep structures of the brain the body's sense of time, space, consciousness, and emotions are all inseparable patterns of energy that have multiple states of consciousness and dimensions of reality. These patterns can be seen as body auras by those who have developed the gifts for this empathic-intuitive ability.

Brennan (1987) points to the work of Albert Einstein's special theory of relativity published in 1905 to illustrate how neuroscientists have taken a new look at the connection between one's mind, body, and spirit. She explains how Einstein confronted the current thinking of his day regarding Newtonian physics and avowed that space is not a three-dimensional entity. Rather, time and space together form a fourth dimension; hence, the space–time continuum. In other words, time is not a linear or absolute concept. Time is relative to the observer. So if two independent observers observe the same event happening at the same time (e.g., speed of light) within the same general physical space, they will order the event differently as to when the event actually occurred. This is especially true if each person moves at a different velocity relative to the observed event. As Hawking (1988) states parsimoniously, "Since the speed of light is just the distance it has traveled divided by the time it has taken, different observers would measure different speeds for the light" (p. 21). Thus, in the theory of relativity, all observers must agree on how fast light travels. They still, however, may not agree on the distance with which light travels and the time it takes to travel such a distance.

The point being is that Einstein's theory of relativity basically put an end to earlier ideas suggesting that time is an absolute concept. Thus, there was a major consciousness shift in our thinking and philosophy about who our ultimate Creator or Supreme Being is, where we came from, and where we are going after we die. Likewise, dissecting and measuring brain cell activity in laboratory animals can no longer provide neuroscientists with answers on how the human brain functions in terms of emotions (e.g., love, fear, compassion), mood (e.g., sad, excited), intelligence, or behaviors (e.g., laziness, anger). We cannot consign human beings to a physical or biological entity.

The consciousness shift on the event horizon is that there is enormous capacity to develop our mind, body, and spirit for healing the emotions associated with stress and trauma. This integral connection is much like gravity. Gravity is an unseen form of energy that keeps us earthbound. We hardly notice gravity until we trip and fall to the ground. As other quantum physicists describe gravity, ". . . gravity is mysterious. It is a grand force permeating the life of the cosmos, but it is elusive and ethereal" (Greene, 1999, p. 61). Thus, it requires integral approaches in mind–body research with consideration given to the existential and spiritual aspects of human beings to understand the true emotional capacity of the brain.

This very brief discussion of the cosmos and quantum physics is a metaphor for the new paradigm shift in consciousness, transpersonal, and brain research studies. Such a discussion is required today because most states of consciousness were viewed as pathological and related to specific states such as being intoxicated, psychotic, or homicidal. Today, many therapists have experienced a special type of empathic awareness and intuitiveness with clients (Sollod, 2005). Although conventional psychotherapeutic approaches also emphasize the importance of focusing on understanding the client's thoughts and feelings and responding empathically, empathic intuitiveness is at a much deeper level of consciousness and has sparked interest among mind–body researchers. Thus, we may be on the event horizon of understanding how human emotions are communicated through intentional and intuitive mind, body, and spiritual work. There are many positive aspects to understanding personal emotions at a deeper level.

## CONCLUDING REMARKS

The scientific paradigm and manifestations of transpersonal psychology and other metaphysical events should not be disciplines that work independent of each other. Rather, blending the scientific paradigm (i.e., neuroscience) with transpersonal psychology and mysticism has been a developing area of research that has expanded within the past 20 years in psychology, theology, philosophy, and other specialty areas. Interestingly, when we study some time-honored healing traditions (e.g., shamanic drumming, native chants, dance, meditation, yoga) perhaps we have come full circle in our quest for understanding both ordinary and nonordinary states of consciousness. Such indigenous practices facilitated by mystics, healers, and folk medicine men and women could provide a model for achieving higher levels of intuitiveness and empathic states of consciousness for professional counselors. The synthesis of conventional counseling and psychotherapy with indigenous healing approaches can only enrich our understanding of the brain's profound capabilities for deeper levels of compassion and empathy.

## REFERENCES

Ader, R. (1990). *Psychoneuroimmunology* (2nd ed.). San Diego, CA: Academic Press.

Bar-On, R., & Parker, J. D. (2000). *The handbook of emotional intelligence: Theory, development, assessment, and application at home, school, and in the workplace.* San Francisco, CA: Jossey-Bass.

Barrett, L. F., Moreau, E. B., Duncan, S. L., Rauch, S. L., & Wright, C. I. (2007). The amygdala and the experience of affect. *Social Cognitive and Affective Neuroscience, 2*(2), 73–83.

Brennan, B. A. (1987). *Hands of light: A guide to healing through the human energy field.* New York, NY: Bantam Books.

Brother, L. (1989). A biological perspective on empathy. *American Journal of Psychiatry, 146*(1), 1–16.

Cann, R. I., Stoneking, M., & Wilson, A. C. (1987). Mitochondrial DNA and human evolution. *Nature, 325,* 31–36.

Eagle, R. (2003). *Native American spirituality: A walk in the woods.* Zanesfield, OH: Rainbow Light.

Frankl, V. E. (1963). *Man's search for meaning.* New York, NY: Pocket Books.

Genome News Network. (2016). Genome variations. Retrieved from http://www.genomenewsnetwork .org/resources/whats_a_genome/Chp4_1.shtml

Goleman, D. (2003). *Healing emotions: Conversations with the Dalai Lama on mindfulness, emotions, and health.* Boston, MA: Shambhala.

Greene, B. (1999). *The elegant universe: Superstrings, hidden dimensions, and the quest for the ultimate theory*. New York, NY: W. W. Norton.

Harner, M. (1990). *The way of the shaman*. San Francisco, CA: Harper San Francisco.

Hawking, S. (1988). *A brief history of time: From the big bang to black holes*. New York, NY: Bantam Books.

Hubbard, B. M. (2015). *Conscious evolution: Awakening the power of our social potential*. Novato, CA: New World Library.

Huther, G. (2006). Neurobiological approaches to a better understanding of human nature and human values. Retrieved from http://www.gerald-huether.de/pdf/nature_and_values.pdf

Kabat-Zinn, J. (1990). *Full catastrophe living: Using the wisdom of your body and mind to face stress, pain, and illness*. New York, NY: Dell Publishing.

Kitayama, S., Markus, H. R., & Matsumoto, H. (1995). Culture, self, and emotion: A cultural perspective on "self-conscious" emotions. In J. P. Tangney & K. W. Fischer (Eds.), *Self-conscious emotions: The psychology of shame, guilt, embarrassment, and pride* (pp. 439–464). New York, NY: Guilford Press.

Kohrt, B. A., & Hruschka, D. J. (2010). Nepali concepts of psychological trauma: The role of idioms of distress, ethnopsychology and ethnophysiology in alleviating suffering and preventing stigma. *Cultural Medicine Psychiatry, 34*, 322–352.

Lane, R. D. (2000). Levels of emotional awareness: Neurological, psychological, and social perspectives. In R. Bar-On & J. D. Parker (Eds.), *The handbook of emotional intelligence: Theory, development, assessment, and application at home, school, and in the workplace* (pp. 171–214). San Francisco, CA: Jossey-Bass.

Lazarus, R. S. (1999). *Stress and emotions: A new synthesis*. New York, NY: Springer Publishing.

LeDoux, J. E. (1996). *The emotional brain: The mysterious underpinnings of emotional life*. New York, NY: Touchstone.

LeDoux, J. E. (2014). Coming to terms with fear. *Proceedings of the National Academy of Sciences of the United States of America, 111*(8), 2871–2878.

Marci, C. D., Ham, J., Moran, E., & Orr, S. P. (2007). Physiologic correlates of perceived therapist empathy and social-emotional process during psychotherapy. *Journal of Nervous and Mental Disorders, 195*, 103–111.

Mauro, R., Sato, K., & Tucker, J. (1992). The role of appraisal in human emotions: A cross-cultural study. *Journal of Personality and Social Psychology, 62*, 301–317.

Mayne, T. J., & Bonanno, G. A. (2001). *Emotions: Current issues and future directions*. New York, NY: Guilford Press.

Mayne, T. J., & Ramsey, J. (2001). The structure of emotion: A nonlinear dynamic systems approach. In T. J. Mayne and G. A. Bonanno (Eds.), *Emotions: Current issues and future directions* (pp. 1–37). New York, NY: Guilford Press.

Meadows, K. (1991). *Shamanic experience: A practical guide to shamanism for the new millennium*. Boston, MA: Element.

Mehl-Madrona, L. (1997). *Coyote medicine: Lessons from Native American healing*. New York, NY: Fireside.

Pert, C. B., Dreher, H. E., & Ruff, M. R. (2005). The psychosomatic network: Foundations of mind-body medicine. In M. Schlitz, T. Amorok, & M. Micozzi (Eds.), *Consciousness and healing: Integral approaches to mind-body medicine* (pp. 61–78). St. Louis, MO: Elsevier, Churchill, & Livingstone.

Pessoa, L. (2014). Understanding brain networks and brain organization. *Physics of Life Review, 11*(3), 400–435.

Prasad, K. N., & Bondy, S. C. (2015). Common biochemical defects linkage between post-traumatic stress disorders, mild traumatic brain injury (TBI) and penetrating TBI. *Brain Research, 1599*, 103–114.

Sankararaman, S., Mallick, S., Donnemann, M., Prufer, K., Kelso, J., Paabo, S., . . . Reich, D. (2014). The genomic landscape of Neanderthal ancestry in present-day humans. *Nature, 507*, 354–357. http://dx.doi.org/10.1038/nature12961

Sapolsky, R. M. (1998). *Why zebras don't get ulcers: An updated guide to stress, stress-related diseases, and coping.* New York, NY: W. H. Freeman.

Schlitz, M., Amorok, T., & Micozzi, M. S. (2005). *Consciousness and healing: Integral approaches to mind-body medicine.* St. Louis, MO: Elsevier, Churchill Livingstone.

Selye, H. (1976). *The stress of life.* New York, NY: McGraw-Hill.

Sollod, R. N. (2005). Spiritual and healing approaches in psychotherapeutic practice. In R. Moodley & W. West (Eds.), *Integrating traditional healing practices into counseling and psychotherapy* (pp. 270–281). Thousand Oaks, CA: Sage Publications.

Tart, C. T. (2000). *States of consciousness.* Lincoln, NE: iUniverse.com.

The Tech Museum of Innovation. (2016). People are not as alike as scientists once thought. Retrieved from http://genetics.thetech.org/original_news/news38

Touroutoglou, A., Lindquist, K. A., Dickerson, B. C., & Barrett, L. F. (2015). Intrinsic connectivity in the human brain does not reveal networks for "basic" emotions. *Scan, 10*, 1257–1265.

Tracy, J. L., & Randles, D. (2011). Four models of basic emotions: A review of Ekman and Cordaro, Izard, Levenson, and Panksepp and Watt. *Emotion Review, 3*, 397–405.

Vasterling, J. J., & Brewin, C. R. (2005). *Neuropsychology of PTSD: Biological, cognitive, and clinical perspectives.* New York, NY: Guilford Press.

Vasterling, J. J., & Verfaellie, M. (2009). Posttraumatic stress disorder: A neurocognitive perspective. *Journal of the International Neurobiological Society, 15*, 826–829.

Wachen, J. S., Shipherd, J. C., Suvak, M., Vogt, D., King, L. A., & King, D. W. (2013). Posttraumatic stress symptomatology as a mediator of the relationship between warzone exposure and physical health symptoms in men and women. *Journal of Traumatic Stress, 26*, 319–328.

Walsh, R., & Vaughan, F. (1993). *Paths beyond ego: The transpersonal vision.* New York, NY: Jeremy P. Tarcher/Putnam.

Warren, R. (2002). *The purpose driven life.* Grand Rapids, MI: Zondervan.

Weil, A. (1995). *Spontaneous healing.* New York, NY: Ballantine.

Wilber, K. (1996). *A brief history of everything.* Boston, MA: Shambhala.

Wilson, A. J. (2013). Where did we come from? Retrieved from http://www.christianitytoday.com/ct/2013/october/where-did-we-come-from.html?start=2

# CHAPTER 5

# Empathy First Aid and Disaster Mental Health Counseling*

Disaster mental health counseling is both the same as and different from traditional mental health counseling. One distinct and obvious difference is that in times immediately following a disaster, mental health counselors do not facilitate counseling and psychotherapeutic approaches such as occurs in a clinical setting that concludes with a 45-minute session. This may occur weeks or months later in the follow-up sessions devoted to treating the person's posttraumatic stress symptoms. Typically in disaster mental health deployments, at the onset, there is very little structure and routine that mimic the traditional psychotherapeutic process. Rather, disaster mental health counselors provide short-term services to disaster survivors in shelters, tent cities, disaster recovery centers, school gymnasiums, and community centers.

The disaster mental health counselor's goals in disaster response are to normalize the person's traumatic response as a normal reaction to an abnormal critical event and to try and bring back to balance the individual's internal and external resources. Accordingly, the use of empathy as a sort of first-aid intervention is essential in forming a core relationship with disaster survivors. The concept of "first aid" as applied by medical practitioners is easily understood. There are many hands-on medical protocols and various physiological measures that emergency medical personnel use as a tool to stabilize the individual from a medical/physical status. However, utilizing mental health, empathy, or psychological first aid is quite different. Empathy as a first-aid tool extends the notion that there are beginning-level interventions required to intervene in times of mental health disaster response (e.g., listening, attending, empathic responding). Compassion alone does not set the stage for trauma recovery. Rather, empathic attunement and connection is required as a first-aid approach in order to work competently with trauma survivors before any mental health screenings, evaluation, and interventions are facilitated.

---

*Adapted in part from material appearing in Chapters 3 and 5 from Stebnicki (2008), *Empathy Fatigue,* © Springer Publishing Company.

The loss, grief, death, and dying associated with natural and person-made disasters require empathy as the essential element of developing the therapeutic relationship. Thus, disaster empathy training is an important construct to understand so that its approaches can be facilitated by skilled and competent counselors. So the question is: *What is the role of empathy first aid in disaster mental health response?* The following sections help delineate some of these issues.

## BRIEF HISTORY OF EMPATHY

The conceptual underpinnings of empathy can be traced back long before its modern application in research and practice as described by Carl Rogers (1902–1987) when he published his seminal work, *Client-Centered Therapy* in 1951. Barrett-Lennard (1981) suggests that modern usage of the meaning and concept of empathy was dated by R. L. Katz in 1963. Katz noted that the nonclinical use of empathy was first conceptualized in 1897 by Theodore Lipps (1851–1914). Jackson's (1992) research into the origins of the foundational aspects of the theory and practice of empathy can in fact be traced to Theodore Lipps and his concept of *Einfuhlung*. Lipps used the Germanic term *Einfuhlung* to refer to the process of becoming totally absorbed in an external object, or projecting oneself into an esthetic object such as a form of art. Later, Lipps and a colleague, Robert Vischer (1847–1933), suggested that *Einfuhlung* is a particular emotion that can manifest as one's appreciation for the feelings and attitudes of another person. Sigmund Freud referred to Lipps's concept of *Einfuhlung* in his *Jokes and Their Relation to the Unconscious* in 1905 (as cited in Katz, 1963). Although Freud did not infer the clinical application of this concept, he suggested that this emotion produced a feeling of projecting oneself into the psychological state of another person.

By 1909, the expression "empathy" became the accepted translation in Western psychoanalytic theory through the suggestion of Edward B. Titchener (1867–1927). Barrett-Lennard (1981) suggests that as E. B. Titchener introduced empathy as the English equivalent of *Einfuhlung*, its meaning and usage advanced in theory. The concept of empathy advanced significantly into experimental and clinical practice during the 1940s and 1950s through the separate, often unacknowledged scholarly work of Roy Schafer (1922–present); Heinz Kohut (1913–1981); and Ralph R. Greenson (1911–1979).

Among the early pioneers of empathy is Alfred Adler (1931), who simply stated that if we are genuinely interested in the other person, then "we must be able to see with his eyes and listen with his ears" (p. 172). Barrett-Lennard (1981) suggests that empathy was not brought to prominence in counseling theory and practice until the work of such thinkers as Rogers and Katz. These individuals made the primary distinction that empathy was a process of "feeling into" the other person in a deeply responsive way and that one must experience this awareness. Today, most research studies concerned with the clinical application of empathy have accepted, incorporated, and credited the lifework of Carl Rogers's *Client-Centered Therapy* (e.g., empathic attending, listening, understanding, responding) as the primary contribution to the 20th and 21st century of this therapeutic facilitative approach.

## EMPATHY AS META-COMMUNICATION

Throughout the history of the helping profession, the most fundamental approach for communicating with others has been rooted in compassion or empathy. Empathy has been discussed in the counseling and psychology literature as a skill that can be both developed and learned if facilitated by a competent professional (Barone et al., 2005). Empathy as a way of being (Rogers, 1980) is also a form of communication that involves attending, listening, observing, understanding, responding to the concerns of others with a deep respect, and genuineness. In fact, much of what we communicate to one another is done nonverbally. Empathy involves being aware of the other's meta-communication through eye contact, body language, silence, tone of voice, gestures, facial expressions, and physical space, as well as many other ways. Empathic communication cannot be understated in the helping relationship. It is a tool to build the foundation for a trusting, genuine, and therapeutic relationship. Its intention is to build a strong working alliance with others.

Empathy is often a misunderstood concept that is often confused with sympathy. Recent studies suggest that, from a prosocial perspective, people express more sympathy for disaster survivors and rarely do they sense empathic concerns from others (Banfield & Dovidio, 2012). Sympathy, as an emotional reaction to another person's life event, is essentially stating: "I'm sorry this has happened to you." Conversely, empathy communicates verbally and nonverbally to others by affirming: "I'm sorry this has happened to you—it has to be very difficult for you; what can I do to help?" Accordingly, empathy requires the professional helper to be an active participant during therapeutic interactions and be deeply involved with others in a powerful way.

If we expect our clients to have the capacity to understand; express their thoughts openly, honestly, and directly; resolve problems on their own; and make good decisions in life, then a high level of empathic communication must be at the foundation of the therapeutic alliance. It is vital that helping professionals model this deep level of awareness, understanding, and responding during person-centered interactions. Accordingly, to be a competent and effective communicator, it is essential that professional helpers: (a) hold positive beliefs about themselves and their clients, (b) have a healthy self-concept, (c) embrace and express values that respect other people and cultures, (d) are able to fully listen and understand others, and (e) possess the skills of empathy. If the skills of empathy are not present within person-centered interactions, there will likely be very little respect, understanding, or compassion communicated to the individuals who we are trying to help. Otherwise, there is risk that the therapist would likely respond with an attitude of indifference, apathy, and overall lack of concern for others.

## EMPATHY AS THERAPEUTIC LEVERAGE

Despite numerous problems of research design within the study of empathy, the core conditions of empathy as it relates to positive therapeutic outcome have been enthusiastically supported in most studies conducted between 1960 and 1989 (Duan & Hill, 1996;

Patterson, 1984). Paying attention to and sensing the other person's wants and needs is the focal point of any client-centered relationship. Attending, listening, and responding to others in a way that they know they have been understood and heard is perhaps one of the oldest and most powerful tools for understanding the human experience and others' worldview (Corey & Corey, 2016; Egan, 2014). Skilled helpers such as professional counselors use empathy to build the foundation of a trusting relationship for the purpose of establishing an effective working alliance with others. Thus, empathy can be used as therapeutic leverage.

Psychologist and founder of the person-centered therapy movement, Dr. Carl Rogers (1957), introduced the concept of empathy as a *necessary and sufficient condition* required for the therapeutic change to occur. He hypothesized that there are core conditions that apply to all psychotherapy: (a) counselor congruence or genuineness within the therapeutic relationship, (b) unconditional positive regard for the client, (c) the ability of the counselor to empathize with the client in this relationship, (d) communication of empathy, and (e) expressing unconditional positive regard toward the client. Rogers (1980) talked passionately about empathy and empathic listening as "a way of being." He was known as a deeply intuitive man and provided a description of empathy:

> It means entering the private perceptual world of the other and becoming thoroughly at home in it. It involves being sensitive, moment by moment, to the changing felt meanings which flow in this other person, to the fear or rage or tenderness or confusion or whatever that he or she is experiencing. It means temporarily living in the other's life, moving about in it delicately without making judgments. (p. 142)

The richness of using a basic- and advanced-level empathy builds a relationship that is open and honest. It is particularly essential during disaster mental health response to develop a relationship that is built on trust and rapport. If facilitated appropriately, and timing of its use is appropriate, then empathy can increase the disaster survivor's self-awareness, be an impetus for personal growth and change, and spark new ways of thinking and learning that move the person beyond the "victim status." Equally important is the fact that the more we are open and honest in modeling our own emotions with clients, the better we are able to communicate and show them that we are also human. The intentional and conscious use of empathy during disaster survivor interactions appears to be integral to the helper's way of being both verbally and nonverbally.

Empathy transcends more than just attending, listening, observing, and responding to another person with unconditional positive regard. Egan (2014) suggests that many individuals feel empathy toward others, but few know how to put it into words. Empathy as a way to communicate understanding is not often experienced in everyday life. Many in the counseling field suggest that possessing the skills of empathy is a prerequisite for becoming a competent helper. It is a person-centered approach used as a means of increasing the practitioner's interpersonal effectiveness and enhancing outcomes with his or her clients (Corey & Corey, 2016; Egan, 2014; Ivey, Bradford Ivey, & Zalaquett, 2014; Truax & Carkhuff, 1967).

## THE SHADOW SIDE OF EMPATHY

There appears to be a "shadow side" of empathy (Egan, 2014) as the helper enters the client's world deeply enough to understand issues that may be related to extraordinary stressful and traumatic events. Consequently, some of the client's experiences, content, and emotions may become distorted as the counselor organizes issues into his or her own schema and worldview. Because of the heavy reliance in counselor education on the basic and advanced skills of empathy, it is paramount that cultivating the practice and application of empathic communication be facilitated in a culturally competent manner.

Empathy is not simply responding to what the other person feels; we can never really totally understand and sense another's pain and suffering from his or her disaster or traumatic experiences. The underlying premise of acting empathically is that our compassion for another human being moves us so deeply that we instinctually have a desire to help that individual. However, communicating empathically obviously has limitations with some individuals in certain settings. This is especially relevant if the individual may have to be confronted about his or her negative and high risk-taking behaviors (e.g., adolescent substance abusers, conduct disorders, borderline personality disorders). Despite the shadow side of empathy, we can continue to facilitate therapeutic interactions in a compassionate manner. We can do so by understanding the individual's personality and behavioral traits, the sociocultural environment in which the person may be forced to exist, or the realities of his or her external struggles and barriers he or she may encounter (e.g., severe physical or mental disabilities, racial/ethnic prejudices, job discrimination). If our compassion is our true motivation to help others, then we can act compassionately using the skills of empathy. Even though we can never totally experience the other person's grief, pain, or loss, it is critical that we form an understanding and working definition of the individual's unique emotional experiences as they relate to his or her life.

## CULTURAL ASPECTS OF EMPATHY

Empathy has been discussed in the counseling and psychology literature for the past 125 years and has been conceptualized as a skill that can be both developed and learned if facilitated properly (Barone et al., 2005). Empathy has a rich history of being at the foundation of most theoretical orientations within counselor education programs. However, the concept of empathy has brought a new meaning to its theoretical and practical use in cross-cultural counseling settings. For instance, cultural empathy (Ivey et al., 2014; Ridley & Lingle, 1996), empathic multicultural awareness (Junn, Morton, & Yee, 1995), cultural role taking (Scott & Borodovsky, 1990), ethnotherapeutic empathy (Parson, 1993), and ethnocultural empathy (Wang et al., 2003) have all been used interchangeably to delineate both the same and different constructs of cultural empathy. There is little doubt that in the past 10 years or so, multicultural counseling issues have been at the forefront of the counseling profession. This is because of the changing demographics in the United States and the projections that some time between 2030 and 2050 racial and ethnic minorities will become the majority population in the United States. (Sue, 1996).

In regard to the more general term *cultural specific empathy* as described by some multicultural counseling theorists (Ponterotto & Bensesch, 1998; Ridley, 1995; Ridley, Mendoza, & Kanitz, 1994), empathy is seen as a skill that is pancultural or universal. If empathy can be facilitated in a culturally sensitive manner, this should help strengthen the therapeutic relationship (Ibrahim, 1991). Ridley (1995) suggests that cultural empathy has two dimensions: understanding and communication. Understanding requires that the counselor try and synthesize the idiographic meaning of his or her client's stories, and then respond with the accurate meaning of what the client has communicated to the counselor. Accordingly, all therapy can be culturally contextualized and a positive therapeutic outcome can be enhanced by the skills of a culturally competent counselor.

Some authors have criticized traditional counseling approaches that place a heavy reliance on empathic communication that is not culturally sensitive (Freeman, 1993; Pedersen, 2000; Sue & Sue, 1990; Usher, 1989). If the expectations of therapy are that clients should disclose emotions at a deep level during session, then stepping inside the private world of the culturally different client may be perceived as being too intrusive or offensive. Lee and Richardson (1991) suggest that if the discipline of multicultural counseling is to have any therapeutic value in the counseling relationship, then we must go beyond training counselors in the broad conceptualizations of developing more than just cultural awareness and knowledge. Having an understanding of different cultures alone does not allow us to develop competent practitioners who can apply the skills of cultural empathy. It requires strategies and approaches that are culturally specific and relevant so as to help build a strong trusting relationship and form a therapeutic alliance.

Ridley and Lingle's (1996) model of cultural empathy has defined this construct as a "learned ability" that is interpersonally focused and has many dimensions. This model proposes that there are three processes that underlie cultural empathy: (a) cognitive process (cultural perspective taking and differentiating self from others), (b) affective process (vicarious feelings and empathy expression of concern for others), and (c) communicative process (probing for insight, expression of accurate understanding).

Corey and Corey (2016) suggest that a self-assessment and exploration of both compassion and empathy are important for beginning-level counselors so that they may become aware of their clients' needs from different cultural backgrounds and respond with care, concern, and understanding. Lazarus (1999) views compassion as a double-edged sword, however. He suggests that having too much compassion toward another person can impair our ability to help others. He further states that "we must learn how to distance ourselves emotionally from the emotional significance of their suffering, so it does not overwhelm us" (p. 246). There are others who feel compassion has been left out of training programs in Western psychology, counseling, and medical education (Goleman, 2003). This may be because compassion itself has different ideologies and religious beliefs attached to its meaning. However, competent and ethical counselors should consistently evaluate the impact that their belief systems have on client–counselor sessions and how interventions that use empathy and compassion might be perceived by their clients (Corey & Corey, 2016; Egan, 2014; Ivey et al., 2014).

Compassion, as opposed to empathy or sympathy, as described by the Dalai Lama (see Goleman, 2003) is a quality "that needs to be naturally drawn from within one's own inner resources" (p. 245). His Holiness places a paramount importance on promoting the values of compassion, loving kindness, and altruism as a significant human quality to cultivate at a very early age in life. Even though compassion is a highly desirable and healthy human emotion, it does not appear to be a skill that we can teach in traditional counselor education programs they way we train counselors in the skills of empathy. Intentional acts of compassion, if approached in a culturally sensitive manner, appear to be an unquestionably desirable human attribute that can potentially strengthen the client–counselor therapeutic relationship.

Throughout the history of the helping profession, both compassion and empathy have been the wellspring of establishing a rapport, building a relationship, and achieving optimal levels of therapeutic functioning with clients/consumers. If we could measure compassion and empathy as facilitated by highly developed professionals, then perhaps counselor educators and supervisors could train preprofessionals on how to model such therapeutic interactions with clients/consumers. However, measuring therapeutic interactions using empathy and compassion as the dependent variable can become quite challenging for researchers. The amount, level, degree, and quality of empathy expressed within therapeutic interactions vary depending on the observer, the professional, and the client/consumer. Considering the interchange of emotions during therapeutic interactions, it may be useful to examine how empathy and compassion are experienced by the counselor, client, and outside observer.

In order to use empathy as a first-aid approach during disaster mental health response, counselor educators, supervisors, and researchers could benefit from developing theories and conceptual models that measure empathy first aid. Critical areas to address for interventions might evaluate the complex interplay between (a) personal traits, (b) situation-specific critical events, (c) cognitive-affective states, and (d) general facilitative communication skills (e.g., attending, listening, empathy responses, use of therapeutic touch, spatial distance) of the disaster mental health professional with the intention of facilitating a high level of empathy.

Because empathy is used for (a) therapeutic leverage in rapport building with clients, (b) strengthening the client–counselor relationship, and (c) improving client outcomes, it should be of interest to researchers to measure such variables within the therapeutic setting. Most importantly, measuring such a construct can assist other researchers in developing screening and functional assessment instruments to deal with the constellation of professional fatigue syndromes and issues related to counselor impairment. Ultimately, the goal should be to develop prevention strategies and self-care approaches.

## MEASURING EMPATHY

Empathy is a unique and complex area of study within the expanding discipline of counseling and psychology. It is a multidimensional construct because of the way it is operationally defined in the literature, as well as the philosophical and theoretical differences posed within the profession itself. Thus, measuring empathy can become quite challenging for some researchers. Many have suggested that empathy is qualitatively distinct from other emotions experienced and expressed by the therapist (e.g., compassion, sympathy). This is because there are multiple variables that mediate a therapeutic relationship between the giver and the receiver of empathy. The perceptual differences in the amount, level, degree, and quality of empathy expressed within the client–counselor session also seem to vary. Accordingly, perceptions of empathy are dependent on who is measuring or rating this experience: the professional counselor (self-ratings of empathic competence), the client/consumer (client ratings of his or her counselor), or a counselor educator/clinical supervisor (expert observer ratings).

Considering the interchange of emotions during disaster mental health response, it would be useful to investigate how empathy is experienced by the counselor, client, and outside observer. It is this experience of empathic attunement where the research falls short. The lack of knowledge concerning the professional's motivation to help others, as well as the emotional, physical, and spiritual involvement during therapeutic interactions, could provide an understanding of why some practitioners may be unconsciously reluctant or purposely avoiding clients who have stories of stress, trauma, grief, and loss.

## Defining the Phenomenon of Interest

Throughout most of the 1960s, the counseling and psychotherapy literature has confirmed Rogers's views and definition of empathy as a *necessary and sufficient* condition that should be facilitated during therapeutic interactions (see Carkhuff, 1969; Truax, 1963). Greenberg, Watson, Elliott, and Bohart (2001) suggest that the clearest operational definition of Rogerian-style empathy includes Barrett-Lennard's (1981) delineation of the three components and perspectives of measuring empathy: (a) the therapist's experience (*empathic resonance*), (b) the observer's view (*expressive empathy*), and (c) the client's experience (*received empathy*). As a result of studying empathy from these three perspectives, instruments were developed so that such a facilitative approach could be observed and measured.

Other theories and models in the literature that have conceptualized empathy for the purpose of measurement (Duan & Hill, 1996) have characterized empathy as a: (a) personality trait, (b) situation-specific event, (c) cognitive-affective state, or (d) general competence and tool of the helper. Empathy has also been commonly defined as a vicarious response to a stimulus or an emphasis on the emotional aspects of a relationship (Stotland, 1969), a motivational state of the individual helper (Duan, 2000), and a cognitive phenomenon with a focus on the intellectual processes of forming an accurate perception of others (Dymond, 1949; Kerr & Speroff, 1954, as cited in Davis, 1983).

Despite the disagreements in the literature on the definition and experience of empathy, Davis et al. (1999) suggest that there is general agreement in two areas: (a) the domain of empathy includes both cognitive and affective dimensions, and (b) affective dimensions encompass a variety of important emotional responses by the professional to the individual (i.e., client/consumer) who is distressed by a significant life event. There is a plethora of evidence in the research regarding the role and value of empathy for therapeutic settings. However, most studies have focused on the elements of the therapeutic alliance between the counselor and the client, or the core conditions that are facilitated by the counselor within the counseling relationship (Feller & Cottone, 2003).

## Empathy as a Trait or State

In personality theory, the construct of empathy has been widely studied from both the trait and state levels. The preponderance of studies on individual differences in empathic styles of communication suggests that empathy is a personality trait. However, more contemporary research designs have analyzed empathy from both the trait and state levels, measuring the interaction effects that exist between daily psychological states of functioning, moods, and specific daily events. Nezlek, Feist, Wilson, and Plesko (2001) note that few studies have been done that measure the variability of empathy as expressed by the individual (nonprofessionals) on a day-to-day basis. This group of researchers in a well-designed study assessed a group of introductory psychology students' daily psychological state of empathy and evaluated how it covaried with state mood and the positive and negative events that occurred in conjunction with the person's state of empathy.

Based on the data, it was suggested that students adjusted their day-to-day empathic response based on more positive interactions with others rather than negative interactions. How empathic a person perceived himself or herself to be on a particular day was a function of individual personality traits and states. It was suggested that people generally tend to feel and express the same affective states that others are experiencing and expressing. In other words, there is an emotional contagion that affects how empathy is expressed person to person. This is confirmed by other studies that have shown that people likely feel what others around them are feeling and therefore are more likely to empathize with them.

Few studies have claimed to actually measure the degree, level, or quality of empathy that is expressed within the client–counselor relationship. This is primarily because empathy may be both qualitatively and quantitatively different from other theoretical approaches. Thus, gaining an understanding of the correlates of empathy may provide others with insight into the multidimensional characteristics of the theoretical aspects of empathy as a first-aid approach. Ultimately, this should serve as a research agenda for those interested in developing disaster mental health approaches for survivors of extraordinary stressful and traumatic events.

## THE ROLE OF EMPATHY IN DISASTER MENTAL HEALTH

Recent investigations have shown that, socially, nonprofessionals who work outside the epicenter of disaster express more sympathy than empathy for disaster survivors (Banfield & Dovidio, 2012; Cameron & Payne, 2011; Kogut & Ritov, 2005). As alluded to earlier in this chapter, sympathy reactions are more passive expressions of disaster "victims," whereas empathic responses are more intentional and active expressions of disaster "survivors." The psychological advantage of being a "survivor" at the epicenter of trauma and disaster is that of resiliency, coping, and hardiness. The survivor is independent, takes responsibility for healing his or her own trauma, and he or she knows how to bounce back from adversity. Accordingly, empathy, as a trait variable, creates the difference between "active helping" (active empathy) and "helping intentions" (sympathy; Banfield & Dovidio, 2012).

Indeed, there is a strong link between empathy and helping behavior when it comes to disaster response (Wayment, 2006). Wilson and Brwynn Thomas (2004) offer a model of empathy in trauma work. The model describes a complex set of dynamic variables (e.g., trauma and stress response patterns, defense mechanisms, trauma transmission, empathic balance, and empathic attunement) that influence the process of healing stress and trauma after disaster. The model suggests that the use of empathy in trauma work begins with an understanding of the complexities that posttraumatic states of stress and trauma have on the individual. Accordingly, skilled and competent trauma therapists have the ability to decode the client's trauma experience, understand the symbolic manifestations of stored traumatic memories, and understand emotional reactions of the client in response to the acquired traumatic experience. So, the nature of disaster mental health counseling itself may be found in the counselor's ability for empathic attunement to persons who have been at the epicenter of disaster.

The literature is replete with narrative, conceptual, qualitative, and quantitative studies on empathy. These studies apply various definitions and conceptualizations of the states, traits, and skills of empathy. There are also a plethora of studies that have observed client–therapist interactions involved in facilitating empathic approaches. The degree, frequency, and nature of empathic engagements tend to fluctuate on a scale of optimal states of accurate empathy to suboptimal states of disengagement. However, the use of empathy by mental health counselors, the quality with which it is facilitated, and the way in which the therapist attunes oneself to the trauma survivor are critical in responding optimally to the client's trauma experience (Banfield & Dovidio, 2012). Overall, facilitating empathic approaches with trauma survivors should come as a natural "way of being" with mental health professionals. Many have viewed the states and traits of empathic engagement as accessible to everyone. Thus, when the trained therapist uses these skills, it can be a powerful combination of healing one's trauma experience.

## CONCLUDING REMARKS

The concepts of "first aid" as applied by medical practitioners are easily understood in the field. However, the medical protocols and physiological measures common to emergency medicine have not been translated for use in disaster mental health response. The constructs based on stress debriefing and psychological and mental health first aid could offer guidelines as a first-level response to stabilize the disaster survivor psychologically and emotionally. Empathy as an approach in mental health therapy is both the same and different as for those in crisis. The foundations of the helping profession have been based on the notions of attending, listening, and empathic responding for the purpose of cultivating the client relationship. Thus, the use of empathy as a first-aid approach by disaster mental health counselors can be helpful if professionals attune themselves to trauma survivors; understand their wounded spirit, pain, and suffering; and respond to these critical events in a way so that survivors understand they have been heard. Empathy as a first-aid tool has the potential to transform the disaster "victim" into a "survivor." More research in this area is needed to develop the essential tools for intervention.

## REFERENCES

Adler, A. (1931). *What life should mean to you.* New York, NY: Little, Brown.

Banfield, J. C., & Dovidio, J. F. (2012). The role of empathy in responding to natural disasters: Comment on "Who helps natural disaster victims?" *Analyses of Social Issues and Public Policy, 12*(1), 276–279.

Barone, D. F., Hutchings, P. S., Kimmel, H. J., Traub, H. L., Cooper, J. T., & Marshall, C. M. (2005). Increasing empathic accuracy through practice and feedback in a clinical interviewing course. *Journal of Social and Clinical Psychology, 24*(2), 156–171.

Barrett-Lennard, G. T. (1981). The empathy cycle: Refinement of a nuclear concept. *Journal of Counseling Psychology, 26*(2), 91–100.

Cameron, C. D., & Payne, B. K. (2011). Escaping affect: How motivated emotion regulation creates insensitivity to mass suffering. *Journal of Personality and Social Psychology, 100*, 1–15.

Carkhuff, R. (1969). *Helping and human relations: A primer for lay and professional helpers* (Vol. 1). New York, NY: Holt.

Corey, M. S., & Corey, G. (2016). *Becoming a helper.* Belmont, CA: Brooks/Cole.

Davis, M. H. (1983). Measuring individual differences in empathy: Evidence for a multidimensional approach. *Journal of Personality and Social Psychology, 44*(1), 113–126.

Davis, M. H., Mitchell, K. V., Hall, J. A., Lothert, J., Snapp, T., & Meyer, M. (1999). Empathy, expectations, and situational preferences: Personality influences on the decision to participate in volunteer helping behaviors. *Journal of Personality, 67*(3), 469–503.

Duan, C. (2000). Being empathic: The role of motivation to empathize and the nature of target emotions. *Motivation and Emotion, 24*(1), 29–49.

Duan, C., & Hill, C. E. (1996). The current state of empathy research. *Journal of Counseling Psychology, 43*, 261–274.

Dymond, R. F. (1949). A scale of measurement of empathy ability. *Journal of Consulting Psychology, 13*(2), 127–133.

Egan, G. (2014). *The skilled helper: A problem-management and opportunity-development approach to helping* (10th ed.). Belmont, CA: Brooks/Cole.

Feller, C. P., & Cottone, R. R. (2003). The importance of empathy in the therapeutic alliance. *Journal of Humanistic Counseling, Education, and Development, 42*, 53–60.

Freeman, S. C. (1993). Client-centered therapy with diverse populations: The universal within the specific. *Journal of Multicultural Counseling and Development, 21*(1), 248–254.

Goleman, D. (2003). *Healing emotions: Conversations with the Dalai Lama on mindfulness, emotions, and health.* Boston, MA: Shambhala.

Greenberg, L. S., Watson, J. C., Elliott, R., & Bohart, A. C. (2001). Empathy. *Psychotherapy, 38*(4), 380–384.

Ibrahim, F. (1991). Contribution of cultural world view to generic counseling and development. *Journal of Counseling & Development, 70*, 13–19.

Ivey, A. E., Bradford Ivey, M., & Zalaquett, C. P. (2014). *Intentional interviewing and counseling: Facilitating client development in a multicultural society* (8th ed.). Belmont, CA: Brooks/Cole.

Jackson, S. W. (1992). The listening healer in the history of psychological healing. *American Journal of Psychiatry, 149*, 1623–1632.

Junn, E. N., Morton, K. R., & Yee, I. (1995). The "Gibberish" exercise: Facilitating empathetic multicultural awareness. *Journal of Instructional Psychology, 22*, 324–329.

Katz, R. L. (1963). *Empathy: Its nature and uses.* New York, NY: Free Press.

Kogut, T., & Ritov, I. (2005). The singularity effect of identified victims in separate and joint evaluations. *Organizational Behavior and Human Decision Processes, 97*, 106–116.

Lazarus, R. S. (1999). *Stress and emotion: A new synthesis.* New York, NY: Springer Publishing.

Lee, C. C., & Richardson, B. L. (1991). *Multicultural issues in counseling: New approaches to diversity.* Alexandria, VA: American Counseling Association.

Nezlek, J. B., Feist, G. J., Wilson, C., & Plesko, R. M. (2001). Day-to-day variability in empathy as a function of daily events and mood. *Journal of Research in Personality, 35*, 401–423.

Parson, E. R. (1993). Ethnotherapeutic empathy (EthE): II, Techniques in interpersonal cognition and vicarious experience across cultures. *Journal of Contemporary Psychotherapy, 23*, 171–182.

Patterson, C. H. (1984). Empathy, warmth, and genuineness: A review of reviews. *Psychotherapy, 21*, 431–438.

Pedersen, P. (2000). *A handbook for developing multicultural awareness* (3rd ed.). Alexandria, VA: American Counseling Association.

Ponterotto, J. G., & Bensesch, K. F. (1998). An organizational framework for understanding the role of culture in counseling. *Journal of Counseling & Development, 66*, 237–241.

Ridley, C. R. (1995). *Overcoming unintentional racism in counseling and therapy: A practitioner's guide to intentional intervention.* Thousand Oaks, CA: Sage Publications.

Ridley, C. R., & Lingle, D. W. (1996). Cultural empathy in multicultural counseling: A multidimensional process model. In P. B. Pederson & J. G. Draguns (Eds.), *Counseling across cultures* (4th ed., pp. 21–46). Thousand Oaks, CA: Sage Publications.

Ridley, C. R., Mendoza, D. W., & Kanitz, B. E. (1994). Multicultural training: Reexamination, operationalization, and integration. *The Counseling Psychologist, 22*, 227–289.

Rogers, C. R. (1951). *Client-centered therapy: Its current practice, implications, and theory.* Boston, MA: Houghton Mifflin.

Rogers, C. R. (1957). The necessary and sufficient conditions of therapeutic personality change. *Journal of Consulting Psychology, 21*, 95–103.

Rogers, C. R. (1980). *A way of being.* Boston, MA: Houghton Mifflin.

Scott, N. E., & Borodovsky, L. (1990). Effective use of cultural role taking. *Professional Psychology: Research and Practice, 21*, 167–170.

Stebnicki, M. A. (2008). *Empathy fatigue: Healing the mind, body, and spirit of professional counselors.* New York, NY: Springer Publishing.

Stotland, E. (1969). Exploratory studies of empathy. In L. Berkowitz (Ed.), *Advances in experimental social psychology* (Vol. 4, pp. 271–314). New York, NY: Academic Press.

Sue, D. W. (1996). Ethical issues in multicultural counseling. In B. Herlihy & G. Corey (Eds.), *ACA ethical standards casebook* (5th ed., pp. 193–200). Alexandria, VA: American Counseling Association.

Sue, D. W., & Sue, D. (1990). *Counseling the culturally different* (2nd ed.). New York, NY: Wiley.

Truax, C. B. (1963). Effective ingredients in psychotherapy: An approach to unraveling the patient-therapist interaction. *Journal of Counseling Psychology, 10,* 256–263.

Truax, C. B., & Carkhuff, R. R. (1967). *Towards effective counseling and psychotherapy.* Chicago, IL: Aldine-Atherton.

Usher, C. H. (1989). Recognizing cultural bias in counseling theory and practice: The case of Rogers. *Journal of Multicultural Counseling and Development, 17,* 62–71.

Wang, Y., Davidson, M. M., Yakushko, O. F., Savoy, H. B., Tan, J. A., & Bleier, J. K. (2003). The scale of ethnocultural empathy: Development, validation, and reliability. *Journal of Counseling Psychology, 50*(2), 221–234.

Wayment, H. A. (2006). Attachment style, empathy, and helping following a collective loss: Evidence from the September 11th terrorist attacks. *Attachment and Human Development, 8*(1), 1–9.

Wilson, J. P., & Brwynn Thomas, R. (2004). *Empathy and the treatment of trauma and PTSD.* New York, NY: Brunner-Routledge.

# CHAPTER 6

# Cultural Empathy and Disaster Mental Health Counseling

Within the past 20 years, we have been in the midst of a cultural revitalization movement that has had a tremendous impact on counselor education, training, research, and the mental health profession as a whole. To enhance interpersonal cross-cultural communications during disaster mental health response, we are constantly mindful of those who differ from ourselves in regard to color, language, gender, sexual orientation, religious or spiritual beliefs, disabilities, and the many other ways in which a person may identify or define himself or herself. Whether disaster mental health counselors are facilitating therapeutic interactions in their regions, homelands, or some other geographic areas of the world, cultural sensitivity, awareness, knowledge, and skills must be at the foundation of developing a working alliance. Mental health counselors who fail to recognize some of the unique cultural differences between Western empathy—as it is applied to counseling and psychotherapy practices—and the concept of cultural empathy may be stereotyping others by using broad-spectrum therapeutic approaches that may not generalize well to a particular culture. Accordingly, this chapter offers guidelines as to how to integrate traditional mental health counseling approaches in disaster mental health response with culturally different individuals.

## CULTURAL EMPATHY

The term *cultural-specific empathy* as described by multicultural counseling theorists (Ponterotto & Bensesch, 1988; Ridley, 1995; Ridley, Mendoza, & Kanitz, 1994) is understood as a skill that is pancultural or universal. Cultural empathy, if facilitated in a culturally oriented and sensitive manner, can strengthen the therapeutic relationship with culturally different individuals (Ibrahim, 1991). Ridley (1995) suggests that cultural empathy has two dimensions: understanding and communication. Understanding requires counselors to try and synthesize the idiographic meaning of their clients' stories and then respond to the accurate meaning of what has been communicated by clients. Accordingly, all interactions can be culturally contextualized and a positive therapeutic outcome can be enhanced by the skills of cultural empathy.

Empathy is relationship-oriented and is particularly enriched through therapeutic relationships that are multicultural centered (Egan, 2014). Pedersen, Crethar, and Carlson's (2008) construct of "inclusive cultural empathy" suggests that professional helpers need to be attuned to clients' underlying thoughts, feelings, behaviors, and overall worldview within a cultural contextual meaning. The natural therapeutic relationship between two culturally different individuals is what "drives" the session. It is not necessarily the strategies, skills, or tools associated with empathy. Rather, inclusive cultural empathy facilitates empathy as a natural way of being, and the intention of its principles should permeate all multicultural interactions.

Much of the research in multicultural counseling has shown that there is an overdependence on general information about a person's cultural background that may perpetuate cultural stereotypes (Harley, Stebnicki, & Rollins, 2001; Stebnicki & Cubero, 2008; Stebnicki, Rubin, Rollins, & Turner, 1999; Sue, 2008). A key criticism of advocates from the cultural revitalization movement is the way in which traditional helping relationships are formed through the diagnosis and assessment process, whereby solution-focused objectives are formed. Additionally, there appears to be a heavy reliance on the traditional Western principles of counseling theories and strategies that dominate the professional practice of counseling and psychotherapy. Recognition of the person's unique culture characteristics (e.g., languages spoken, spiritual/religious practices, traditional healing rituals) is minimally addressed across the counselor education curriculum unless, of course, you are enrolled in a multicultural course or have other counselor supervision, training, and educational development opportunities (Stebnicki & Cubero, 2008).

Clearly, Western models of counseling and psychotherapy have a dependence on talk therapies. However, mental health professionals who facilitate the appropriate use of *cultural empathy* find that silence, listening, gestures, and other forms of metacommunication are equally vital in developing a rapport and working alliance with a culturally different individual. Even though there are some universal commonalities that all human beings share with one another (e.g., biological characteristics, languages spoken, geographic locations, religious and spiritual beliefs, health and healing modalities), mental health professionals must recognize that individuals are not simply representatives of a single cultural group. Rather, they are members of different cultural groups that can be described as having multiple, simultaneous, and ever-shifting identities that influence all forms of interaction. Thus, developing multicultural awareness is critical in understanding the intracultural (within-group) and intercultural (between-group) differences that exist during helping interactions. This increases the likelihood of optimal cross-cultural communications and produces more meaningful and effective outcomes with culturally different individuals (Pedersen, 2000).

Developing cultural competence requires intentional awareness, knowledge, and skills, which has been described as a continuous process of self-examination and maintaining cognitive flexibility (Corey & Corey, 2016; Egan, 2014; Lee, 2014; Pedersen, 2000). Being mindful of how individuals communicate and perceive themselves within their cultural environments can be complex because it requires a global mind change that is characterized by a respect for others' cultural values and an appreciation of diversity. Mental health professionals who are aware of the impact that their personal worldviews and cultures has during therapeutic interactions increase their opportunities to gain trusting relationships and working alliances with culturally different individuals.

## DEVELOPING CULTURAL EMPATHY AWARENESS

Throughout the history of the helping professions, the most fundamental approach for communicating with others has been rooted in compassion or empathy. Ridley (1995) suggests that counselors first and foremost synthesize the idiographic meaning of their clients' stories so that they can understand the meaning and interpretation within a cultural context. The use of cultural empathy is a form of communication that can be adapted within a cultural meaning. It requires professional counselors to attend, listen, observe, understand, and respond to the cultural concerns of others with a deep respect, understanding, and genuineness. Developing cultural empathy also includes being aware of how others who are culturally different communicate nonverbally through eye contact, body language, silence, tone of voice, gestures, facial expressions, and physical space (Corey & Corey, 2016; Egan, 2014; Ivey, Bradford Ivey, & Zalaquett, 2014).

Many experts in counseling and psychology believe that therapists themselves can model empathy within the cultural context of their clients. The impact of modeling empathy itself has the potential to increase a common language, both verbally and nonverbally. In other words, if therapists can facilitate their clients' capacity for understanding and expressing their thoughts, feelings, and experiences from a cultural perspective, then this can enrich therapeutic interactions and become a growth opportunity for both the client and the counselor.

Empathy often becomes confused with sympathy. Sympathy, as an emotional experience, is basically saying to the person: "I'm sorry this has happened to you." Empathy, as a tool for verbal and nonverbal communication, essentially states to the person: "I'm sorry this has happened to you, I can't understand what you must be feeling right now, what can I do to help?" Accordingly, the use of empathy can be a very powerful technique for change and requires simply listening (verbally/nonverbally) and responding to others (verbally/nonverbally) in a way so that the person understands that his or her feelings, thoughts, and experiences have been heard.

Psychologists suggest that persons who communicate a high level of empathy also possess a high degree of social and emotional intelligence (IQ; Bar-On & Parker, 2000; Goleman, 2006; Meyer & Geher, 1996; Salovey & Mayer, 1990). Some researchers suggest that individuals who possess this special type of "intelligence" have an advantage in life because they exhibit excellent interpersonal communication skills. Persons high in social and emotional IQ also typically have the ability to understand others' emotions and experiences. Additionally, they have a mastery of how to work effectively and cooperatively with others. Individuals who have a high social and emotional IQ know how to motivate others, and many have successful careers as salespersons, politicians, teachers, counselors, and spiritual/religious leaders. Indeed, possessing this level of interpersonal communication is essential for connecting with individuals who are culturally different.

Empathy, in the mental health counseling setting, is a way to build a foundation of trust and establish an effective working alliance with clients. The focal point of empathy is the skill of active listening and attending. It is one of the oldest and perhaps most powerful tools for understanding another person's experience and worldview (Corey & Corey, 2016; Egan, 2014; Ivey et al., 2014). Even though psychologists and counselors who were trained early on in their career learned how to facilitate person-centered talk therapies, the therapeutic use of empathy and the skill of listening can be learned and applied by almost anyone in a relatively brief period of time.

Psychologist and founder of the person-centered therapy movement, Dr. Carl Rogers, introduced the concept of empathic listening. Rogers (1980), known as a deeply intuitive man, provided a description of empathy:

> It means entering the private perceptual world of the other and becoming thoroughly at home in it. It involves being sensitive, moment by moment, to the changing felt meanings which flow in this other person, to the fear or rage or tenderness or confusion or whatever that he or she is experiencing. It means temporarily living in the other's life, moving about in it delicately without making judgments. (p. 142)

Overall, if the skills of cultural empathy are not present within person-centered relationships, there may be very little respect, understanding, or compassion communicated, both verbally and nonverbally. Thus, it is critical for mental health counselors to understand the cultural experiences of individuals they serve. Professional counselors may have to adapt their skills of empathy when it comes to perceiving the thoughts, feelings, emotions, and extraordinary stressful and traumatic experiences of their culturally different clients. The following seven guidelines are offered as a way to intentionally increase the facilitative effectiveness of cultural empathy awareness with clients who have experienced extraordinary stressful and traumatic events:

1. Realize that your clients' experiences, thoughts, and feelings may be the same as or different from yours. People from different cultures may see an interconnectedness between their mind, body, and spirit that can affect their physical, mental, and spiritual functioning.

2. Some individuals impacted by disasters have a natural distrust of mental health interactions. If the interaction is not related to food, shelter, clothing, or physical health-related needs, the culturally different individual may not respond well to mental health-related interventions and screenings. Mental health professionals should view this as natural reluctance, rather than resistance or defensiveness.

3. Communicate to clients that (a) all thoughts, feelings, and emotions are naturally transpiring experiences that are okay to embrace; (b) thoughts, feelings, or emotions that have arisen from traumatic experiences are natural, because we are humans; (c) there are not good–bad emotions or thoughts (e.g., feelings of survivor guilt) and we should not place "conditions" on good–bad emotions, thoughts, or how we "should feel"; and (d) the way in which we bring meaning to a traumatic

experience is important and verbal expression is not necessary; rather, it is important to be mindful of how our thoughts, feelings, and experiences manifest in healthy (e.g., bringing meaning to a critical event) and unhealthy (e.g., anger, violence, substance abuse) ways.

4. It is okay for clients to have negative, hurtful, and painful thoughts or feelings. This is all just "unwanted energy." Just because you have these thoughts or feelings does not mean that there is something wrong with you, or that you are going crazy. This is a natural cue that our mind, body, and spirit may have something to offer in terms of healing energy.

5. Verbalizing thoughts and feelings to others that you trust and are close to assists in the healthy release of your trauma experience. Verbalizing thoughts and feelings helps you feel centered or back to balance. This may take some time, but be patient. Remember that expressing your thoughts, feelings, and experiences to others does not mean that you are weak. Everyone needs help from others throughout his or her life.

6. It is important that you ask others for help. We generally do not live in environments in which we are totally independent, unless of course you are a survivalist. It is okay to accept help and support from others for a while until you feel more in balance. Remember that even professional counselors and psychologists need someone to talk with for help in problem-solving some critical life issues.

7. It may take multiple attempts to try and get in touch with your thoughts and feelings and express these in a culturally appropriate manner. As time goes on, it becomes easier for you based on your cultural healing values, principles, philosophy, and beliefs.

## DEVELOPING THE CULTURAL SKILLS OF EMPATHY

It is generally recognized within the foundations of counselor education, training, and research that about 75% of what we communicate to one another is done nonverbally. Communicating with others using facilitative empathy is not just the verbalization of thoughts, feelings, and experiences. Rather, empathy requires us to pay attention nonverbally through a meta-communication channel. This includes, but is not limited to, posture, hand gestures, facial expressions, and voice intonation. Nonverbal behaviors usually communicate specific thoughts, feelings, or emotions that are important to the individual. Thus, the following is a description of several nonverbal communication skills that can be facilitated in therapeutic relationships that enhance cultural empathy. These have been summarized using the acronym MOM:

*Maintain culturally appropriate eye contact and body language:* Do not stare at the other person. Based on the individual's background, he or she may interpret this action as hostility, anger, or that you are challenging or confronting him or her. Appropriate eye contact is culturally based and conveys that you are interested in and concerned with what others have to say (verbally/nonverbally). Adjust your posture for the degree of direct eye-to-eye contact versus viewing the person from your peripheral vision. Observe how the other person uses eye contact, then adjust your level of directness and gaze as you sense his or her level of comfort.

*Open and relaxed posture:* An open and relaxed posture generally communicates to others that you are open and accessible to them. This helps the other person relax because you are nonverbally communicating a high level of interest, accessibility, and attentiveness. You may not want to mirror your clients' body language at the outset because he or she may initially be reluctant to assist with the helping process. Be mindful of your posture through internal self-observation.

*Movement of body-spatial distance:* Body movement and spatial distance can communicate different cultural messages. Make sure that you are familiar with the other person's culture as it relates to body movement and spatial distance before you lean toward him or her or interact within his or her physical space. Violating "personal space" may prompt an emotional or physical reaction by the other person that you had not anticipated or did not intend to create. Being too distant may also communicate that you are not interested in what the other person has to communicate (verbally/nonverbally). Be acutely aware of opposite gender therapeutic interactions as male clients may be reluctant or resistant to discuss emotions and experiences openly with a female counselor.

## Attending and Listening: Talker–Listener Activity

The purpose of this activity is to practice your attending and listening skills with others so that you can build a rapport and establish a trusting working relationship with others. Because everyone has a culture, attending and listening to the other person may bring about some degree of cultural awareness. To gain the maximum benefit from this activity, break into groups of two or three in a quiet place. *Person One* in the group is the listener (he or she should *only listen* to what the other person is saying). *Person Two* is the talker (he or she should *talk about* three things he or she likes and three things he or she does not like about himself or herself), and *Person Three* is the primary observer who provides feedback to the talker and the listener. If time allows, each person in the group should have an opportunity to participate in each of the three roles as a listener, talker, and observer. Remember that the talker only talks, the listener only listens, and the observer observes and leads the feedback with the talker and the listener. Allow about 4 to 5 minutes for the talker and the listener to interact. The observer should then facilitate the following questions in the triad. After the feedback session, participants may switch roles so everyone has an opportunity to be in the role of the talker, listener, and observer:

*Questions for the Talker*

1. How effective was your listener as you were talking about your three likes/dislikes?

2. What were some of the things that the listener was doing that you perceived to be most effective in allowing you to talk?

3. What specific nonverbal cues was your listener communicating to you as you were talking?

4. How effectively did your listener use MOM? Were there times during this interaction that you felt you were not being heard or understood?

5. How natural or relaxed was your listener? Were there any times that you sensed your listener was not being himself or herself?

6. From an attending and listening point of view, what other feedback could you give to your listener so he or she can be more effective with talkers?

*Questions for the Listener*

1. How effective did you perceive yourself to be in your role as a listener?

2. In the listener role, were there times during your interaction that you felt like you were not attending and listening effectively?

3. Was it difficult for you to only be able to attend and listen for the 3- to 4-minute session? Describe this experience.

4. How natural did you feel? Were there times when you felt more natural or unnatural in your attending and listening?

5. What types of nonverbal communication did you observe in the talker? Describe what you were experiencing.

6. What could you do to become more effective with your attending and listening skills?

## Listening Empathically to the Core Message

There are many other things communicated between two individuals than what is described in MOM. However, the talker–listener activity described in the previous section demonstrates that listening can be a difficult activity for some. Effective cross-cultural communication involves more than MOM, but it is foundational to building a trusting and genuine relationship with others. The quality of person-centered connections can be enhanced by a higher level of empathic listening (verbally/nonverbally) and responding within a cultural context.

From a cultural perspective, it is crucial that we organize the important components of listening so that the talker's core message can be fully understood. Implicit in understanding what the other person is saying is that we must listen without being judgmental, so that we can understand the person's: (a) core content of the message, (b) cultural meaning behind his or her thoughts or cognitions, (c) emotions and feelings, (d) covert or overt behaviors that may hinder his or her interpersonal effectiveness with others, and (e) overall experience within a cultural context. In essence, listening and responding to another person's story or personal testimonial requires more than just listening to the content. It requires us to fully understand what others are saying about themselves and how they express their cultural experience or meaning of a critical event.

## CULTURAL EMPATHIC LEVELS OF LISTENING (CELL): A THEORETICAL MODEL OF CULTURAL UNDERSTANDING

The CELL, as outlined in the next section, is a theoretical model that offers guidelines to disaster mental health counselors who seek a deeper meaning of the survivor's disaster or trauma experience from a cultural perspective. Each level of the CELL Model (Levels I–V) offers benchmarks for optimal levels of functioning as competent and skilled multicultural counselors in the use of cultural empathy. The CELL Model is based on the hypothesis that cultural empathy and communication begin at an initial level of cultural unawareness and listening. Theoretically, this ranges on a continuum of cultural awareness, understanding, and insight by mental health counselors who want to gain a deeper level of cultural communication. Ultimately, heightened cultural insight and awareness occur through intense listening whereby the mental health professional accurately interprets cultural meaning of the trauma or disaster survivor's expression and experience of a critical incident.

Hypothetically, the competent and skilled mental health professional begins by using cultural empathy at Level I (Listening to the Content), then as trust and rapport are built with the person the counselor progresses to Level V (Listening for Experience and Meaning). Depending on a variety of variables (e.g., the client's cultural background, geographical setting in which services are provided, type of disaster scenario, previous experience with a particular culture) the counselor typically begins an intervention at Level I and moves through each of the levels, which ultimately cultivates into a higher level of cultural understanding, awareness, and meaning of the survivor's experiences.

Competent and skilled mental health counselors first cultivate a strong foundation for cultural empathy and rapport. After this process, the skilled professional begins working in higher levels of cultural awareness, as depicted in Levels I to IV. To achieve Level V, the competent multicultural counselor has a strong working alliance and therapeutic relationship built so he or she may facilitate other therapeutic approaches (e.g., facilitating client meaning of critical event, connecting with resources, providing trauma interventions that are culturally relevant). The overall intention of the CELL Model is to achieve Level V, where it is anticipated that the therapeutic relationship is optimal.

The CELL theoretical model should be differentiated from other models or scales that measure empathy, communication, and understanding. This model considers a constellation of cultural communication, states, traits, behaviors, and meta-communication, as well as other factors, by viewing individuals as both a reflection of their specific cultural group and other cultures that they may identify. This cannot be discovered solely on an intake interview of demographic variables (e.g., racial/ethnic identity, sexual orientation, religious/spiritual beliefs). Rather, the CELL Model assumes that the person has multiple cultural identities. The use of cultural empathy and person-centered interactions guides counselors through this cultural identity process. It assists counselors in finding the cultural meaning of a variety of issues such as daily hassles (e.g., projected needs for self-sustaining resources), life adjustment issues (e.g., health, relationships, transition), or exposure to extraordinary stressful and traumatic events.

## CELL Theoretical Model

### Level I—Listening to the Content

Many persons/clients communicate a description of people, things, or events that they have experienced in their past. Individuals typically tell their stories from a culturally specific point of view. In some instances, persons/clients may communicate their needs for immediate things (e.g., food, shelter, clothing). They may communicate their basic intentions for how they plan to actively or not actively change their situations, problem-solve a critical situation, or utilize certain resources.

The goals for professional helpers in Level I is to use MOM as well as cultural empathy for the purpose of gaining a better understanding of persons'/clients' immediate needs within a cultural context and what they might be trying to communicate to you indirectly. In disaster mental health response, professional helpers typically listen to basic information about persons'/clients' cultures and how they (a) experienced their extraordinary stressful or traumatic events; (b) acculturate, assimilate, or accept life as citizens within their homelands or geographic areas and how they perceive others outside their cultures; and (c) talk about specific events, rituals, or experiences that are part of their overall system of health, healing, and wellness.

At this level of cultural awareness, communication may be strained if counselors do not use cultural empathy, cultural sensitivity, and basic attending and listening skills, or if they expect client disclosure too soon.

### Level II—Listening to Thoughts and Cognitive Style

Most persons/clients have a unique way of expressing how they experience other people, things, or critical events within their cultures. Feelings may not be recognized, discussed, or expressed directly by the individual. Some persons/clients may be disorganized as they tell their stories in regard to their thoughts because they may be feeling overwhelmed by a particular trauma experience. They may have a concrete or abstract way in which they tell their stories or may talk about things in a realistic-rational, unrealistic-irrational, or negative-pessimistic manner. Regardless of the persons'/clients' thoughts or cognitive style of perceiving the world around them, effective helpers must listen for the frequency and level of intensity that occurs as persons/clients talk about their thoughts and cognitions.

The goals for professional helpers in Level II are to listen to the person's/client's thoughts, cognitions, and perceptions that provide information on the process of his or her thinking, feeling, and experiencing people, things, and traumatic events. Competent and skilled helpers are open and flexible as they relate to the person's/client's style of thinking. They try to connect the person's/client's thoughts and cognitions as they relate to a critical event from a cultural perspective. Professional helpers at Level II are effective listeners but may misinterpret or not fully grasp the person's/client's patterns of thinking. Cultural misunderstanding may occur when the professional helper listens to the person/client from a Western mental health counseling perspective, which may sound irrational, dysfunctional, and unhealthy in the person's life.

In Level II, effective helpers begin to listen for the person's/client's resiliency traits and coping skills or initial signs of positivity, hopefulness, and ability to adapt. Effective helpers assist the person/client to begin the search for personal meaning of the trauma or disaster experience.

## Level III—Listening for Behaviors and Experiences

Behaviors expressed by the person/client may be communicated verbally (i.e., a strained vocal quality or the person stating, "I had to fight for my life"); nonverbally (i.e., any number of facial expressions, making a fist, tensing other body parts); or in the present moment (i.e., expression of physical psychomotor behaviors of irritability, agitation, or anger). Verbal and nonverbal behaviors that are expressed by persons/clients are important because they typically have a connection with the core content of their stories. Behaviors that are expressed either negatively or positively by the person/client should be interpreted within the cultural context of the person's/client's experience.

The goals for professional helpers in Level III are to build on the skills from Levels I and II and make sure that they accurately reflect the person's/client's behavior and experience. These include actions that are exhibited or communicated by the person/client, which can be easily observed by others who are familiar with the person. Competent and skilled helpers think about the cultural interpretation of the persons'/clients' critical events and their motivation for behavior(s) that may be unhealthy, impulsive, or irrational. To further achieve the listening goals in Level III, effective helpers remain open-minded and do not express any value judgments at this point. Professional helpers are also keenly aware of their own body language that may communicate displeasure, distrust, or some negativity. In cases of lethality or life-threatening emergencies (i.e., the direct or indirect expression by the person that he or she may harm himself or herself or others), competent and skilled professional helpers respond with some urgency and obtain the assistance of other skilled professionals (e.g., MD psychiatrist, law enforcement personnel) to handle such matters to make sure the person is in a safe environment. A suicide contract may be warranted if a suicide threat becomes evident. It is critical, however, that professional helpers not overreact to a threat of suicide. They need to balance the level of lethality with the cultural expression of harm to self and others versus intense anger. Also, some cultures do not express specific degrees of lethality that may be communicated more indirectly.

## Level IV—Affect or Feelings

At the heart of Western models of counselor education and training are the expectations that competent and skilled helpers facilitate client disclosure of feelings and emotions. However, it is critical to facilitate cultural empathy and the person's/client's cultural expression of feeling and emotion, which may be disclosed verbally (i.e., "I was very angry at him for doing that to me") and/or nonverbally (i.e., facial expressions of sadness, shame, withdrawal). Western models of counseling and psychotherapy generally suggest that verbalizing and disclosure of feelings and emotions are healthy and required for personal awareness, insight, growth, and development. However, if persons/clients did not grow up in a culture where this was present (especially disclosing feelings/emotions to strangers or mental health professionals), then this would be counter to their belief system on health, healing, and wellness. Many feelings such as stress and anxiety come from our perception of specific events (i.e., intimidation, physical assault). Feelings expressed by the person may range from no emotion to very little emotion expressed at all, to feelings that overwhelm persons to the degree and intensity that they cannot cope with life and they may prefer death to life.

The goals for professional helpers in Level IV are to integrate Levels I to III so that the persons/clients can recognize emotions, thoughts, behaviors, and experiences from their own unique cultural point of view. Accordingly, it is of paramount importance that professional helpers understand the cultural style of expressing (or not expressing) emotions, thoughts, behaviors, and experiences and use all the facilitative skills of cultural empathy to reflect, clarify, respond empathically, summarize, and check for the specific cultural meaning and interpretation of the person's/client's issues.

## Level V—Listening for Experience and Meaning

In Level V, the professional helper ties together the person's/client's story, feelings, thoughts, behaviors, and experiences. The goals for professional helpers in Level V are to have a much clearer understanding of persons'/clients' culture as they define what happened to them, how they make sense and meaning from a critical event, and their expression of feelings, thoughts, behaviors, and experiences as they communicate these from a cultural orientation.

In Level V, professional helpers have a more complete understanding of the critical impact that a specific critical incident has on the person's/client's past, present, and future. Persons/clients in Level V take on a more active role in communicating their wants and needs with professional helpers. Competent and skilled helpers do not give advice or problem-solve issues for persons/clients. There is a shared responsibility for cultivating resources for a critical incident.

Overall, the professional helper in Level V focuses on effective communication skills that promote the development and facilitate a plan of action with a high degree of cultural sensitivity and awareness, one that empowers the person/client with as many resources as are available to him or her.

## CELL Summary

Overall, it is hypothesized that professional helpers have opportunities to gain insight, awareness, and cultural skills through serving persons/clients from a diversity of backgrounds. From a professional helping perspective, we can enhance cultural empathy by paying attention and being mindful of verbal and nonverbal interactions, as well as other meta-communication that takes place between two individuals. Laying the groundwork for multicultural counseling interactions goes beyond Western models of counseling theories and psychotherapeutic approaches. Indeed, disaster mental health response requires first and foremost a robust working alliance. Accordingly, to be an effective, competent, ethical, and skilled mental health counselor, cultural empathy is the platform by which to build multicultural relationships for healing in the aftermath of disaster.

## EMPATHIC RESPONDING: BECOMING A CULTURALLY SKILLED PROFESSIONAL

Mental health professionals are culturally effective when they are able to do more with less effort because this would indicate that the person/client is becoming more of an active participant in the helping–receiving process. To become more proficient and effective in the use of cultural empathy and to become intentional in your style of cultural communication, basic empathic listening requires basic empathic responding within a cultural context. This section helps you become familiar with using the helping skills of continuing responses, permission statements, use of open-ended questions, probes, paraphrasing, clarifying, summarizing, and other basic empathic responses. The use of these skills is framed within a multicultural context. Consideration is given to multicultural competencies that provide a pancultural approach yet honors the within- and between-group differences from a variety of cultures. Given the focus and intention of this chapter, it is recommended that mental health professionals engage in cultural immersion activities such as those outlined later in the chapter. It is in these environments where one can grow personally and professionally so as to function optimally as a competent and skilled multicultural counselor.

The skills that follow lay the foundation for developing increased levels of cultural empathy and other necessary skills to become culturally competent. Indeed, we communicate with others through our body posture, facial expressions, gestures, voice quality, and in other culturally specific mannerisms. Thus, before engaging in any helping relationship, it is important to be mindful of the following points:

1. *Responding with cultural empathy is not the same as sympathy:* Sympathy is very passive, while empathy communicates to the other person that you understand what he or she is saying, feeling, and experiencing. Responding empathically to others suggests that you or someone else may be able to help them deal with their problems in a different or more effective way.

2. *Cultural empathic communication skills can be used by everyone:* The skills of cultural empathy are not reserved exclusively for mental health professionals. These skills are taught to many people such as company executives, managers and administrators, customer relations personnel, travel agents, parks and recreation personnel, lay clergy and pastors, and many other groups interested in achieving a higher level of communication with others who are culturally different.

3. *Cultural empathy is not the same as advice-giving or problem-solving:* It is critical that people take responsibility for their own lives because there are many allures that keep individuals off-balance and not focused on positive goals. Professional helpers can assist others by empowering individuals to acquire all the support and

resources that are available to them both inside and outside their indigenous cultural groups. Mostly anyone can give advice or be overnurturing, protective, or sympathetic. However, not everyone has acquired the skills of cultural empathy that can be used to facilitating awareness, personal growth, and problem-solving strategies with others.

4. *Do not take on more than you can competently handle:* If you are feeling overwhelmed by the person you are trying to help, this may become a stressor for you. It may be time to reexamine your relationship with this particular culture and find other professionals who can offer assistance. Let your physical, cognitive, and emotional intuition be your guide in your ability to competently and ethically serve the person/ client. Also, be aware that if you do not possess the clinical training, experience, and supervision in working with persons/clients who are culturally different, then a cultural immersion activity may be practical. Regardless of your training and expertise in multicultural counseling, there are many cultures to explore.

5. *Be open, honest, and genuine:* The most effective therapeutic relationships are those that are open, honest, upfront, and genuine. Despite the fact that you cannot help every individual, it is important to become familiar with some referral sources that can provide other resources and support within the context of your client's particular culture.

## BASIC EMPATHY: RESPONDING WITHIN A CULTURAL CONTEXT

Basic empathy is an honest, direct, intentional, and conscious way of communicating with others. Cultural empathy requires that mental health professionals use the facilitative skills of empathy through their clients' cultural lens or worldview. Thus, the use of cultural empathy invites professional counselors to accurately understand the person's/ client's "story" as it relates to the content, feelings, thoughts, behaviors, and experiences, but within a particular cultural group that is defined by the person/client.

Empathic communication skills are the foundation of the helping process in person-centered models of counseling (Corey & Corey, 2016; Egan, 2014; Ivey, Bradford Ivey, & Zalaquett, 2014; Murphy & Dillion, 2015). Effective helping within a multicultural counseling context requires awareness, knowledge, and skills to work with persons who are culturally different. Some readers may discover that the foundational skills that follow look familiar and have been acquired early on in your counselor education and training. It is assumed that the reader has a foundational knowledge of the definitions, concepts, and use of the skills of empathy, reflection, use of continuing responses, clarification statements, open-/closed-ended questions, summary statements, and other essential facilitative skills. Thus, the intent is to reframe some of the basic foundational counseling skills within a cultural context. Many multicultural theorists, researchers, and practitioners report that some skills of empathy can be facilitated across many different cultures. Other skills require an adaptation such as described in the MOM Model of attending and listening.

## CASE STUDY: AMIRA AND AAMINAH

Consider the scenario "Best Friends Talk," where two Middle Eastern international college students, Amira and Aaminah, are best friends and are talking about their difficulty with acculturating and transitioning to the United States from their war-torn countries. Amira and Aaminah are first-year doctoral students in a doctoral of physical therapy (DPT) program at a state university in North Carolina. Amira and Aaminah are talking about some arguments they have each had lately. They have heard about on-campus mental health services and are both thinking about making an appointment. They have seen other students in their DPT program visit the campus counseling center, so they feel making an appointment might benefit them, too.

### Best Friends Talk

**Amira:** "I don't know what got into me! I am such a disrespectful daughter. I was yelling at my mother because she kept putting pressure on me about my grades just like she always does. I hope she doesn't tell my father about our argument—he may make me return to Port Said (northeast Egypt along the Mediterranean Sea). She kept nagging at me the way she always does, asking me why I don't call her more often. She wouldn't get off my case; it made me more and more angry. (Amira looks down at floor sadly, tearfully.) I finally began screaming at her and I said to her *Ya Sharmouta* (American translation "you bitch") then hung up on her. (Amira puts hands over face and shakes her head.) I can't believe I actually called her that name. Things are going so bad in my life now with school and trying to adjust to life in North Carolina. . . . I don't know what I should do any more. . . ."

**Aaminah:** (looking shocked at the level of agitation Amira is exhibiting) "Oh . . . Oh . . . maybe it is time we talk to the campus counseling services . . . like the other students do. I'm worried about you Amira. I also am feeling somewhat stressed . . . perhaps we can make an appointment and go together.

### Questions for Discussion

▶ What is Amira experiencing at this moment?
▶ Identify some of Amira's key behaviors that she is exhibiting and reporting to her best friend Aaminah.
▶ What are the cultural implications of showing this level of agitation and anger to a parent from a Middle Eastern culture?
▶ Discuss some of Amira's feelings and emotions that she is communicating to Aaminah. What are the cultural implications?
▶ What is the etiology of this level of stress and emotion? Family issues? Poor grades? Or something else?
▶ What impact does acculturative stress have on Amira? On Aaminah?

*(continued)*

## CASE STUDY: AMIRA AND AAMINAH (*continued*)

- ▶ As a mental health counselor, would you also invite Amira's best friend, Aaminah, to the same brief counseling session to act as an extended family member?
- ▶ What would be the cultural impact on Amira and Aaminah of facilitating brief counseling approaches using a male versus female mental health professional?

### Cultural Analysis From the Basic Cultural Empathy Perspective

- ▶ *Key experience (what the person sees happening to him or her):* Amira is experiencing her mother nagging at her.
- ▶ *Key behavior (behaviors that are observable by others):* Losing her temper, yelling *Ya Sharmouta*, hanging up the phone abruptly, holding her face in her hands.
- ▶ *Key feelings/emotions (any mood, tone, or sensation arising from experiences and behaviors):* Amira feels a wide range of emotions—embarrassment, shame, guilt from yelling at her mother and abruptly hanging up the phone, being overwhelmed by school, living in North Carolina, fear of her future.

### The Basic Cultural Empathic Response

*Basic cultural empathic response* (Assuming that Amira is attending her first session with a White female mental health counselor who specializes in working with international students, the mental health counselor uses the response formula of placing emotion first and experience or content second [see Egan, 2014]): "It sounds like *you're feeling* overwhelmed *because* of the way things are going on at home, school, and your transition to North Carolina."

The mental health counselor uses the basic empathic response formula of "You feel" [state correct emotion here] "because" [indicate the correct experiences and behaviors that result from the person's feelings/emotions] (see Egan, 2014). The importance of responding with basic empathy (as opposed to "uh-huh," "ah," "I see") is that we are communicating to the client that we understand what he or she is feeling and experiencing. For this response to be genuine and effective, it is important that the professional counselor vary his or her empathic responses so as to avoid repetition or restating what the client has already stated. It is important to note that the counselor is using some foundational facilitative skills as taught in traditional Western schools of counselor education and training. However, the difference is that the counselor is not drawing any conclusions here in this case study of Amira and is somewhere between Levels I and IV of the CELL Model. The following are some examples for varying the use of empathic responses using cultural sensitivity to approach the client in a nonjudgmental way:

"I think I hear you saying that you're feeling [insert feeling word] because of _____."

"So you're feeling _____ because _____."

"It _____ because of [insert content and/or experience]."

"If I understand you correctly, it sounds like you're feeling _____ because of _____."

As Gerald Egan (2014) suggests, if professional helpers truly understand how the skills of empathy can be applied within a multicultural context, then this will enhance the counselors' knowledge and skills in working with a diverse group of clients. He goes on to note that over the course of one's career, professional helpers can come to understand a great deal about the characteristics and attributes of specific cultural groups with whom they work. However, the basic skills of empathy within a cultural context help build client rapport so that an optimal working alliance can be formed.

The following empathic communication tools can be utilized in a helping session that should assist you in helping clients reflect, continue to talk, and bring some meaning to the problems they are experiencing within a cultural context.

## Continuing Responses and Permission Statements

Continuing responses and permission statements simply "give permission" for the other person to verbalize or disclose an issue that has some significance in his or her life. These types of responses help build trust with the other person because you are showing him or her that you are interested and present emotionally and cognitively. Continuing responses and permission statements communicate to the other person that you care about him or her and support his or her needs to disclose issues that may be very personal in nature. Such statements are used as prompts to help others continue to verbalize. They usually take the form of: "It's OK . . . I know this must be difficult for you to talk about. . . . Yes. . . . Go on. . . . I understand what you are saying. . . . Tell me more." The foundational point for effective use of continuing responses and permission statements is to incorporate culturally competent approaches in your interpersonal interactions. Attunement to the multicultural counseling skills related to spatial distance, nonverbal communication, and reinforcing or the use of cultural assumptions or negative stereotypes can help or hinder the working and therapeutic alliance with culturally different clients.

## Effective Use of Questioning

Open-ended questions help facilitate persons/clients to elaborate and provide a clearer understanding of their functional limitations. Closed-ended questions are useful if you attempt to elicit a concrete response (i.e., "How many years did it take to finally find your biological father?"). However, closed-ended questions provide only limited information, especially if you are trying to gather a lot of data in a short period of time. Open-ended questions are the essence of effective interpersonal communication skills and assist professional counselors in assessing the person's/client's problems. Consider asking some of the following open-ended questions:

"Could you tell me more about that?"

"How did it feel when you . . . ?"

"Given what you said, what would be your ideal solution to . . . ?"

"What have we missed so far?"

"What else comes to mind as you describe . . . ?"

Oftentimes, using specific questions leads to predictable responses. For example:

"What" questions most often lead to the person stating facts about a situation.

"What happened?"

"What are you going to do?"

"How" questions most often lead to a discussion about processes or sequences.

"How could that be explained?"

"Why" questions most often lead to a discussion of reasons.

"Why did you allow that to happen?"

"Why do you choose to do that?"

Questions that incorporate "could" such as "Could you tell me more about your family?" have the advantage of allowing the client to say whatever comes to his or her consciousness. The client chooses the direction in which to take the cultural conversation. Foundationally, it is essential that skilled professionals know the difference between reluctance, resistance, and defensiveness from a cultural sense. Skilled multicultural counseling professionals have a good sense for these behaviors, particularly when they may be asking too many questions from their clients.

## Clarifying

Clarification is an important skill in communication because it allows professional helpers to conceptually grasp and define the person's/client's problem issues. Many individuals are vague or ambiguous in their communication with others because they may have some anxiety about disclosing personal information about themselves or others. Other persons may have such complex issues to disclose that they do not know where to begin disclosing. Thus, they may be somewhat disorganized in their thoughts and feelings about a particular issue. If the skilled professional has a sense that there is a "hidden meaning" or "hidden emotions" behind what the person/client is saying, then it may be beneficial for the counselor to clarify what the person/client is only half-saying or what he or she is trying to say in a vague or ambiguous way. Culturally, it is critical that counselors do not use their own cultural meaning to interpret what their clients are attempting to express.

## Summarizing

The skill of summarizing assists professional helpers in pulling together the person's/client's major content issues, themes, emotions, and verbal and nonverbal patterns of communication. Basically, summarizing is a conclusion that is given at the end of a session. It is different from all of the communication skills because the professional helper provides a brief, but comprehensive summary of the primary content issues, emotions, themes, and experiences. From a cultural viewpoint, checking, clarifying, and understanding the meaning of client–counselor interactions is first and foremost required to move on into other vital areas that require attention.

## Cultural Checklist (CC)

The following checklist of verbal and nonverbal behaviors and observations can be utilized in several ways. For instance, if you have an opportunity to videotape yourself during a therapeutic interaction with a culturally different client, then the CC could be used as a self-reflection and evaluation measure. Clinical supervisors may find the CC a helpful checklist to guide feedback during supervisory sessions. Lastly, the CC could be utilized in peer supervision sessions where an objective, third person could address the professional helper's level of cultural competence from verbal and nonverbal perspectives.

### Nonverbal Checklist

1. *Eye contact:* How well did the counselor initiate and maintain culturally appropriate eye contact throughout the session?

2. *Vocal qualities:* Were there any changes in the counselor's tone, volume, or vocal quality during the session? Were there any hesitations with specific words or phrases? Were some words emphasized more than others with a particular vocal quality?

3. *Body language:* Describe the professional counselor's general physical posture. Was it open or closed? Did you notice any tension? Were there any shifts in posture during the session? What did the professional counselor's breathing pattern and spatial distance communicate to you?

4. *Nonverbal discrepancies:* Did the professional counselor's body language communicate anything that appeared to be inconsistent with his or her vocal responses? What other meta-communication did you observe that enhanced cultural empathy?

### Verbal Checklist

1. *Verbal tracking and attending:* Did the professional counselor respond to the client's cultural concerns in a consistent manner? and Did it make cultural sense what the counselor was trying to communicate when he or she used a reflective response? Were any of the professional counselor's responses abstract or did they lose any cultural meaning?

2. *Continuing responses:* Did the professional counselor use good continuing responses that put the client at ease and encouraged the client to discuss cultural concerns?

3. *Reflection of feeling:* Did the professional counselor accurately reflect the essence of emotion and cultural empathy at the same level of intensity that you felt during the session?

4. *Open-ended questions:* Did the professional counselor use appropriate and purposeful open-ended questions/probes that were culturally appropriate—ones that you felt helped explore the client's concerns?

5. *Paraphrase/summarize:* Did the professional counselor paraphrase and summarize the different sections of the session in an accurate manner?

6. *Assessment of overall effectiveness:* Was the overall atmosphere comfortable for the client? Did the client feel like this session addressed his or her concerns adequately given the limited time available? Did this session accomplish anything in particular?

## PERSONAL HISTORY CULTURAL PERSPECTIVE: THE INTAKE INTERVIEW

It is important to recognize that everyone has a culture. The purpose of the personal history cultural intake is to (a) gain insight into and understanding of your client's cultural roots, (b) challenge you with researching your own cultural roots through family interviews and/or other historical records, and (c) communicate and reflect on your client's own cultural identity. The questions and guidelines offered should assist mental health counselors to understand culturally different clients at a deeper level of description, understand the cultural significance and personal meaning of a potential traumatic experience, and understand the social–emotional, sociopolitical, family lifestyle, and other traits that are culturally relevant in your clients' lives. It may be helpful to have your clients discuss hardships, barriers, or prejudices that their cultures or families had to endure (personally, economically, occupationally, and spiritually). Make sure that you are aware of how specific cultural concepts (e.g., cultural assumptions, cultural assimilation, within-group family differences, any racism, ethnic prejudices encountered) are integrated into your clients' expression of their mental, physical, and spiritual well-being.

The 13 questions listed in the next section are guidelines for a personal interview with culturally different clients. It is best to interview the person in his or her own environment if possible (home, tent, safe outdoor area). Please assure clients that any information they share is confidential (unless, of course, they are a danger to self or others). Be mindful that before you begin your interview you should have an appropriate cultural rapport built. Remind your clients that they may talk to you at the level they most feel comfortable; you are not requiring them to reveal any "family secrets" or any information that may be of a personally deep nature. It is recommended that you develop cultural questions related to specific cultures that you serve. The following are offered to begin an exploration of your culturally different client's background that can be helpful with developing resources and other treatment approaches.

### Suggested Questions

1. How would you describe your family or cultural background?
2. Describe your cultural beliefs, philosophy, or values from a holistic perspective.
3. When did you first become aware or begin to practice some of your cultural value beliefs?
4. Can you remember how you initially felt—emotionally, physically, or spiritually—when you first became aware of your cultural identity?
5. Did your culture or family experience any prejudice or discrimination based on your race, ethnicity, religious, or spiritual beliefs?

6. What were some of the ways in which this prejudice or discrimination was expressed or communicated toward you and your culture?

7. Were there any negative attitudes, barriers, prejudices, or stereotypes that your family members or culture expressed toward other groups?

8. How do your cultural beliefs or values affect how you live in your everyday life (emotionally, physically, cognitively, spiritually, occupationally, financially)?

9. What parts of your culture or family traditions (rituals, rules, beliefs, philosophy) do you feel positive about and have carried on with other family members?

10. What parts of your culture or family traditions/values/practices would you like to give up, get away from, ignore, or not be reminded of?

11. Are there any parts of your culture that you have been confused about or have you been uncertain about where these values, beliefs, and practices originated?

12. Have your family members borrowed any practices, beliefs, or other things from other cultures? How were these integrated?

13. If you had some advice to give to others from your culture or your family, what would you tell them?

## CULTURAL IMMERSION ACTIVITY

To become more aware, knowledgeable, comfortable, and skilled in working with persons who are culturally different from you, spend some time interacting with others in a culture that is different from your own. It is recommended that professional counselors interested in increasing their personal and professional growth spend some time throughout the week or month with an individual and/or group that is culturally different. Instead of participating as a detached outside observer, you will need to connect with the "host" culture. The relationships that you develop with others may affect your own cultural worldview in terms of your personal or cultural identity. For you to gain understanding, awareness, knowledge, and skills in working with others who are culturally different from you, you should be immersed as a participant observer in an experience that is out of your ordinary daily routine and structure. There are as many cultural immersion activities as there are cultures globally. Many who have reported life-enriching and transcended experiences have been culturally immersed in activities such as engaging in shamanic, Reiki, and yoga training; mindfulness meditation retreats; sweat lodge ceremonies; attendance at African American church services; and many other positive experiences that enhanced one's personal and professional growth.

Cultural immersion activities use the framework of *ethnography*: a social science and cultural anthropological research field of study. Ethnographers spend many weeks or months of observation and interaction within different geographic regions and cultures of the world gathering qualitative data from a variety of culturally different individuals and groups. Ethnographers generally begin their research by generating a specific set of open-ended questions to guide their research. Questions are based on the individuals and groups of people that are of interest to the researcher. The purpose of this type of research is to develop an understanding of different cultural characteristics, traits, values, and beliefs that is based on an "insider's" point of view. Various government agencies (e.g., NSA, CIA, FBI) use these "intelligence gathering" techniques overtly and covertly to collect information about different cultures that could compromise our personal, political, economic, technological, biological, or physical security in the United States. The intent for professional counselors would be much different in that the "intel" collected about various cultures would be used for a psychological benefit to the individual.

To have a meaningful cultural experience, you will need to develop a set of meaningful questions. You may use the same or similar questions to the 13 samples provided in the "Personal History Cultural Perspective: The Intake Interview" section in this chapter. These sample questions go beyond the closed-ended demographic questions used in traditional counseling and psychotherapy. The cultural questions provide you with an insider's view of the "culture of interest." You may want to keep a journal related to your cultural experiences so that you can reflect and synthesize such attributes as the culture's philosophical beliefs; how the typical person reacts emotionally, socially, cognitively, physically, and spiritually; and what types of occupations persons within the cultures do, as well as consider many other characteristics.

## CONCLUDING REMARKS

This chapter offers a description, discussion, and applied approach to the use of cultural empathy. If facilitated in a culturally relevant manner, the use of cultural empathy can strengthen the therapeutic relationship with culturally different individuals. It has been estimated that 75% of what we communicate is done nonverbally. Thus, interpretation of one's cultural identity, the meaning of his or her experiences, thoughts, feelings, and actions within a cultural context, is essential to build a trust and rapport before progressing to the working alliance with culturally different clients. Application of culturally relevant approaches should become second nature with practice. First and foremost, mental health professionals must have the openness to achieve basic awareness, knowledge, and skillful interactions with clients who are culturally different.

## REFERENCES

Bar-On, R., & Parker, J. (2000). *The handbook of emotional intelligence: Theory, development, assessment, and application at home, school, and the workplace.* San Francisco, CA: Jossey-Bass.

Corey, M. S., & Corey, G. (2016). *Becoming a helper.* Belmont, CA: Brooks/Cole.

Egan, G. (2014). *The skilled helper: A problem-management and opportunity-development approach to helping* (10th ed.). Belmont, CA: Brooks/Cole.

Goleman, D. (2006). *Emotional intelligence: Why it can matter more than IQ.* New York, NY: Bantam Books.

Harley, D. A., Stebnicki, M. A., & Rollins, C. (2001). Applying empowerment evaluation as a tool for self-improvement and community development with culturally diverse populations [Special Issue on Community Development Practice for Diverse Populations]. *Journal of the Community Development Society, 31*(2), 34–38.

Ibrahim, F. (1991). Contribution of cultural world view to generic counseling and development. *Journal of Counseling & Development, 70*, 13–19.

Ivey, A. E., Bradford Ivey, M., & Zalaquett, C. P. (2014). *Intentional interviewing and counseling: Facilitating client development in a multicultural society* (8th ed.). Belmont, CA: Brooks/Cole.

Lee, C. C. (2014). *Multicultural issues in counseling: A new approach to diversity.* New York, NY: Wiley.

Meyer, J. D., & Geher, G. (1996). Emotional intelligence and the identification of emotion. *Intelligence, 22*(2), 89–113.

Murphy, B. C., & Dillion, C. (2015). *Interviewing in action in a multicultural world* (5th ed.). Boston, MA: Cengage.

Pedersen, P. (2000). *A handbook for developing multicultural awareness* (3rd ed.). Alexandria, VA: American Counseling Association.

Pedersen, P., Crethar, H., & Carlson, J. (2008). *Inclusive cultural empathy: Making relationships central in counseling and psychotherapy.* Washington, DC: American Psychological Association.

Ponterotto, J. G., & Bensesch, K. F. (1988). An organizational framework for understanding the role of culture in counseling. *Journal of Counseling & Development, 66*, 237–241.

Ridley, C. R. (1995). *Overcoming unintentional racism in counseling and therapy: A practitioner's guide to intentional intervention.* Thousand Oaks, CA: Sage Publications.

Ridley, C. R., Mendoza, D. W., & Kanitz, B. E. (1994). Multicultural training: Reexamination, operationalization, and integration. *The Counseling Psychologist, 22*, 227–289.

Rogers, C. R. (1980). *A way of being.* Boston, MA: Houghton Mifflin.

Salovey, P., & Mayer, J. D. (1990). Emotional intelligence. *Imagination, Cognition, and Personality, 9*(3), 185–211.

Stebnicki, M. A., & Cubero, C. (2008). A content analysis of multicultural counseling syllabi from rehabilitation counseling programs. *Rehabilitation Education, 22*(2), 89–99.

Stebnicki, M. A., Rubin, S. E., Rollins, C., & Turner, T. N. (1999). A holistic approach to multicultural rehabilitation counseling. *Journal of Applied Rehabilitation Counseling, 30*(2), 3–6.

Sue, D. W. (2008). *Counseling the culturally different: Theory and practice* (5th ed.). New York, NY: Wiley.

# CHAPTER 7

# Multicultural Perspectives in Disaster Mental Health Counseling

There is little doubt that in the past 20 years multicultural counseling issues have been at the forefront of counselor education and training (Harley, Stebnicki, & Rollins, 2001; Stebnicki & Cubero, 2008; Stebnicki, Rubin, Rollins, & Turner, 1999). The changing demographics in the United States require counselors to cultivate increased awareness, knowledge, and skills in working with diverse racial and ethnic groups during disaster mental health response. The U.S. population as a whole is expected to grow from 319 million to 417 million by 2051 (U.S. Census Bureau, 2015). More specifically, the foreign-born population of immigrants is expected to outgrow native-born Americans by 20% between the years 2010 and 2020. Currently, White non-Hispanic individuals comprise over 50% of the U.S. total population. By 2060, it is estimated that White non-Hispanics will comprise only about 44% of the U.S. population. Accordingly, racial and ethnic minorities will become the majority population in the United States (Sue, 2008; U.S. Census Bureau, 2015).

In the United States today, there have been philosophical, ideological, and political conflicts fought over issues of language, inclusiveness, and legal and civil protections for different groups of individuals that have ultimately divided the population and galvanized some Americans' attitudes toward favoring isolationism and segregation. The cost of waging war on our philosophical, ideological, and political positions is that we may have lost some of our compassion for humanity in this process. Thus, looking outside the cultural borders of the United States requires us to look outside ourselves and understand the biological fact that roughly 99% of our DNA is identical for us all. We are all human beings living on the same planet, revolving around the same sun, in one specific solar system, and are invited guests among Earth's billions of other cultures and unidentified entities in the universe.

My intention for this chapter is to support the view that for multicultural counseling approaches to be successful, there must be a strong consideration for race, ethnicity, and biracial/ethnic identity; attributes of age (e.g., children, adolescents, older adults), gender (e.g., men and women), gender fluidity (e.g., lesbian, gay, bisexual, transgender), disability (e.g., spinal cord injury, deafness, neurocognitive disorder), social, economic, educational, rural, urban, and geographic identity (e.g., Northerner, Southerner, Californian, New Englander); country of origin (e.g., Africa, Columbia, Mexico, Syria); and other ethnographic variables that define individuals and groups by nationality, ethnicity, languages, and spiritual and religious identity. In addition, there has to be an awareness that many cultures do not endorse counseling and psychotherapy approaches. Mental health counseling is not natural to many indigenous populations in rural and urban geographic locations of the United States and throughout the globe.

## DEFINING MULTICUTURAL COUNSELING

Defining *multicultural counseling* has eluded many counseling and psychology experts in this specialty area because of the difficulties in defining (a) what correlates comprise the concept of culture, (b) factors related to within-group differences, (c) what particular attributes constitute culture, and (d) literature that discusses cultural concepts purely from either a nonculturally specific or universal perspective (etic) and literature whose primary focus is from a culturally specific or pure-cultural perspective (emic). These definitions, constructs, and models already exist and have been described by a distinguished group of experts in this area (e.g., Corey & Corey, 2016; Fukuyama, 1990; Ivey, Bradford Ivey, & Zalaquett, 2014; Lee, 2013; Lee & Richardson, 1991; Moodley & West, 2005; Pedersen, 2000; Ponterotto & Casas, 1991; Sue, 2008). It is particularly a challenge for disaster mental health counselors to provide mental health services to culturally different populations if they have had little training.

Redefining multicultural counseling by integrating indigenous healing practices promotes personal and professional growth and assists in the ailing multicultural counseling movement that seems to focus primarily on integrating traditional counseling and psychotherapy approaches (Moodley & West, 2005). Thus, it is not the intention of this chapter to recycle definitions and constructs of Western-style multicultural counseling. Rather, I attempt to interpret core constructs in multicultural counseling and offer guidelines as to how to apply such approaches with indigenous cultural groups that reach beyond the U.S. borders. This is necessary because professional counseling associations have organized volunteers and provided disaster mental health relief opportunities for counselors who want to serve on disaster sites internationally.

There are indeed debatable differences in models of multicultural counseling. Part of the challenge is because of the Eurocentric nature of contemporary counseling and psychotherapy that has influenced the multicultural counseling field. Other challenges are the lack of understanding and training opportunities in healing practices used among indigenous cultural groups (e.g., Ayurveda, Sweat Lodge ceremonies, mindfulness meditation). Such indigenous approaches do not always meet the criterion for evidence-based practices. So, defining multicultural counseling and its accompanying constructs is quite a commitment.

## BECOMING A CULTURALLY COMPETENT MENTAL HEALTH COUNSELOR

Becoming a culturally competent trauma counselor is first and foremost an ethical responsibility of the counselor (Cottone & Tarvydas, 2007) whereby the counselor is obligated to be mindful of his or her client's traumatic experience from a cultural lens (Tarvydas & Ng, 2012). Effective mental health counselors understand how their own cultural conditioning, values, beliefs, identity, and patterns of nonverbal and verbal communication can affect relationships with those who are culturally different (Corey & Corey, 2016; Egan, 2014; Ivey et al., 2014). The process of becoming a culturally competent mental health counselor requires development of the essential awareness, knowledge, and skills to work with a diversity of clients in trauma-related issues. Accordingly, effective mental health counselors are obligated to acquire the competencies to work with groups and individuals that may be located overseas in remote geographic locations globally.

Culturally competent counselors in general know how to facilitate culturally appropriate rapport and empathy by taking time to understand their clients' worldview. Counselors who take on this challenge have opportunities to gain insight into the richness of the client's culturally specific perception about self and others. Thus, it is essential that disaster mental health professionals understand and interpret how culturally different clients express and communicate emotions, feelings, cognitions, and behaviors both verbally and nonverbally. Ultimately, understanding clients from their cultural perspectives provides a rich understanding of how they record, transpose, replicate, express, and persistently reproduce trauma experiences.

## EXPRESSION OF TRAUMA FROM A CULTURAL PERSPECTIVE

Because of the heavy reliance on talk therapies in the West, it may be difficult to understand the client's expression of trauma. Many cultures use nonverbal styles of communication more frequently (gestures, eye contact, spatial distance) and may view this as more relevant. Additionally, disclosing personal issues to a mental health practitioner, rather than consulting with an older family member, spiritual leader, or those within their inner circle of trust, is typically not done. The point is that understanding the cultural expression of disaster and trauma is important from both the biopsychosocial and cultural viewpoints. It brings clarity to the communication and expression of individual emotions as a whole.

Mental health counselors who understand how their clients process, feel, and express the emotions of stress and trauma may have a therapeutic advantage. The implications for cultural understanding reach far beyond the expression of thoughts, feelings, and behaviors. Rather, this level of intuitive knowing can help mental health professionals understand cultural differences in the client's expression of ordinary and nonordinary states of consciousness and how they relate to transpersonal, metaphysical, and supernatural healing experiences (Walsh & Vaughn, 1993).

## Integrating Indigenous Healing Practices

Integrating indigenous healing practices into mental health practice transcends the boundaries of models and paradigms in traditional counseling theories. Having an appreciation of the humanistic, transpersonal, and cultural expression of how clients express stress and trauma has enormous cross-cultural significance. In the past two decades, the fields of science, religion, and spirituality have merged into a new dimension of cross-disciplinary collaborative research. The highly specialized fields of quantum physics, biochemistry, physiology, transpersonal psychology, and complementary medicine have shown that human consciousness is now an integral part of the mind, body, and spirit (Gordon, 1996; Seaward, 1997, 2006; Weil, 2009).

Moodley and West (2005) suggest that the respect for indigenous practices, philosophies, and belief systems such as found in Christianity (i.e., faith-based counseling and prayer), Buddhism (i.e., mindfulness meditation), or shamanic traditions (i.e., drumming rituals, journeying for spiritual helpers and power animals) has been ignored by some researchers and practitioners within the fields of counseling and psychology. This may be because there is a strong bias toward quantitative experimental designs that can hypothesize, predict, control, and manipulate variables with the intent to produce evidence-based treatment models.

Qualitative researchers who have studied integrative approaches such as prayer, yoga, Reiki, and meditation practices do not always garner the same support from their colleagues in the scientific community. Overall, this may become problematic for evaluating indigenous healing practices within a multicultural context because of the constraints of evidence-based practices, third-party payers, and the need to diagnose and treat mental health conditions using diagnostic and clinical protocols and symptomatology (i.e., *Diagnostic and Statistical Manual of Mental Disorders* [5th ed.; *DSM-5*; American Psychiatric Association, 2013]). Thus, mental health professionals who have been trained in Western models of disaster mental health response may not have the awareness, knowledge, and skills to work with a variety of cultural groups coming to the United States, such as asylum seekers, immigrants, and refugees.

## USE OF EMPATHY IN DISASTER MENTAL HEALTH COUNSELING

At the core of most humanistic theoretical orientations in the helping profession is the therapeutic use of empathy and compassion. The use of core principles in empathetic communication can assist mental health professionals in building a strong rapport and working alliance in disaster and trauma response if facilitated in a culturally sensitive manner. There is a rich history in the use of empathy during therapeutic interactions as seen in Western counseling and psychotherapy. Possessing the skills of empathy during person-centered therapeutic interactions is seen by many as a prerequisite for becoming a skilled and competent helper (Corey & Corey, 2016; Egan, 2014; Ivey et al., 2014; Truax & Carkhuff, 1967). Culturally appropriate empathy, if facilitated competently by the therapist, can assist in building a strong connection with a variety of clients from different cultural backgrounds (Moodley & West, 2005).

The conceptual underpinnings of empathy can be traced back in the modern application of empathy research and practice as described by Carl Rogers (1902–1987) when he published his seminal work, *Client-Centered Therapy* in 1951. A psychologist and founder of the person-centered therapy movement, Rogers (1957) introduced the concept of empathy as a *necessary and sufficient condition* for the therapeutic change to occur. He hypothesized that there are core conditions that apply to all psychotherapy: (a) counselor congruence or genuineness within the therapeutic relationship, (b) unconditional positive regard for the client, (c) the ability of the counselor to empathize with the client in this relationship, (d) communication of empathy, and (e) expressing unconditional positive regard toward the client. Rogers (1980) talked passionately about empathy and empathic listening as "a way of being." He was known as a deeply intuitive man and provided a description of empathy:

> It means entering the private perceptual world of the other and becoming thoroughly at home in it. It involves being sensitive, moment by moment, to the changing felt meanings which flow in this other person, to the fear or rage or tenderness or confusion or whatever that he or she is experiencing. It means temporarily living in the other's life, moving about in it delicately without making judgments. (p. 142)

Today, most research studies concerned with the clinical application of empathy have accepted, incorporated, and credited the lifework of Rogers's client-centered therapy approaches as the primary contributor to 20th- and 21st-century counseling and psychotherapy. The richness of using a basic- and advanced-level empathy in disaster mental health response builds a relationship that is open and honest. If facilitated in a culturally appropriate manner, empathy can build the client meaning of one's trauma experience and be an impetus for posttraumatic growth. Empathy can also be used as a facilitative tool to spark new ways of thinking and learning in solution-focused therapeutic environments. Thus, the intentional and conscious use of empathy during client–counselor interactions appears to be integral to the helper's way of being with the client both verbally and nonverbally.

Empathy has been discussed in the counseling and psychology literature as a skill that can be both developed and learned if facilitated properly by a competent professional (Barone et al., 2005). Empathy as a way of being (Rogers, 1980) is also a form of communication that involves attending, listening, observing, understanding, and responding to the concerns of others with a deep respect and genuineness. Oftentimes across different styles of cultural communication we communicate with one another nonverbally. Accordingly, empathy involves being aware of other's meta-communication through eye contact, body language, silence, tone of voice, gestures, facial expressions, physical space, and in many other ways.

Empathy is often a misunderstood concept; it is often confused with sympathy. Sympathy, as an emotional reaction to another person's life event, is essentially stating: "I'm sorry this has happened to you." Conversely, empathy communicates verbally and non-verbally to others by affirming: "I'm sorry this has happened to you—this has to be very difficult for you; what can I do to help?" Accordingly, empathy requires the mental health professional to be an active participant during therapeutic interactions and be deeply involved with others in a powerful way.

## CULTURAL EMPATHY

Empathy has been discussed in the counseling and psychology literature for the past 125 years and has been conceptualized as a skill that can be both developed and learned if facilitated properly (Barone et al., 2005). Empathy has a rich history of being at the foundation of most theoretical orientations within counselor education training programs. However, the concept of empathy has brought a new meaning to its theoretical and practical use in cross-cultural counseling settings. For instance, cultural empathy (Ivey et al., 2014; Ridley & Lingle, 1996), empathic multicultural awareness (Junn, Morton, & Yee, 1995), cultural role taking (Scott & Borodovsky, 1990), ethnotherapeutic empathy (Parson, 1993), and ethnocultural empathy (Wang et al., 2003) have all been used interchangeably to delineate both the same and different constructs of cultural empathy.

In regard to the more general term *cultural specific empathy* as described by some multicultural counseling theorists (Ponterotto & Bensesch, 1988; Ridley, 1995; Ridley, Mendoza, & Kanitz, 1994), empathy is seen as a skill that is pancultural or universal. If empathy can be facilitated in a culturally sensitive manner, this should help strengthen the therapeutic relationship (Ibrahim, 1991). Ridley (1995) suggests that cultural empathy has two dimensions: understanding and communication. Understanding requires that the counselor try and synthesize the idiographic meaning of his or her client's stories, and then respond with the accurate meaning of what the client has communicated to the counselor. Accordingly, all therapy can be culturally contextualized and a positive therapeutic outcome can be enhanced by the skills of a culturally competent counselor.

Some authors have criticized traditional counseling approaches that place a heavy reliance on empathic communication that is not culturally sensitive (Freeman, 1993; Pedersen, 2000; Sue, 2008; Usher, 1989). If the expectations of therapy are that clients should disclose emotions at a deep level during session, then stepping inside the private world of the culturally different client may be perceived as being too intrusive or offensive. Lee and Richardson (1991) suggest that if the discipline of multicultural counseling is to have any therapeutic value in the counseling relationship, then we must go beyond training counselors in the broad conceptualizations of developing more than just cultural awareness and knowledge. Having an understanding of different cultures alone does not allow us to develop competent practitioners who can apply the skills of cultural empathy. It requires strategies and approaches that are culturally specific and relevant so as to help build a strong trusting relationship and form a therapeutic alliance.

Ridley and Lingle's (1996) model of cultural empathy has defined this construct as a "learned ability" that is interpersonally focused and has many dimensions. This model proposes that there are three processes that underlie cultural empathy: (a) cognitive process (cultural perspective taking and differentiating self from others), (b) affective process (vicarious feelings and empathy expression of concern for others), and (c) communicative process (probing for insight, expression of accurate understanding).

Corey and Corey (2016) suggest that a self-assessment and exploration of both compassion and empathy are important for beginning-level counselors so that they may become aware of their clients' needs from different cultural backgrounds and respond with care, concern, and understanding. Lazarus (1999) views compassion as a double-edged sword, however. He suggests that having too much compassion toward another person can impair our ability to help others. He further states that "we must learn how to distance ourselves emotionally from the emotional significance of their suffering, so it does not overwhelm us" (p. 246). There are others who feel compassion has been left out of training programs in Western psychology, counseling, and medical education (Goleman, 2003). This may be because compassion itself has different ideologies and religious beliefs attached to its meaning. However, competent and ethical counselors should consistently evaluate the impact that their belief systems have on client–counselor sessions and how interventions that use empathy and compassion might be perceived by their clients (Corey & Corey, 2016; Egan, 2014; Ivey et al., 2014).

Compassion, as opposed to empathy or sympathy, as described by the Dalai Lama is a quality "that needs to be naturally drawn from within one's own inner resources" (Goleman, 2003, p. 245). His Holiness places a paramount importance on promoting the values of compassion, loving kindness, and altruism as a significant human quality to cultivate at a very early age in life. Even though compassion is a highly desirable and healthy human emotion, it does not appear to be a skill that we can teach in traditional counselor education programs the way we train counselors in the skills of empathy. Intentional acts of compassion, if approached in a culturally sensitive manner during disaster mental health response, appear to be an unquestionably desirable human attribute that can potentially strengthen the client–counselor therapeutic relationship.

## CULTURAL RESPONSE TO TRAUMA

Kohrt and Hruschka (2010) report that in the aftermath of a 10-year Maoist civil war in Nepal and the relocation of thousands of Bhutanese refugees from Nepal to Western countries, there was a significant growth of mental health and psychosocial support programs to treat posttraumatic stress symptoms. Each culture has its own unique way of expressing the human trauma associated with horrific events experienced. In the case of Nepal, the trauma survivors felt blamed for experiencing the extraordinary stressful and traumatic events. Some viewed these atrocities as *karma* brought on by past life sins or sins committed by family members. As a result, some cultural groups were reluctant to seek mental health and psychosocial support for the fear of revealing their bad *karma* and shame. Indeed, stigma of seeking assistance from mental health professionals is problematic from Western models of mental and physical health treatment.

This is much like the stigma attached to American military personnel who seek treatment for issues of posttraumatic stress symptoms, depression, anxiety, and substance use disorders (Stebnicki, 2016). Indeed, there are consequences that include loss of rank, status, confidence in the ability to lead, and security clearance, just to name a few concerns. Depending on the diagnosis and severity of symptoms (e.g., substance addiction, severe posttraumatic stress disorder [PTSD]), military personnel could be dishonorably discharged, or have a less-than-honorable discharge.

Many indigenous populations have a great sense of soul loss after extraordinary stressful and traumatic events, which is a type of invisible wound. It can cause a range of symptoms and behaviors that also include insomnia, nightmares, anger, rage, flashbacks, hypervigilance, and difficulty with concentration and focus. Soul loss can occur both individually and collectively, affecting the cultural groups as a whole. This is one explanation in the literature related to historical trauma (e.g., Native North American Indian tribes, colonial slaves, ethnic cleansing) where traumatic events are passed down through generations of families where the mental, physical, cognitive, social, emotional, and psychological effects of trauma are culturally transmitted. Thus, most cultural groups have healing rituals, which is a natural part of their healing system. In the condition related to soul loss, many indigenous groups use traditional healing rituals such as *soul retrieval* (Ingerman, 1991), which is necessary to bring the soul back to balance with the mind, body, and spirit.

Hinton, Nickerson, and Bryant (2011) studied the psychological histories of Cambodian refugees who fought a brutal civil war in 1975. The war was between the Khmer Rouge who took power, leaving 500,000 Cambodians dead, disabled, displaced, and impoverished. Over the next three-and-a-half years, the Khmer Rouge, a group of Maoist-inspired radicals led by Pol Pot, implemented a series of radical socioeconomic reforms in an attempt to gain power and control of Cambodia. By January 1979, the Khmer Rouge was overthrown and almost eight million Cambodians died of disease, starvation, overwork, and execution.

Studies relating to this person-made disaster describe the severe mental health–related symptoms that exist even 40 years after experiencing the trauma and atrocities of the Khmer Rouge killing fields. The Cambodian refugees of these horrific events currently report severe posttraumatic stress symptoms and experience feelings of extreme vulnerability, constant threats to their physical and emotional safety because of reoccurring memories, preoccupation, and cognitions of these catastrophic events. Based on the clinical work of Hinton et al. (2011), Cambodian refugees have frequent panic attacks and chronic worry related to multiple perceived and potential threats. It was found that the panic reaction triggers multiple other psychological and physical reactions that worsen the symptoms related to posttraumatic stress.

Indigenous refugee populations coming from other countries have multiple worries that include financial and housing issues, health care for their children and families, jobs, and education. Current studies that include populations exposed to historically traumatic events suggest that it is critical to address the trauma survivor's adaptation and chain of reactions that trigger the posttraumatic stress symptoms and psychopathological reactions. In theory, having a poor ability to regulate mood, affect, and thoughts/cognitions of worry clearly relates to the person's general ability to regulate affect and cope with posttraumatic stress symptoms. Thus, disaster mental health interventions that can translate mental health symptoms into culturally appropriate interventions have the potential for healing trauma.

Epidemiological studies of similar trauma have increased over the past 15 years in the literature, particularly since September 11, 2001. Other case studies of disaster frequently seen in the literature are that of natural disasters. For example, the devastating Asian tsunami that occurred December 26, 2004, where a massive earthquake struck near the Indonesian island of Sumatra, resulted in the deaths of more than 2.8 million people, the displacement of more than one million people, and the significant disruption of more than five million other lives. The long-term psychological impact is widespread. Survivors of this traumatic event have unique individual, social, cultural, and spiritual coping strategies that have required more than formal mental health services (Rajkumar, Premkumar, & Tharyan, 2008). The overall result reported by Rajkumar et al. (2008) suggests that the prevalence of posttraumatic stress symptoms, 9 months following the tsunami, was 6.4%, which is considerably lower than predicted based on other studies of natural disasters. The outpouring of support internationally assisted in increased coping abilities of the tsunami survivors. There were little changes in the spiritual beliefs and their attitude toward the sea. Indeed, the hardiness and resiliency they experienced made them cherish their survivor-hood as a gift from God. Inherent in the indigenous populations within this region of the world is the meager expectation about occupations, careers, striving for financial wealth, and other variables that suggest materialism was not a perceived loss.

In tsunami-affected Sri Lanka, family support, strong attachment between parents and children, and optimal mental health functioning, particularly among the mothers and women of Sri Lanka, were resiliency factors that reduced posttraumatic stress symptoms (Wickrama & Kaspar, 2007). Preliminary studies in culture and trauma point to the culturally specific resiliency factors that can be integrated with Western mental health interventions. Specifically, family-focused interventions, social and economic recovery activities, and mental health and wellness can be integrated with a combination of the individual, family, and culture in healing trauma.

## TRANSITION FROM TRADITIONAL COUNSELING TO INDIGENOUS HEALING

Anderson (2005) and others have a unique body of research that discusses the cultural role of counseling and psychotherapy as a ritual in Western cultures. Almost all cultures, at times, have experiences of psychological and emotional distress and each has established its own system for dealing with these problems (McLeod, 2001). Thus, disaster mental health response forms a sort of ritual that provides a social framework for the resolution of grief, loss, and extraordinary stressful and traumatic events. Contemporary mental health counseling theories provide the core foundation for the intention and logic to implement disaster mental health counseling strategies and techniques. The system (ritual) that we know as mental health assessment, diagnosis, and treatment was established in the counseling profession between the 19th and 20th centuries. Accordingly, contemporary models of counseling and psychotherapy are a ritual of sorts and are based on a Western cultural understanding of healing psychologically and emotionally after being at the epicenter of disaster and trauma.

Some of the early indigenous cultures (premedical and mental health models of healing) developed their healing system based on their own unique cultural beliefs, values, and philosophy. For instance, shamanism has been practiced in most cultures for more than 5,000 years and involves various rituals, ceremonies, and practices to heal the mind, body, and spirit. Long before there were physicians, psychiatrists, mental health counselors, pharmaceutical products, and medical technology, there was the shaman. The shaman had to be skilled in all arts and health sciences to heal physical, mental, emotional, and spiritual bodies (Harner, 1990). Thus, common to multiple health and healing systems is a form of ritual where the person anticipates that if he or she engages in some type of healing ritual, there is a therapeutic outcome that transforms his or her mental, physical, emotional, psychological, and spiritual health. Cohen (1985) and others discuss the importance of rituals in terms of symbolism that lies at the heart of religious, spiritual, and ideological belief systems in various cultures. Thus, the symbolic meaning that takes place between the person and culture with which he or she lives brings about health, healing, and mental and physical wellness, which is congruent with healing one's extraordinary stressful and traumatic experiences.

## Cultural Transition: Acculturation Versus Assimilation

Chapter 8 offers mental health practitioners culturally specific ways that integrate the foundations of mind, body, and spirit that are congruent with one's cultural belief system. However, this chapter offers mental health practitioners culturally competent skills that help translate theoretical models into multicultural counseling. Accordingly, there are many ways that individuals express their cultural values that for many do not remain static. They are expressed in dynamic ways based on one's cultural identity, assimilation, acculturation, and many other ways. The intent of this section is not to comprehensively discuss all constructs typically found in a multicultural counseling text. Rather, the interested reader should consult the References section for further reading on the foundational models and constructs in this area of study. However, there are two constructs important in multiculturalism that are important to discuss (acculturation and assimilation) that relate to how individuals transition and form their unique cultural identities. More specifically, understanding the person's level of acculturation or cultural identity can be a gauge for the types of Western-style mental health interventions that could potentially be integrated within a therapeutic encounter. First, there are two important concepts that relate to cultural transition.

*Acculturation:* In this situation, two or more cultures come into contact with each other and the minority (or indigenous) culture acquires the cultural values, norms, language, and behaviors of the dominant society (sometimes by choice, sometimes not). Some individuals from minority or indigenous groups adopt the cultural values of the majority culture. At times, this can be observed as necessary, forced, involuntary, or mandatory (i.e., adopting a language in order to find work, purchase food, acquire shelter or clothing).

*Assimilation:* Some indigenous-minority groups "give up" their own identities, attitudes, and behaviors in favor of the identity, attitudes, and behaviors of the dominant culture.

Cultural transition can be complex for many individuals. For instance, there are associated physical, mental, psychological, social, and emotional stressors in cultural transition. There is the perception that one must act or behave according to cultural rituals of the majority culture. There are many world populations that are forced into cultural transition. Thus, the following observations are offered to mental health counselors as a way to view and perhaps assess their clients' cultural transition:

1. What types of behavioral shift do you observe the individual from the minority/indigenous culture make who voluntarily/involuntarily acculturated to the majority culture or healing system?

2. What is the psychosocial response (socially, emotionally, psychologically, medically–physically, spiritually) that minority/indigenous persons made, or plan to make, in their transition to acculturate into the majority society?

3. What are some coping skills, supports, or resources the minority/indigenous person uses while going through the acculturation process?

4. What is the process of becoming an "American" or a member of the majority culture? Which generation is this individual from: first, second, or third generation?

## THE CULTURAL INTAKE INTERVIEW

The traditional intake interview in mental health practice acquires information related to a range of cultural attributes such as race/ethnicity, religious/spiritual beliefs, gender, sexual orientation, marital status, and other demographic variables. The problem with this approach is that it is a gathering of information by the client who is one dimensional. The following sample of 13 questions offers a greater cultural dimension to mental health professionals and provides a means of getting at both the same, yet different information during an initial interview and subsequent sessions. The questions that follow have the ability to uncover important information related to cultural identity, identity development, assimilation, acculturation, gender fluidity, and, most importantly, the system of health, healing, and wellness the individual endorses. The mental health practitioner may want to rephrase some of these questions in terms of the person's own cultural expressions and use of English.

1. How would you describe your family or cultural background?

2. Describe your cultural beliefs, philosophy, or values from a holistic perspective.

3. When did you first become aware or begin to practice some of your cultural value beliefs?

4. Can you remember how you initially felt—emotionally, physically, or spiritually—when you first became aware of your cultural identity?

5. Did your culture or family experience any prejudice or discrimination based on your race, ethnicity, or religious/spiritual beliefs?

6. What were some of the ways in which this prejudice or discrimination was expressed or communicated toward you and your culture?

7. Were there any negative attitudes, barriers, prejudices, or stereotypes that your family members or culture expressed toward other groups?

8. How do your cultural beliefs or values affect how you live in your everyday life (emotionally, physically, cognitively, spiritually, occupationally, financially)?

9. What parts of your culture or family traditions (rituals, rules, beliefs, philosophy) do you feel positive about and have you carried on with other family members?

10. What parts of your culture or family traditions/values/practices would you like to give up, get away from, ignore, or not be reminded of?

11. Are there any parts of your culture that you have been confused about or uncertain regarding where these values, beliefs, or practices originated?

12. Have your family members borrowed any practices, beliefs, or other things from other cultures? How were these integrated?

13. If you had some advice to give to others from your culture or your family, what would you tell them?

## CULTURAL OBSERVATIONS

A cultural shift has emerged since the early 1990s where there was an emphasis on culturally specific characteristics and attributes such as gender, sexual orientation, race, ethnicity, and other salient traits that define the whole person (Moodley & West, 2005). The positive effects of being culturally attuned support mental health counselors in building a strong client rapport from a multicultural counseling framework. To truly understand the stories of trauma and disaster survivors it is of paramount importance to have an increased level of awareness, knowledge, and skills that are both universal and culturally specific. This enhances your work with culturally different individuals and groups.

Pedersen (2000) suggests that the functions of counseling have been practiced for thousands of years and are not merely an invention in modern counseling and psychotherapy. Contemporary counseling practice has rediscovered many of the principles and practices in indigenous healing from a non–Western-centric viewpoint. This has been achieved by practitioners attuning themselves to the salient attributes that comprise an individual's culture. The following informal assessment items are offered with the intention of facilitating follow-up observations and questions that may be pursued with clients who live in different geographic regions of the world outside the United States. Disaster mental health professionals trained in the West are sometimes deployed to different geographic regions of the world, which places the practitioner at a disadvantage. Thus, the following information can be asked directly from the individual or through an interpreter–translator or can be observed in the natural environment.

1. What is the name of your tribe or cultural group?

2. Describe your personal history.

3. What are some unique cultural characteristics related to your group's cultural identity? Within the majority or other minority groups within your culture?

4. How would you describe your style and pattern of verbal or nonverbal communication, time orientation, or spatial distance? As an outsider, what would I notice different about your culture that sets apart your culture from any other cultures?

5. How would you describe your religious and/or spiritual belief system?

6. What are some unique characteristics about the geographic region in which you live?

7. What form of government do you have? What particular rules, codes, laws, and/or standards does your culture have that guide you in everyday life?

8. Describe the types of occupations you have in your culture, as well as the educational system, the labor market, industries, or technological characteristics that separate your culture from others.

9. Describe the specific gender roles, sexual orientations, and/or other lifestyle factors that are unique to your culture.

10. What are the unique racial, ethnic, or specific physical characteristics of your culture?

11. Has your culture ever been forced or voluntarily had to acculturate or assimilate to another culture, or adopt the majority's cultural values, beliefs, or form of government?

12. What are some specific epidemiology mental or physical health characteristics unique to your culture?

## PROCESSING CRITICAL CULTURAL INFORMATION

Disaster mental health professionals who provide disaster relief globally may be inexperienced with a variety of different cultural groups. For many, these exchanges, patterns of verbal and nonverbal communication, and other encounters can occur naturally or through the guidance and direction of other experienced team members. Thus, it is essential that the practitioner new to an indigenous cultural group work alongside a more seasoned professional familiar with that particular culture. Skilled and competent multicultural counselors welcome opportunities for personal and professional growth. These experiences can be recorded in a journal through multiple means, including, but not limited to, (a) written self-expression, (b) written communication from others in the natural environment, or (c) recording of symbols, artwork, and other culturally relevant ways. The intended value is primarily for personal reflection, observation, recording important aspects of cultural communication, and use in processing with your critical incident team or with others from the host or indigenous culture.

Mental health professionals should strive to be culturally sensitive and respectful at all times. Some examples that would violate or disrespect cultural traditions may include taking pictures of indigenous peoples, rituals, or sacred environments while on deployment; taking "souvenirs" or cultural artifacts; dressing inappropriately for a particular culture; using cultural communication (verbal and nonverbal) that could be misinterpreted; and other behaviors that would break trust and cultural rapport.

The following guidelines are offered to disaster mental health counselors and disaster relief teams that may be useful in processing or debriefing one another in the relief, recovery, and reintegration efforts.

1. *Personal self-reflections from each team member:* These comments should be based on the personal self-reflections of each team member and the activities and experiences gained throughout the deployment. Asking for and receiving feedback from the tribal or cultural leader may be important feedback to the team to improve communication, cultivate indigenous resources, and develop outside or natural supports. You may want to note any within-group differences or similarities you perceived/experienced as a team member.

2. *Dynamics of team itself:* These comments should be communicated collectively among team members. For example, your team may reflect upon any interpersonal strain as observed by other team members, by tribal or indigenous cultural group members, or through any relationship strain or conflicts that developed within (or outside of) your team. Resolution should focus on decreasing or eliminating team member conflict and achieving a supportive, balanced, and unified team.

3. *The team members struggle toward cultural dependence–independence:* Because many disaster survivors become dependent on disaster relief teams, it may be difficult to facilitate approaches that foster independence. Team members should process how the organization and implementation of disaster relief strategies may actually reinforce dependent behaviors on the culture. Team leaders should discuss how to manage and fade assistance at appropriate intervals and how the team's own cultural identity may be interfering with that of the indigenous cultural group.

4. *The team's ability to successfully deal, achieve, or resolve conflict inside and outside of the team:* Discuss and process how your team members did (or did not) achieve resolution, peace, and harmony, or how any alliances may have been formed with indigenous cultural members.

5. *The indigenous group's natural coping abilities and resiliency traits:* Discuss and process with team members specific indigenous cultural traits that lead to positive coping and resiliency.

6. *Any other significant reflections:* Discuss any other significant issues based on your team's experiences that relate to optimal effectiveness in this critical incident response and how these efforts could be applied to other cultural groups.

# CULTURAL CREATION ACTIVITY: CREATION OF CULTURAL GROUP/TRIBE

## Intent of Activity

The purpose of this cultural creation activity is to integrate knowledge and skills acquired within multicultural counseling for the purpose of creating your own culture. Using the cultural guidelines listed in this section, your tribe/group/culture develops specific characteristics to establish a culture that may or may not be based on another existing cultural group. After your culture has been established, you engage in face-to-face interactions and activities with members of other cultural groups (participating in this activity) to explore the inter/intrapersonal communication dynamics and to problem-solve different scenarios posed by the group facilitator. Each cultural group has to coexist in one geographic location because its present environment is uninhabitable due to a natural disaster. Assume that there is enough food, shelter, and clothing for everyone and that the new geographic location is welcoming and hospitable to accommodate all cultural groups.

*Provide a description of your cultural group:*

1. Name of your tribe or cultural group (e.g., The Rainbox People, People of the Americas, The Flat Landers, The Water World People, People of the Rainforest):

2. Indigenous geographic characteristics of your culture (e.g., people of the mountain, forest, islands, ocean, lakes, river, desert, canyon):

3. Personal history (e.g., "We were all born from the same mother-father"; "We were forced to acculturate with a majority culture"; "We left our birthplace and moved geographically to have a better way of life"):

4. Cultural characteristics related to your group's cultural identity and any unique characteristics (e.g., biologically, physically, racially/ethnically, sexual orientation):

5. Style and pattern of verbal or nonverbal communication, greetings, time orientation, or spatial distance, eye contact, or other meta-communication:

6. Specific religious and/or spiritual belief system (e.g., based on Native American beliefs, Christianity, Judaism, Buddhism, Hinduism, Sufism, Islam):

7. Form of governance, rules, ethics, laws, and/or standards that guide your culture in everyday life (e.g., type of sociopolitical system, military service, health and human services programs):

8. Occupational, educational, labor market, industrial, or technological characteristics (e.g., farming, fishing, arts/crafts, typical level of academic education, high tech):

## Activity Rules

► All cultural development activities can be developed either before or during this cultural group activity. Groups participating should be able to delineate the cultural characteristics 1 to 8 mentioned in the previous section in less than 30 minutes.

▶ All participants are encouraged to actively participate as group members. If they feel more comfortable in another cultural group, the group facilitator should allow participants to change to a different cultural group, but only at the beginning of the activity.

▶ If any group member senses that a member of its tribe/culture did not participate in the development of its tribe or culture at equivalent levels of participation as the other tribal members, then an individual or individuals within the group itself should take the necessary steps to communicate and resolve this issue with the group member who is reluctant, resistant, or defensive to the process.

## Part One: Interactions Between Cultures

▶ *Cultural greeting:* Participants will mingle with other cultures for a cultural greeting.

▶ *Cultural observations:* Participants make specific notes on the various cultural characteristics set forth previously, then discuss these observations among their cultural group/tribe members.

▶ *Cultural process:* A spokesperson displays his or her own fact sheet on the document cam and (a) introduces his or her own culture and (b) describes what he or she observed (first impressions) among the other cultural groups.

## Part Two: Choose One Cultural Group That Closely Aligns With Your Culture

▶ Based on interactions with all other cultural groups, participants choose one cultural group that aligns with its beliefs and values to develop a solution and problem-solve the "casino" issues as described in Part Three. Some groups may feel connected to more than one group to engage in problem-solving activity.

## Part Three: Casino Vote

▶ Assume that several years have passed and your cultural group has incurred significant amounts of mental and physical health problems, as well as high rates of unemployment, poverty, and poor housing.

▶ The nation's ruler has allowed each cultural group to build a $180 million full-service land-based casino (alcohol, food, entertainment) funded totally by the ruling government. The casino is anticipated/projected to make at least $80 million in its first year of operation.

▶ Assume that after the first year of casino operation and the financial benefits, this could empower your cultural group with hope for a better future.

▶ Draft a response to report to the other group members about your cultural group's decision on the casino.

► Make sure and address the following issues: What impact will the casino have on the culture? What are the short-term and long-term benefits, if any, to your culture? Discuss any environmental impact or any other associated cost to your culture. Provide a general statement of impact.

## CONCLUDING REMARKS

Redefining multicultural counseling by integrating indigenous healing practices promotes personal and professional growth. Contemporary counseling practice has rediscovered many of the principles and practices in indigenous healing from a non–Western-centric viewpoint. There are multiple culturally enriching opportunities to work with culturally different persons geographically in the United States and those who volunteer overseas for humanitarian assistance. Disaster mental health professionals should strive to be culturally sensitive and respectful at all times. Chapter 14 on working with immigrants, refugees, and asylum seekers provides a good example of Western mental health counselors integrating best practices in two worlds: one's own cultural practice and the indigenous culture they are serving.

## REFERENCES

American Psychiatric Association. (2013). *Diagnostic and statistical manual of mental disorders* (5th ed.). Arlington, VA: American Psychiatric Publishing.

Anderson, M. (2005). Psychotherapy as a ritual: Connecting the concrete with the symbolic. In R. Moodley & W. West (Eds.), *Integrating traditional healing practices into counseling and psychotherapy* (pp. 282–292). Thousand Oaks, CA: Sage Publications.

Barone, D. F., Hutchings, P. S., Kimmel, H. J., Traub, H. L., Cooper, J. T., & Marshall, C. M. (2005). Increasing empathic accuracy through practice and feedback in a clinical interviewing course. *Journal of Social and Clinical Psychology, 24*(2), 156–171.

Cohen, A. P. (1985). *The symbolic construction of community.* London, United Kingdom: Routledge.

Corey, M. S., & Corey, G. (2016). *Becoming a helper.* Belmont, CA: Brooks/Cole.

Cottone, R. R., & Tarvydas, V. M. (2007). *Counseling ethics and decision making* (3rd ed.). Upper Saddle River, NJ: Pearson/Merrill Prentice-Hall.

Egan, G. (2014). *The skilled helper: A problem-management and opportunity-development approach to helping* (10th ed.). Belmont, CA: Brooks/Cole.

Freeman, S. C. (1993). Client-centered therapy with diverse populations: The universal within the specific. *Journal of Multicultural Counseling and Development, 21*(1), 248–254.

Fukuyama, M. A. (1990). Taking a universal approach to multicultural counseling. *Counselor Education and Supervision, 30*, 6–17.

Goleman, D. (2003). *Healing emotions: Conversations with the Dalai Lama on mindfulness, emotions, and health.* Boston, MA: Shambhala.

Gordon, J. S. (1996). *Manifesto for a new medicine: Your guide to healing partnerships and the wise use of alternative therapies.* Reading, MA: Perseus Books

Harley, D. A., Stebnicki, M. A., & Rollins, C. (2001). Applying empowerment evaluation as a tool for self-improvement and community development with culturally diverse populations [Special Issue on Community Development Practice for Diverse Populations]. *Journal of the Community Development Society, 31*(2), 34–38.

Harner, M. (1990). *The way of the shaman.* San Francisco, CA: Harper San Francisco.

Hinton, D. E., Nickerson, A., & Bryant, R. A. (2011). Worry, worry attacks, and PTSD among Cambodian refugees: A path analysis investigation. *Social Science & Medicine, 72,* 1817–1825.

Ibrahim, F. (1991). Contribution of cultural world view to generic counseling and development. *Journal of Counseling & Development, 70,* 13–19.

Ingerman, S. (1991). *Soul retrieval: Mending the fragmented self.* San Francisco, CA: Harper San Francisco.

Ivey, A. E., Bradford Ivey, M., & Zalaquett, C. P. (2014). *Intentional interviewing and counseling: Facilitating client development in a multicultural society* (8th ed.). Belmont, CA: Brooks/Cole.

Junn, E. N., Morton, K. R., & Yee, I. (1995). The "Gibberish" exercise: Facilitating empathetic multicultural awareness. *Journal of Instructional Psychology, 22,* 324–329.

Kohrt, B. A., & Hruschka, D. J. (2010). Nepali concepts of psychological trauma: The role of idioms of distress, ethnopsychology and ethnophysiology in alleviating suffering and preventing stigma. *Cultural Medicine Psychiatry, 34,* 322–352.

Lazarus, R. S. (1999). *Stress and emotion: A new synthesis.* New York, NY: Springer Publishing.

Lee, C. C. (Ed.). (2013). *Multicultural issues in counseling: New approach to diversity* (4th ed.). Hoboken, NJ: Wiley and American Counseling Association.

Lee, C. C., & Richardson, B. L. (Eds.). (1991). *Multicultural issues in counseling: New approaches to diversity.* Alexandria, VA: American Counseling Association.

McLeod, J. (2001). *An introduction to counselling.* Buckingham, United Kingdom: Open University Press.

Moodley, R., & West, W. (2005). *Integrating traditional healing practices into counseling and psychotherapy.* Thousand Oaks, CA: Sage Publications.

Parson, E. R. (1993). Ethnotherapeutic empathy (EthE): II, Techniques in interpersonal cognition and vicarious experience across cultures. *Journal of Contemporary Psychotherapy, 23,* 171–182.

Pedersen, P. (2000). *A handbook for developing multicultural awareness* (3rd ed.). Alexandria, VA: American Counseling Association.

Ponterotto, J. G., & Bensesch, K. F. (1988). An organizational framework for understanding the role of culture in counseling. *Journal of Counseling & Development, 66,* 237–241.

Ponterotto, J. G., & Casas, J. M. (1991). *Handbook of racial/ethnic minority counseling research.* Springfield, IL: Charles C. Thomas.

Rajkumar, A. P., Premkumar, T. S., & Tharyan, P. (2008). Coping with the Asian tsunami: Perspectives from Tamil Nadu, India on the determinants of resilience in the face of adversity. *Social Science & Medicine, 67,* 844–853.

Ridley, C. R. (1995). *Overcoming unintentional racism in counseling and therapy: A practitioner's guide to intentional intervention.* Thousand Oaks, CA: Sage Publications.

Ridley, C. R., & Lingle, D. W. (1996). Cultural empathy in multicultural counseling: A multidimensional process model. In P. B. Pederson & J. G. Draguns (Eds.), *Counseling across cultures* (4th ed., pp. 21–46). Thousand Oaks, CA: Sage Publications.

Ridley, C. R., Mendoza, D. W., & Kanitz, B. E. (1994). Multicultural training: Reexamination, operationalization, and integration. *The Counseling Psychologist, 22,* 227–289.

Rogers, C. R. (1951). *Client-centered therapy: Its current practice, implication, and theory.* Boston, MA: Houghton Mifflin.

Rogers, C. R. (1957). The necessary and sufficient conditions of therapeutic personality change. *Journal of Consulting Psychology, 21,* 95–103.

Rogers, C. R. (1980). *A way of being.* Boston, MA: Houghton Mifflin.

Scott, N. E., & Borodovsky, L. G. (1990). Effective use of cultural role taking. *Professional Psychology: Research and Practice, 21*(3), 167–170.

Seaward, B. L. (1997). *Stand like mountain, flow like water: Reflections on stress and human spirituality.* Deerfield Beach, FL: Health Communications.

Seaward, B. L. (2006). *Essentials of managing stress.* Boston, MA: Jones & Bartlett.

Stebnicki, M. A. (2016). Military counseling. In I. Marini & M. A. Stebnicki (Eds.), *The professional counselor's desk reference* (2nd ed., pp. 499–506). New York, NY: Springer Publishing.

Stebnicki, M. A., & Cubero, C. (2008). A content analysis of multicultural counseling syllabi from rehabilitation counseling programs. *Rehabilitation Education, 22*(2), 89–99.

Stebnicki, M. A., Rubin, S. E., Rollins, C., & Turner, T. N. (1999). A holistic approach to multicultural rehabilitation counseling. *Journal of Applied Rehabilitation Counseling, 30*(2), 3–6.

Sue, D. W. (2008). *Counseling the culturally different: Theory and practice* (5th ed.). New York, NY: Wiley.

Tarvydas, V. M., & Ng, H. (2012). Ethical perspectives in trauma work. In L. L. Levers (Ed.), *Trauma counseling: Theories and interventions* (pp. 521–539). New York, NY: Springer Publishing.

Truax, C. B., & Carkhuff, R. R. (1967). *Toward effective counseling and psychotherapy.* Chicago, IL: Aldine.

U.S. Census Bureau. (2015). Projections of the size and composition of the U.S. population 2014–2060: Current populations report 2015. Retrieved from https://www.census.gov/content/dam/Census/library/publications/2015/demo/p25-1143.pdf

Usher, C. H. (1989). Recognizing cultural bias in counseling theory and practice: The case of Rogers. *Journal of Multicultural Counseling and Development, 17,* 62–71.

Walsh, R., & Vaughn, F. (1993). *Paths beyond ego: A transpersonal vision.* New York, NY: Putnam.

Wang, Y., Davidson, M. M., Yakushko, O. F., Savoy, H. B., Tan, J. A., & Bleier, J. K. (2003). The scale of ethnocultural empathy: Development, validation, and reliability. *Journal of Counseling Psychology, 50*(2), 221–234.

Weil, A. (2009). *Why our health matters: A vision of medicine that can transform our future.* New York, NY: Penguin Books.

Wickrama, K. A. S., & Kaspar, V. (2007). Family context of mental health risk in tsunami-exposed adolescents: Findings from a pilot study in Sri Lanka. *Social Science & Medicine, 64,* 713–723.

# CHAPTER 8

# Integrating Culture Into Disaster Mental Health Counseling: Foundations of Mind, Body, and Spirit*

The challenge for today's disaster mental health counseling and trauma specialists is how to integrate culturally relevant therapeutic interactions with a diversity of clients. This especially becomes problematic with the constraints of evidence-based practices, third-party payers, and the need to diagnose and treat mental health conditions using clinical protocols and symptomatology (i.e., *Diagnostic and Statistical Manual of Mental Disorders* [5th ed.; *DSM-5*; American Psychiatric Association, 2013]). Mental health counselors who have been trained in Western models of disaster response may not have the awareness, knowledge, and skills to work with a variety of cultural groups coming to the United States, such as asylum seekers, immigrants, and refugees. This chapter draws on 30 foundational beliefs, philosophies, and examples of ancient wisdom commonly found in many cultures throughout the world. A comprehensive exploration of literature in counseling, psychology, theology, and spirituality, as well as complementary, alternative, and integrated medicine approaches, is offered to the reader that advocates building awareness, knowledge, and skills to work competently with individuals from a variety of cultural backgrounds. Sacred texts, koans, and scriptures are not included in this chapter because many are based on a particular religious and spiritual belief system. Although they are foundational to the mind, body, and spirit, the interpretation is best left to a particular cultural belief system in which to interpret or debate theologically.

Almost all indigenous healing practices maintain some forms, structures, and rituals for health and healing. Many culturally relevant systems of health and healing may look similar yet significantly different from Western models of mental health treatment. For

*Adapted with newly written material for mental health counselors from Chapter 90, Stebnicki (2016), in *The Professional Counselor's Desk Reference* (2nd ed.), © Springer Publishing Company.

instance, in Western models of disaster mental health response, traditional person-centered empathetic-oriented approaches typically do not translate well to indigenous healing practices because of the emphasis on talk therapies. Combining these two systems of traditional Western talk therapies with indigenous practices can provide a powerful experience for both clients and counselors.

At the core of most humanistic theoretical orientations in the helping profession is the therapeutic use of empathy and compassion. There is a rich history in the United States based on core principles within humanistic theoretical orientations. Possessing the skills of empathy and integrating this in person-centered therapeutic environments are seen by many as a prerequisite for becoming a skilled and competent helper (Corey & Corey, 2016; Egan, 2014; Ivey, Bradford Ivey, & Zalaquett, 2014; Truax & Carkhuff, 1967). Culturally appropriate empathy, if facilitated competently by the therapist, can assist in building a strong connection with a variety of clients from different cultural backgrounds (Moodley & West, 2005).

Pedersen (2005) suggests that "the functions of counseling have been practiced for thousands of years and are not merely an invention of the last century or two" (p. xi). Pedersen and many others advocate that to truly facilitate multicultural counseling approaches we must look beyond counseling models proposed by a small constituency of dedicated scholars in the counseling and psychology professions. Accordingly, counseling models that advocate knowledge, awareness, and skills may not be enough to understand true cultural indigenous practices. Mental health counselors who have little exposure or experience with indigenous health and healing practices (e.g., Ayurveda, shamanism, Buddhist, African-centered, and/or Latin American healing traditions) may be missing opportunities to facilitate culturally appropriate trauma interventions that enhance the mental and physical well-being of their culturally different clients.

## THE CONSCIOUSNESS SHIFT IN DISASTER MENTAL HEALTH COUNSELING

The multicultural counseling literature suggests that to truly facilitate culturally centered therapeutic approaches we must be open to a diversity of thoughts, perceptions of reality, and belief systems about culturally different health and healing systems. Understanding the medical, physical, psychological, emotional, and psychosocial impact of disaster requires mental health practitioners to view disaster through their culturally different client's worldview. Indeed, there is a population shift in the United States to more diverse racial, ethnic, and cultural groups. This requires disaster mental health professionals to shift their consciousness as it relates to providing disaster mental health services. The respect for such indigenous practices, philosophies, and belief systems such as those found in Christianity (i.e., faith-based counseling and prayer), Buddhism (i.e., mindfulness meditation), or shamanic traditions (i.e., drumming rituals, journeying for spiritual helpers and power animals) has been ignored by some within the fields of counseling and psychology (Moodley & West, 2005). This may be because there is a strong bias toward quantitative experimental designs that can hypothesize, predict, control, and manipulate variables with the intent to produce evidence-based treatment models.

Qualitative designs that study integrative approaches such as prayer, yoga, and meditation practices many times do not garner the same support in the scientific community.

We are at a time in our history where the collective wisdom of some of the planet's tribal elders, wisdom keepers, new-age scientists, spiritual-religious teachers, cultural leaders, and prophets are available to provide rich opportunities for integrating mind, body, and spiritual work within therapeutic interactions. Many of these traditions have been lost within the cultures where they once existed. This is partly because they may have only been communicated verbally or by ritualistic practices within the culture, and the language itself and the tribal leaders may no longer exist. Thus, enriching opportunities abound if we are open to other culturally relevant belief systems in health and healing.

## What Is Integrative Medicine?

The term *integrative* for the most part has replaced the terms and constructs of *holistic*, *complementary*, and *alternative* within the fields of medicine, mental health, counseling, and psychology. These terms are used interchangeably in the literature; however, some would argue there are unique differences. For instance, most individuals in the West do not purely use alternative approaches when treating a mental or physical condition. Likewise, most individuals engage in what they perceive to be complementary approaches (e.g., vitamins, supplements, herbal remedies, exercise, dieting) to health and wellness based on what fits within their belief systems. Many complementary approaches are not endorsed by the medical literature, yet many consumers integrate these within their daily health care routines.

Complementary, alternative, and holistic models of care are deeply rooted in 20th- and 21st-century theories and practices within Western medicine, counseling, and psychology. Some of these models do not give recognition to the cultural roots of such indigenous practices. For example, breathing, meditation, or visualization has existed for thousands of years and has been used throughout many different cultural health and healing systems. Despite the routine use of such approaches, many current practitioners in the West may lack the recognition of its origin, cultural roots, or intended application.

The National Institutes of Health (NIH) has recognized the research needs of integrative approaches and created the Office of Alternative Medicine, renamed in 1999 as the National Center for Complementary and Alternative Medicine. Medical historians have widely viewed 20th-century medicine as a turning point for a variety of epidemiological, case review, case control, population, prospective, and retrospective studies, especially in cancer treatment (American Cancer Society, 2000). Weil (2009) states that we need to change *how* and *what* we research in terms of integrative health approaches. He strongly advocates for NIH to create a National Institute for Health and Healing so that we can research the body's natural healing systems as opposed to our current heavy reliance on discovering new medical technology and pharmaceutical products. Duke Integrative Medicine (2016) is one example of a comprehensive research and training center that integrates the body's natural healing system using integrative approaches in the subtle interactions of the mind, body, and spirit. There are many other centers and clinics in the United States that now integrate indigenous healing approaches as a routine part of their systems of healing and treatment.

Overall, the constructs presented within the Western paradigm of complementary, alternative, and holistic medicine appear to have the restrictions of being deeply rooted in Western models of medicine, counseling, and psychology. Many times the indigenous healers themselves are not included within research designs. Rarely do indigenous healers partner with the training center's faculty or instructors. This may require mental health practitioners to become involved in cultural immersion activities within various indigenous groups. Accordingly, the methods and approaches applied may be the researcher's or practitioner's perception of how such indigenous approaches should be facilitated; thus, not totally possessing a cultural consciousness.

## What Is Mind, Body, and Spiritual Healing?

The term *healing* does not represent an end point, cure, or absence of disease or illness. Individuals with chronic illnesses or disabilities prefer not to be defined by their diseases, disabilities, mental or physical conditions, or functional limitations. Accordingly, most are on a healing journey to maintain an excellent quality of life and live optimally. As a point of orientation for the reader, the following are generally accepted definitions of mind, body, and spirit.

*Mind:* The literature in counseling and psychology has considered that the mind encompasses ordinary states of consciousness, such as the individual's thoughts, beliefs, perceptions, philosophies, attitudes, feelings, and general cognitions. However, Assagioli (1965), Castaneda (1968), Tart (2000), Wilber (1996), and many other integrative practitioners and theorists have suggested that the phenomena of the mind and consciousness include much more than waking or dreaming states of consciousness. Rather, healthy individuals may also express nonordinary states, alternative states, or discrete altered states of consciousness that are not drug induced. It is through these powerful states that individuals may transcend the physical, mental, and spiritual realms into transpersonal experiences. These "peak experiences" can only be understood by living or experiencing such states of consciousness. By definition of the mind, one's spirituality and physical existence have interconnectedness with the body and spirit. Thus, it would be artificial to create boundaries.

*Body:* The physical body is much more comprehensible, logical, and rational to define. This is because medical science has examined, analyzed, and delineated the structure of the human organism from a purely physiological, cellular, and biological state of functioning within each of the body systems. Chinese medicine, shamanism, and many other indigenous belief systems have a much different view of the biological mechanisms of the body. In the indigenous worldview, this structure is not viewed from a system or mechanics point of reference. Rather, the body is expressed as an energy form that consists of *energy vortexes, body chakras, energy blockages, light,* and *body auras.* By definition, one's physiology cannot be separated from thoughts, feelings, or images about one's physical–biological self. Spiritual energy enters or leaves the body through the various chakras or energy centers. Thus, it is artificial from an integrative sense to separate the body from the mind and spirit.

*Spirit:* Much of the literature in spirituality separates this construct from religiosity and describes this primarily as the individual's spiritual experiences, although there are many who would argue that it is artificial to make such a separation because many individuals express their spirituality through religious rituals or ceremonies. For the purposes of definition, it is agreed upon by most that spirituality has come into existence before humankind's creation of world religions, rituals, sacred texts, beliefs in doctrine, and a formal physical structure (e.g., church, temple) by which to hold religious activities. Thus, spirituality is a felt sense of meaning and purpose within the context of a higher power, divine source of energy, God, The Great Spirit, or some other presence not of our physical world. Spirituality cannot be seen but is made up of experiences of faith, hope, comfort, beliefs, philosophies, rituals, and a belief in a divine source of energy that guides our lives. As one might gather, it appears artificial to separate the physical body and mind with spirituality. Spirituality in action requires an explicit state of consciousness, intention, and motivation by which to access the spiritual realm. Additionally, there may be a physical presence, as well as use of body mechanics expressed sometimes as kneeling, folding hands, raising of the arms, bowing, and use of other body movement activities to bring in (or drive out) spiritual energies.

## INTEGRATING TRADITIONAL MENTAL HEALTH COUNSELING WITH INDIGENOUS PRACTICES

Stebnicki (2016) offered a description of 30 specific foundational cultural beliefs and philosophies as documented through an extensive literature review. The cultural principles, thoughts, beliefs, wisdom, and philosophies are an exploratory analysis of common and perhaps universal beliefs about health, healing, meaning, and purpose of life within a cultural context. The literature in counseling, psychology, theology, and spirituality, as well as complementary, alternative, and integrated medicine, clearly points to an alternative level of sociocultural awareness when dealing with the meaning of trauma across different cultures. Mental health counselors may best understand these unique cultural differences by being open to a diversity of cultural leaders who have a deep connection to their own indigenous cultural experiences, some of which have been communicated through tribal elders, shamans, saints, spiritual leaders, mystics, prophets, sacred and spiritual texts, and other means.

Moodley and West (2005), trained in both Western psychotherapy and non-Western indigenous healing traditions, propose a model to integrate talk therapies with indigenous healing approaches using the mind, body, and spirit. Their research suggests that a large number of psychotherapists already integrate mind, body, and spiritual techniques within their person-centered psychotherapy practice. Approaches such as prayer, breathing, meditation, visualization, body energy work, and intuitive healing are already being facilitated by advanced practitioners with clients who have issues related to chronic illness, life-threatening illness, disability, trauma, and addictions.

Mijares (2003) suggests that the teachings, wisdom, and prophecies from the world's spiritual traditions are available to those who seek these approaches. Global communication and transportation systems allow us to connect with one another and form collaborative relationships during a disaster mental health response. It is not my intention to suggest we disregard Western counseling, psychology, theory, and practice in lieu of indigenous approaches. Rather, integrating indigenous practices with traditional counseling and psychotherapy should be viewed by clients and professional counselors as opportunities for activating the body's own natural healing system. Approaches such as breathing, meditation, visualization, and body energy work are already common techniques facilitated in today's psychotherapy practices. These are time-honored traditions in many cultures and should be embraced by 21st-century mental health practices.

Integrating indigenous approaches requires an understanding and openness to different worldviews about health and healing, some of which may be seen by others as paranormal, esoteric, or transpersonal experiences. It is essential for mental health counselors to be open to the testimonials and personal perspectives of indigenous peoples who have experienced healing of the mind, body, and spirit in a nontraditional Western system of health and healing. Indigenous approaches facilitated within the therapeutic environment should be natural, intentional, and a conscious way of being. It may require the coordination and/or participation by indigenous leaders for approaches to have culturally specific meaning for clients. However, for Western therapists, a paradigm shift in the definition of therapy and appreciation of other cultural values and belief systems is necessary when it comes to facilitating and/or coordinating culturally specific approaches (Walsh & Vaughn, 1993).

The literature relating to native and indigenous healers, mystics, shamans, saints, and sages from all cultures has much to offer mental health counselors in terms of responding to mental health disasters. Many native and indigenous healers discovered that optimal living of the mind, body, and spirit came through peak spiritual experiences, various meditation practices, and long journeys of soul searching and self-discovery (Harner, 1990; Rainbow Eagle, 2003). Thus, it is my intention to offer these foundational principles to the readers so they may find ways to introduce these within the therapeutic environment and to perhaps enlist the support of various indigenous leaders to help emulate culturally appropriate healing systems.

## THE CULTURALLY CENTERED INTERVIEW

Building trust and rapport is critical in achieving an optimal therapeutic working alliance with clients who are culturally different. This could take several meetings/sessions before your clients may get some sense that you understand their unique cultural background. It is important to be mindful of how persons who are culturally different communicate. For instance, there is a heavy reliance on nonverbal communication among some cultural groups. Also, silence is viewed by some cultural groups as a sign of respect, whereas in Western counseling interactions the silent client could be viewed as reluctant, resistant, or defensive to therapy. Spatial distance and eye contact are also a consideration when building trust and rapport with others. These issues are discussed in greater detail in the chapters related to cultural communication.

The most parsimonious way to describe a culturally centered interview where the mental health practitioner may want to collect some background information on his or her culturally different client would be to ask your clients the following questions:

- ▶ What cultural (racial/ethnic) groups do you identify yourself with?
- ▶ How would you describe your cultural beliefs, values, philosophies, wisdom, or rituals that you practice?
- ▶ Are there some cultural beliefs, values, philosophies, wisdom, or rituals that you practice or that you combine (integrate) with other cultures?
- ▶ What advice did your family members or your culture give to you about mental and physical health, healing, or wellness?
- ▶ From where did your family members first hear about this particular wisdom?
- ▶ If you could trace your family roots back to its origin, how are you both the same and different compared with your ancestors in terms of your beliefs, philosophies about health, healing, or wellness?

Current scientific thinking suggests that some of our emotions, thoughts, cognitions, and behaviors are recorded in various parts of our anatomy (e.g., brain and nervous system, DNA) and are responsible for how we think, feel, and act. Thus, defining our personality traits, moral and ethical reasoning, physical–biological characteristics, and many other characteristics is influenced from a biopsychosocial perspective. We may not know our family of origin, but theoretically we are likely a combination of the same, similar, yet different traits in how we think, feel, and act.

The point is that belief systems are typically handed down person to person within a culture. They are communicated and experienced many times through storytelling, oral histories, mentoring relationships, guided experiences, expressive arts, rituals, and many other ways. They are not the special property of any one particular culture because cultures have existed for centuries simultaneously despite geographic separation. Knowing and understanding the foundations of your client's cultural background can assist in times of disaster response and trauma interventions. Mental health professionals who increase their awareness, knowledge, and skills as they relate to the foundations of a specific culture increase their opportunities to build an optimal working alliance using culturally sensitive and relevant approaches that are therapeutic in nature.

## FOUNDATIONAL PRINCIPLES

This section is an exploration of the universal and foundational attributes that comprise almost all cultures. Mental health professionals interested in personal and professional growth (a) constantly seek opportunities to work across cultures; (b) continually seek ways in which to communicate, relate, build rapport, and develop a working alliance with a diversity of individuals; and (c) use their clients' unique cultural attributes to integrate trauma therapies within a cultural context. Mental health professionals motivated to transition into the therapist–healer role may find the following foundational cultural attributes essential in constructing meaningful relationships with culturally different individuals. As we have seen in other chapters in the book, exposure to extraordinary stressful and traumatic events is culturally contextualized. Becoming a skilled and competent disaster mental health or trauma therapist requires openness to a diversity of healing systems. It requires us to work intentionally in person-centered and culturally centered environments.

▶ *God:* Almost all cultures and even the world's religious traditions have one Supreme Being or divine source of loving, all-knowing energy that is at the foundation and center of all life in the universe. Some cultures use the terms *God, The Gods, The Great Spirit, The Holy Spirit, The Great One, Mother Earth,* or *the Creator.* God is seen by most cultures as permanent; keeper of all life forms; creator of Heaven, Earth, and the universe; creator of all truths, morals, principles, and physical laws that rule the universe; creator of time as it relates to the past, present, and future; and is the alpha and omega of all things known within human existence.

▶ *Meaning and purpose:* Most cultures acknowledge they cannot possibly know the mind of God because there are scientific, philosophical, spiritual, and theological questions that are a mystery and cannot be totally comprehended by the human experience. Some cultures believe that everything in life happens for a reason, while others believe that we have some level of control. Cultures throughout time have sought meaning, purpose, and spiritual guidance for health and healing through God's presence, which can be accessed through experiences, practices, and rituals integrating the mind, body, and spirit. At the core of all great world religious and spiritual traditions is a God that emphasizes kindness, compassion, and love toward others, loving your neighbor as you would love yourself, and service to others. For some, God is the meaning and purpose of life.

▶ *Why bad things happen:* Bad things happen in life to good people and good things happen to bad people. Some cultures interpret bad things happening in life as God presenting opportunities for personal and spiritual growth (e.g., with crisis comes opportunity). God has the power to send angels, power animals (as noted in shamanic cultures), and other divine sources of energy to intercede, guide, and provide answers or solutions to health and healing of our mind, body, and spirit. The question of why good things happen to bad people is perplexing and each culture has its own interpretation. There are various theological and nontheological explanations that create the foundations for cultural belief systems in regard to *why bad things happen.*

▶ *Miracles and things we cannot control:* Many cultures believe that miracles do not happen in contradiction to nature or our Creator. They are ordinary experiences in an extraordinary universe where we live. Some cultures view the birth of a child, spontaneous remission from an illness or disease, or new plant and animal growth as a miracle. Some degree of skepticism exists within every culture because of within-group differences in the belief of supernatural forces or claims of Christ-like healings. It may not fit within the logical confines of the human brain, especially within the modern world where we currently live. As humans, we try and place conditions and limitations on what God can and cannot do. By doing so, we may only accept or acknowledge God within certain settings or environments (e.g., church or sacred ceremonies versus school or the workplace). This results in the human-like reaction or attitude that "I know what is best for me" or "I can control my own destiny." Overall, most cultural belief systems maintain that miracles still exist and abound throughout the planet. There are unexplained phenomena, life is full of mystery, and there are some things in life that may or may not be able to be controlled.

▶ *Good versus evil:* During the Middle Ages, the world was full of disease, barbaric invasions, poverty, famine, pain, and suffering. Most cultures at the time viewed this as "evil." Currently, there exist wars, disease, poverty, famine, pain, and suffering in the world. Many cultural belief systems still struggle with evil and attached dark spiritual beings (i.e., The Devil in Christianity) that exist in the heart and minds of all humans. Some cultural belief systems interpret this dark energy as moral evil (i.e., sins against humanity) and natural evil (i.e., disease, floods, tsunamis). The existential and spiritual dilemmas that exist throughout most cultures pose the question: "If God is an all-loving God, then why would God allow evil to exist?" Almost all cultural belief systems suggest that no Gods or religions seek to increase misery, suffering, hatred, or hostility. The fundamental qualities of God as the Creator of all life are that God is the ultimate divine source of love and compassion, and invites us to try and be more God-like in our daily lives. The ultimate reward is waiting for us in Heaven, the afterlife, or some other dimension that has no pain and suffering. The ultimate challenge of the human spirit may be this balance of drawing toward the light instead of the dark energy in our internal and external worlds.

▶ *Breathing:* Breathing is foundational to all meditative practice and is integral for mind, body, and spiritual health. Taking a deep cleansing breath has physiological benefits and helps quiet the mind so we can listen to God or "the other side of silence" and receive all spiritual things through our Creator. The breath was given to us by our Divine Creator at birth, so we need to learn how to take care of it on a daily basis.

▶ *Compassion:* Compassion and the expression of compassion through empathy toward self and others are natural to all human beings and lie at the heart of almost all world cultures, religions, and spiritual practices. Some cultures have specific beliefs about "the nature of humankind" (e.g., evil versus good). Unconditional and absolute compassion is found in God, Buddha, and other divine sources of energy. We all possess these characteristics at varying levels. Cultivating increased levels of compassion and empathy toward self and others is a quest for those who desire and choose to have more compassion and empathy in their lives.

▶ *Medicine:* Medicine, a term and practice that dates back to ancient times, has been integral to the health and healing of the mind, body, and spirit of all cultures. In many cultures, religion, spirituality, magic, mysticism, herbals, botanicals, and any element that facilitates health, healing, and cures were not separated into specialty areas. Indigenous healers such as tribal shamans facilitated cultural medicine that "treated" all conditions of the physical body, mental–emotional–psychological health, and the spirit. Most indigenous medicine practices were not shared with anyone outside the culture. Many indigenous medicine practices are not known today because of cultural extinction and loss of languages, and because the practices themselves were handed down by word of mouth.

▶ *Suffering:* Suffering, a complex concept to understand, exists in many cultures as a natural human condition. The experience, such as "dark night of the soul," is described as depression, dryness, futility, or the sense of wandering aimlessly or feeling lost. It is quite natural to experience suffering and dark energy. However, such misery and suffering are viewed as only temporary. Almost all spiritual and religious traditions aim to overcome the temporary state of unhappiness, pain, and suffering. For some, their sufferings may end only by their eventual physical death. The intention is to achieve everlasting life in what some cultures refer to as Heaven. Since we cannot escape suffering, the challenge is to find ways transcending this experience. For some individuals, bringing meaning and purpose to their sufferings is an empowering experience that can mean freedom from suffering and dark energy.

▶ *The journey:* Many cultures believe that achieving balance and wellness of your mind, body, and spirit is a journey, not a goal. All great spiritual leaders throughout history (e.g., Jesus, Buddha, Mother Teresa, the Dalai Lama, Thich Nhat Hanh, Billy Graham, and Native Shaman) pursued a spiritual journey to acquire insight, enlightenment, illumination, meaning, and purpose in life and to try and enhance their spiritual relationships with the Divine Creator or God. A journey has no real definitive beginning or end. For some, optimal mind, body, and spiritual living is a journey that takes place over one's lifetime. Some cultural belief systems suggest that a "journey of a thousand miles begins with the first step"; however, there are many steps that start and stop along the way. Journeying requires constant mindfulness and attention to both your internal and external environments on a daily basis.

▶ *Zen:* Bodhidharma, an Indian Monk and founder of Zen Buddhism in the fifth century, developed this indigenous approach to life based on the principles of Buddhism. Zen is not just a meditation practice or a journey. Rather, the intent is enlightenment or illumination that can only be attained spontaneously. As described by some, Zen is a form of consciousness and practice for everyday life.

There is nothing mystical or esoteric about Zen. Zen has evolved in many Western cultures but has a difficult translation because of the rational thinking, scientific paradigm, and the need to predict and control thoughts, feelings, and actions. Zen requires us to cease ordinary consciousness and thought processes and experience a type of mindful and meditative consciousness while being engaged in such activities as washing dishes, sweeping, chopping wood, going for walks on the beach or in a forest, and so forth.

▶ *Contemplative prayer:* In Christian traditions, contemplative prayer is experienced as a type of deep meditative experience. It is a way to quiet the mind, body, and spirit. Prayer is a gift from God and cannot be earned. Through this all-sensory experience we can be transported to another realm or dimension. It is through this process that we merge with the light or divine presence of God.

▶ *Dreams:* Dreams are a way for us to pay attention and access deeper insight into our mind, body, and spirit. In the fourth century, the great saint and mystic Gregory of Nyssa recognized the art of Christian meditation and the experience of dreaming states of consciousness. Dreams are a gift from the Creator. Many cultures understand the symbolic importance of dreaming as a way to bring meaning, purpose, health, and healing into everyday living. It is also understood that the symbolic meaning within dreams may not come about immediately. Rather, such meaning may take days, weeks, months, and even years.

▶ *Visualization:* Visualization and use of imagery have the possibilities of creating profound changes in thoughts, feelings, and actions. The 20th and 21st centuries have revealed some unprecedented discoveries in technology, health care, space travel, and environmental sciences. These discoveries were first visualized by a human being as an inner reality (e.g., space travel, cures or vaccines for diseases, lifesaving medical procedures). The awakening of visualization and imagination stirs thoughts and emotions, and has the possibilities of propelling someone into action. Visualizations do not have to be actions that contribute to humankind from a global perspective. Rather, humans have the capacity to change something pivotal within their inner worlds. This could be visualizing a career change, new relationship, or how to live optimally with chronic illness or disability. Thus, visualization and use of imagery are gifts from the Creator and have empowering qualities for individuals to make profound changes for optimal living.

▶ *Awakening:* Awakening the mind, body, and spirit does not have to be achieved through experiences of ecstasy or nonordinary states of consciousness, nor a transcendental or deep meditative state. Awakening can be achieved in everyday life through sudden illumination of a thought, feeling, or intuitive senses.

▶ *Mindfulness:* Mindfulness simply means paying attention to your mind, body, and spirit at different levels of awareness within the present here-and-now moment in a nonjudgmental and unconditional way. This kind of attention nurtures and cultivates greater awareness, clarity, and acceptance of self and others on a day-to-day basis.

▶ *Quieting the mind:* Quieting or silencing the mind opens the door to other dimensions, allowing us to listen to the voice of God. This may come in terms of symbolic meaning or through an all-sensory experience of sight, smell, sound, light, feeling, sensing, and/or touching. Quieting the mind and listening from a spiritual perspective is a difficult task for many. The rules of reality, logic, rational thinking, or ordinary states of consciousness do not apply when accessing the "other side of silence." Many indigenous groups suggest that listening through the "third-eye chakra" is vital to awakening the intuitive self. Many cultures believe that God has given us the capacity for intuitiveness. However, most of us do not know how to be silent and quiet our mind because we have "monkey mind" that is a Zen Buddhist expression for a cluttered, disorganized deficit in attention. Thus, quieting the mind and listening are essential to accessing the presence of God, light, or other divine sources of energy.

▶ *Koans, parables, and storytelling:* Koans are indigenous to some Zen Buddhist practices. A koan such as "What is the sound of one hand clapping?" is interpreted not by the rational mind, but rather through a deep meditative state with the intent of illumination or enlightenment on its meaning, which is typically found in its actions. Parables and stories are also seen in many sacred texts, indigenous rituals, and healing ceremonies, and have rich metaphors that require one to reflect and meditate on their meaning. This meaning brings change in one's thoughts, feelings, and actions.

▶ *Attitudinal change:* Each new healthy thought, feeling, or experience has the potential for an attitudinal change that can create a better future. Unhealthy attitudes can disturb the balance within our physiological and biological existence, which can break down the various body and immune systems, creating the risk for illness and disease. Having an attitude of gratitude and compassion, for example, keeps us from focusing on the dark energy. Living within the present, here-and-now moment, as opposed to spending too much time in your past or future, is viewed as healthy. Thus, embracing the "right" attitude within the present moment creates the potential to visualize an attitudinal change.

▶ *Karma:* Karma, a Buddhist concept, is correctly translated as "action" of intention. It is the sum of your life's direction whether it be suffering, happiness, anger, or fear. Karma is created by your past actions, thoughts, and behaviors. Karma is often confused with a person's fixed destiny, but is more of an accumulative pattern of actions, thoughts, and behaviors. Accordingly, you can change your karma by choosing different thoughts, feelings, cognitions, and actions in the present moment, which ultimately affect your future. Thus, being mindful in the "now" moment is what matters most because what you are in the present moment affects every action, thought, and feeling in your future. Changing karma is a conscious choice we make, which spawns attitudinal change, lifestyle changes, and all changes within our mind, body, and spirit.

▶ *Simple life:* To attain balance and wellness of the mind, body, and spirit, many cultures believe that we should look for the most parsimonious practical solutions and wisdom: ones that fit best with who you are as a person and your life. Materialism complicates the human existence and does not allow us to experience the simple life. Some cultural belief systems would suggest that it is not so much the material things we possess; rather, it is the amount of time we spend focusing on such materialism that takes us away from the simple life.

▶ *Judgments and conditions:* There are not "good–bad"; "positive–negative"; or "acceptable–unacceptable" thoughts and feelings. Rather, there are a range of human emotions, behaviors, and experiences we feel and communicate to ourselves and others throughout the day and in a diversity of environments. The natural world is not static; it is constantly evolving. There is up, down, and sideways; North, South, East, and West. Thus, our inner and outer worlds also have many directions, places, and spaces. Placing values, standards, or ideals as a condition for our thoughts, feelings, emotions, behaviors, and experiences can hinder growth and development of our mind, body, and spirit. It is okay to be who you are because you are a unique individual created by a divine source of energy.

▶ *Unconditional love and acceptance:* Loving unconditionally, both self and others, requires the ultimate in patience, devotion, and acceptance. This typically does not occur instantaneously but does require attitudinal change that may take place over many months or years. Having a love and acceptance of oneself and all the limitations we have in the human experience bring about attitudinal change that has the potential for harmonizing our mind, body, and spirit.

▶ *Connections:* A tree cannot survive without its roots. Persons without connections to their roots cannot survive, either. Living alone is an aching stressor. This principle may not necessarily mean reconnecting with your biological roots or family. There are many who have had to endure physical, mental, and sexual abuse or alcoholism within their family roots. Rather, the implication is that we have spiritual ancestors and spiritual families that we can draw to in time of need. Some may refer to this as a social-therapeutic support group (e.g., Alcoholics Anonymous [AA], Narcotics Anonymous [NA]); church family; neighborhood or community support.

▶ *Taking responsibility:* Taking responsibility for your own mind, body, and spirit is essential to stay on the path of your journey. There are some things you will have to give up to God, a higher power, or the universe, but we should be open to the idea that there are some thoughts, feelings, or behaviors that we can change but only if we choose responsibility.

▶ *Higher states of consciousness:* Many cultures practice alterations in their states of consciousness with the intention of accessing God, angels, or power animals. Achieving higher states of mind, body, and spiritual well-being is a desirable characteristic and attribute in many cultures. Being mindful, quieting the mind, and listening to our "inner voice experiences" provide rich opportunities for personal transformation for optimal health.

▶ *Gratitude:* Strive for gratitude, obedience, loyalty, and devotion toward your mind, body, and spirit. Cultivating more love and compassion toward yourself and others leaves less room for unwanted thoughts, feelings, and emotions. Striving for gratitude, obedience, loyalty, and devotion can create true freedom from stress, anxiety, depression, or suffering.

▶ *Attachments:* Becoming aware that you may be holding on to the true experience of your feelings, emotions, thoughts, cognitions, and other levels of consciousness requires higher states of consciousness. We all have attachments to many things in our lives. Reluctance or resistance to become enlightened concerning our attachments or what we may be holding on to does not provide opportunities for optimal growth of your mind, body, and spirit. Letting go has profound effects in health and healing.

▶ *Movement:* Movement activities such as dance, expressive arts, tai chi, yoga, walking meditations, and many other activities reach our deepest nature of human existence. Such activities have the profound power to transform the mind, body, and spirit for health and healing purposes. Epidemiological researchers, when studying longevity "hot spots" of the world, find that physical movement is a protective factor in resiliency against disease and illness. Movement cultivates good overall physical and mental health. In shamanic cultures, various rituals that involved expressive arts (i.e., dancing, drumming) were believed to be able to have the power to change the physical world. Awakening the spirits, soul retrieval, and other shamanic rituals were very physical in nature. Without accessing these ancient movement activities, it is difficult to awaken the healing energies internally and externally. Energy must not be contained for internal use; it should flow freely outward and be shared with others within the culture. Peaceful marches or demonstrations, having cheerleaders at sporting events, and tai chi in the park all invite participation and a vibrational energy that can impact the world outside of oneself.

▶ *Aromas and essential oils:* Essential oils date back thousands of years to ancient Egypt, China, and India, as well as other countries. Aromas and essential oils have always been part of healing rituals and social celebrations. Fragrant substances, or essential oils, distilled from plants and other natural substances have the power to alter mood and affect, reduce pain and stress, and improve overall mental and physical health. A French chemist, René-Maurice Gattefossé, originated modern day aromatherapy. Today, it is common to find over 40 different essential oils that are typically present in massage therapy, yoga, Reiki, and acupuncture practices. In the integrative psychotherapeutic environment, essential oils are used to enhance calm and balanced states of consciousness.

▶ *Sounds:* Sounds such as drumming, waves, wind, rain, animals, person-made, and even high-altitude environments produce frequencies that stimulate the relaxation centers of the brain as modern-day researchers note. Drumming and other sounds have been used since the beginning of human history. Sounds are frequently used for rituals, religious/spiritual ceremonies, celebrations, and many other events to enhance the group's and individual's experience of the ritual itself. Rhythmic drumming with indigenous handmade instruments (rattles, string, wood) is commonly integrated into shamanic and Native American cultures. Drumming and other sound frequencies have the opportunities to produce trances and other altered states of consciousness by which a shaman may journey for his or her power animal.

▶ *Body energy:* Energy from all different forms has been present from the beginning of life. Energy never dies; it continues on into all eternity, a world without end. We are all made from a divine source of energy and our natural environment (plants, animals, and the physical Earth). Subtle energies such as different states of consciousness give birth to new life. This happens every moment of every day from a cellular structure as our body replenishes itself. Our mental, physical, and spiritual health is dependent on this system of energy that is designed to maintain health, wellness, balance, and healing. Ancient traditional writings have identified over 88,000 chakras or energy vortexes connecting all body systems. In Japanese Reiki, there are over 40 energy centers considered to be significant that, if blocked, can cause disease, illness, and imbalances in the mind, body, and spirit. Ki, chi, or qi flows through this invisible meridian system of the body. There are those who can sense the body's energy through various sensory and extrasensory perceptions such as body auras. Body energy healers, such as those attuned in Reiki, shamanism, massage, or other body energy systems of healing, use their intuitive gifts to find these energy blockages and rebalance these areas that are vulnerable to illness and disease. The individual can also facilitate self-healing if attuned to such practices.

▶ *Art:* All cultures have art. There are as many art forms as there are cultures. Art is used to express and communicate cultural identity to others and those within their own cultures. Art forms such as dancing, painting, carving, tattoos, jewelry making, music, and other forms have therapeutic value and contribute to the culture's overall well-being.

▶ *Environment:* Some native cultures view the environment as made up of earth, air, water, wind, and fire that connect all life forms to planet Earth. Our Mother Earth represents all of existence, even before the first human, and this energy connects us with a web to the cosmos and everything else in the universe (e.g., the sun, sunspots, meteor showers, exploding stars, and universes). When cataclysmic events happen on our planet naturally (floods, hurricanes, fires, earthquakes, volcanic eruptions) or unnaturally (person made), our planet must make adjustments to rebalance its energy forces. Because the Creator has provided us with all that exists, we dishonor our Creator when we intentionally upset this balance. Whatever we take from nature, we must give back. This is consistent from a global perspective or to our own geographic area where we live (our town, community, or neighborhood). Environment is also connected to our personal inner space and intertwines with our mind, body, and spirit. Feng Shui, which is a Chinese system of harmonizing everything within the surrounding environment, is one example of feeling and sensing this balance. Feng Shui is a sophisticated system that integrates our architectural surroundings and natural spaces to create an optimal living environment that brings peace to the mind, body, and spirit.

## CONCLUDING REMARKS

The principles, thoughts, beliefs, wisdom, and philosophies of many native and indigenous groups have been offered for consideration when providing disaster mental health services to individuals and groups that may be culturally different than that of the professional counselor. Providing disaster mental health services in a multicultural environment requires the awareness, knowledge, and skills to facilitate resources and strategies that are culturally appropriate. The Foundational Resources chosen are those that represent a deep connection to his or her own indigenous cultural group(s) and/or have been interconnected with the experiences of individuals and groups that identify themselves as tribal elders, shamans, saints, spiritual leaders, mystics, and prophets and have studied sacred and ancient spiritual texts. Indeed, from a multicultural perspective, there are multiple ways of healing. The skilled and competent disaster mental health professional is one who is open to many different cultural perspectives, beliefs, and philosophies so as to develop a culturally sensitive rapport with all individuals.

## REFERENCES

American Cancer Society. (2000). *American Cancer Society's guide to complementary and alternative cancer methods*. Atlanta, GA: Author.

American Psychiatric Association. (2013). *Diagnostic and statistical manual of mental disorders* (5th ed.). Arlington, VA: American Psychiatric Publishing.

Assagioli, R. (1965). *Psychosynthesis*. New York, NY: Viking Press.

Castaneda, C. (1968). *The teachings of Don Juan: A Yaqui way of knowledge*. Berkeley: University of California Press.

Corey, M. S., & Corey, G. (2016). *Becoming a helper* (7th ed.). Belmont, CA: Brooks/Cole, Cengage.

Duke Integrative Medicine. (2016). Home page. Retrieved from http://www.dukeintegrativemedicine.org

Egan, G. (2014). *The skilled helper: A problem-management and opportunity-development approach to helping* (10th ed.). Belmont, CA: Brooks/Cole, Cengage.

Harner, M. (1990). *The way of the shaman*. San Francisco, CA: Harper San Francisco.

Ivey, A. E., Bradford Ivey, M., & Zalaquett, C. P. (2014). *Intentional interviewing and counseling* (8th ed.). Belmont, CA: Brooks/Cole, Cengage.

Mijares, S. G. (2003). *Modern psychology and ancient wisdom: Psychological healing practices from the world's religious traditions*. New York, NY: The Haworth Integrative Healing Press.

Moodley, R., & West, W. (2005). *Integrating traditional healing practices into counseling and psychotherapy*. Thousand Oaks, CA: Sage Publications.

Pedersen, P. (2005). Editor's foreword. In R. Moodley & W. West (Eds.), *Integrating traditional healing practices into counseling and psychotherapy*. Thousand Oaks, CA: Sage Publications.

Rainbow Eagle. (2003). *Native American spirituality: A walk in the woods*. Zanesfield, OH: Rainbow Light and Company.

Stebnicki, M. A. (2016). Integrative approaches in counseling and psychotherapy: Foundations of mind, body, and spirit. In I. Marini & M. A. Stebnicki (Eds.), *The professional counselor's desk reference* (2nd ed., pp. 593–604). New York, NY: Springer Publishing.

Tart, C. (2000). *States of consciousness*. Lincoln, NE: iUniverse.com.

Truax, C. B., & Carkhuff, R. R. (1967). *Toward effective counseling and psychotherapy*. Chicago, IL: Aldine.

Walsh, R., & Vaughan, F. (1993). *Paths beyond ego: The transpersonal vision*. New York, NY: G. P. Putnam's Sons.

Weil, A. (2009). *Why our health matters: A vision of medicine that can transform our future*. New York, NY: Hudson Street Press.

Wilber, K. (1996). *A brief history of everything*. Boston, MA: Shambhala.

## FOUNDATIONAL RESOURCES

Anderson, R. A. (2001). *Clinician's guide to holistic medicine*. New York, NY: McGraw-Hill.

Balch, J. F., & Stengler, M. (2004). *Prescription for natural cures: A self-care guide for treating health problems with natural remedies including diet and nutrition, nutritional supplements, bodywork, and more*. Hoboken, NJ: Wiley.

Batie, H. F. (2007). *Healing body, mind, & spirit: A guide to energy-based healing*. Woodbury, MN: Llewellyn Publications.

Braden, G. (2008). *The spontaneous healing of belief: Shattering the paradigm of false limits*. Carlsbad, CA: Hay House.

Brennan, B. A. (1987). *Hands of light: A guide to healing through the human energy field*. New York, NY: Bantam Books.

Castaneda, C. (1968). *The teachings of Don Juan: A Yaqui way of knowledge*. Berkeley: University of California Press.

Chopra, D. (1995). *The way of the wizard: Twenty spiritual lessons for creating the life you want*. New York, NY: Harmony Books.

Corey, M. S., & Corey, G. (2016). *Becoming a helper*. Belmont, CA: Brooks/Cole.

Eagle, R. (2003). *Native American spirituality: A walk in the woods*. Zanesfield, OH: Rainbow Light.

Eden, D. (1999). *Energy medicine*. New York, NY: Jeremy P. Tarcher/Putnam.

Egan, G. (2014). *The skilled helper: A problem-management and opportunity-development approach to helping* (10th ed.). Belmont, CA: Brooks/Cole.

Eliade, M. (1964). *Shamanism: Archaic techniques of ecstasy*. New York, NY: Pantheon.

Elliott, W. (1996). *Tying rocks to clouds: Meetings and conversations with wise and spiritual people*. New York, NY: Image Books/Double Day.

Emoto, M. (2004). *The hidden messages in water*. Hillsboro, OR: Beyond Words Publishing.

Fanning, P., & McKay, M. (2000). *Family guide to emotional wellness: Proven self-help techniques and exercises for dealing with common problems and building crucial life skills.* Oakland, CA: New Harbinger Publications.

Foundation for Shamanic Studies. (2016). Home page. Retrieved from http://www.shamanism.org/workshops/announcement.php?aid=1

Fox, M., & Sheldrake, R. (1996). *The physics of angels: Exploring the realm where science and spirit meets.* San Francisco, CA: Harper San Francisco.

Frankl, V. E. (1963). *Man's search for meaning.* New York, NY: Pocket Books.

Goleman, D. (2003). *Healing emotions: Conversations with the Dalai Lama on mindfulness, emotions, and health.* Boston, MA: Shambhala.

Gordon, J. S. (1996). *Manifesto for a new medicine: Your guide to healing partnerships and the wise use of alternative therapies.* Reading, MA: Perseus Books.

Haberly, H. J. (1990). *Reiki: Hawayo Takata's story.* Olney, MD: Archedigm Publications.

Hanh, T. N. (1999). *Going home: Jesus and Buddha as brothers.* New York, NY: Riverhead Books.

Harner, M. (1990). *The way of the shaman.* San Francisco, CA: Harper San Francisco.

Ingerman, S. (1991). *Soul retrieval: Mending the fragmented self.* San Francisco, CA: Harper San Francisco.

Institute of Noetic Sciences. (2016). Home page. Retrieved from www.ions.org

International Center for Reiki Training. (2006). Home page. Retrieved from www.reiki.org

Ivey, A. E., Bradford Ivey, M., & Zalaquett, C. P. (2014). *Intentional interviewing and counseling: Facilitating client development in a multicultural society* (8th ed.). Belmont, CA: Brooks/Cole.

Kabat-Zinn, J. (1990). *Full catastrophe living: Using the wisdom of your body and mind to face stress, pain, and illness.* New York, NY: Dell Publishing.

Kabat-Zinn, J. (1994). *Wherever you go there you are: Mindfulness meditation in everyday life.* New York, NY: Hyperion.

Kardec, A. (1989). *The book on mediums: Guide for mediums and invocators.* York Beach, MA: Samuel Weiser.

Kelsey, M. T. (1976). *The other side of silence: A guide to Christian meditation.* New York, NY: Paulist Press.

Kelsey, M. T. (1986). *Transcend: A guide to the spiritual quest.* New York, NY: Crossroad.

Kopp, S. B. (1972). *If you meet the Buddha on the road, kill him!* New York, NY: Bantam Books.

Kushner, H. S. (1980). *When bad things happen to good people.* New York, NY: Avon Books.

Lama, D. (1999). *Ethics for the new millennium.* New York, NY: Riverhead Books/Penguin Putnam.

Lama, D. (2011). *A profound mind: Cultivating wisdom in everyday life.* New York, NY: Harmony Books.

LeShan, L. (1974). *How to meditate: A guide to self-discovery.* New York, NY: Bantam Books.

Levine, S. (1987). *Healing into life and death.* New York, NY: Anchor Books/Doubleday.

MacNutt, F. (1985). *Healing.* Notre Dame, IN: Ave Maria Press.

Maslach, C. (2003). *Burnout: The cost of caring.* Cambridge, MA: Malor Books.

Meadows, K. (1991). *Shamanic experience: A practical guide to shamanism for the new millennium.* Boston, MA: Element Books.

Mehl-Madrona, L. (1997). *Coyote medicine: Lessons from Native American healing.* New York, NY: Fireside/Simon & Schuster.

Merton, T. (1961). *New seeds of contemplation.* New York, NY: New Directions Book.

Mijares, S. G. (2003). *Modern psychology and ancient wisdom: Psychological healing practices from the world's religious traditions.* New York, NY: Haworth Integrative Healing Press.

Mitchell, K. K. (1994). *Reiki: A torch in daylight.* St. Charles, IL: Mind Rivers Publications.

Monaghan, P., & Diereck, E. G. (1999). *Meditation: The complete guide.* Novato, CA: New World Guide.

Moodley, R., & West, W. (2005). *Integrating traditional healing practices into counseling and psychotherapy.* Thousand Oaks, CA: Sage Publications.

Moore, T. (1996). *The re-enchantment of everyday life.* New York, NY: Harper Perennial.

Moore, T. (2004). *Dark nights of the soul: A guide to finding your way through life's ordeals.* New York, NY: Penguin Group.

Myers, J. E., & Sweeney, T. J. (2005). *Counseling for wellness: Theory, research, and practice.* Alexandria, VA: American Counseling Association.

Nouwen, H. J. M. (1972). *The wounded healer.* New York, NY: Doubleday.

Peale, N. V. (1952). *The power of positive thinking: A practical guide to mastering the problems of everyday living.* Englewood Cliffs, NJ: Prentice-Hall.

Rainbow Eagle. (2003). *Native American spirituality: A walk in the woods.* Zanesfield, OH: Rainbow Light and Company.

Schlitz, M., Amorok, T., & Micozzi, M. S. (2005). *Consciousness & healing: Integral approaches to mind-body medicine.* St. Louis, MO: Elsevier Churchill Livingstone.

Schlitz, M. M., Vieten, C., & Amorok, T. (2007). *Living deeply: The art & science of transformation in everyday life.* Oakland, CA: New Harbinger Publications.

Seaward, B. L. (1997). *Stand like mountain flow like water: Reflections on stress and human spirituality.* Deerfield Beach, FL: Health Communications.

Sekida, K. (1985). *Zen training: Methods and philosophy.* Boston, MA: Shambhala.

Sha, Z. G. (2010a). *Divine transformation.* New York, NY: Atria Books.

Sha, Z. G. (2010b). *Tao I: A way of all life.* New York, NY: Heaven's Library Publications Corp.

Siebert, A. (2005). *The resiliency advantage: Master change, thrive under pressure, and bounce back from setbacks.* San Francisco, CA: Berrett-Koehler Publishers.

Stebnicki, M. A. (2008). *Empathy fatigue: Healing the mind, body, and spirit of professional counselors.* New York, NY: Springer Publishing.

Stebnicki, M. A. (2016). Integrative approaches in counseling and psychotherapy: Foundations of mind, body, and spirit. In I. Marini & M. A. Stebnicki (Eds.), *The professional counselor's desk reference* (2nd ed., pp. 593–604). New York, NY: Springer Publishing.

Stella, T. (2001). *The God instinct: Heeding your heart's unrest.* Notre Dame, IN: Sorin Books.

Swerdlow, J. L. (2000). *Nature's medicine: Plants that heal.* Washington, DC: National Geographic.

Tart, C. (1997). *Body, mind, and spirit: Exploring the parapsychology of spirituality.* Charlottesville, VA: Hampton Roads Publishing.

Tart, C. (2000). *States of consciousness.* Lincoln, NE: iUniverse.com.

Thurman, H. (1961). *The inward journey.* Richmond, IN: Friends United Press.

Tillich, P. (1952). *The courage to be.* New Haven, CT: Yale University Press.

Vaughan, F. (1995). *The inward arc: Healing in psychotherapy and spirituality.* Nevada City, CA: Blue Dolphin Publishing.

Walsh, R., & Vaughan, F. (1993). *Paths beyond ego: The transpersonal vision.* New York, NY: G. P. Putnam's Sons.

Webb, H. S. (2004). *Traveling between the worlds: Conversations with contemporary shamans.* Charlottesville, VA: Hampton Roads Publishing.

Weil, A. (1995). *Spontaneous healing.* New York, NY: Ballantine.

Weil, A. (2005). *Healthy aging: A lifelong guide to your physical and spiritual well-being.* New York, NY: Alfred A. Knopf.

Weil, A. (2009). *Why our health matters: A vision of medicine that can transform our future.* New York, NY: Penguin Group.

Weil, A. (2011). *Spontaneous happiness.* New York, NY: Little, Brown.

Wesselman, H. (1998). *Medicine maker: Mystic encounters on the shaman's path.* New York, NY: Bantam Books.

Wilber, K. (1996). *A brief history of everything.* Boston, MA: Shambhala.

Woodham, A., & Peters, D. (1997). *Encyclopedia of healing therapies.* New York, NY: DK Publishing.

Yancey, P. (1990). *Where is God when it hurts?: A comforting, healing guide for coping with hard times.* Grand Rapids, MI: Zondervan.

# CHAPTER 9

# Trauma and Spirituality: Implications for Counselor Educators, Supervisors, and Practitioners*

Integrating spirituality within trauma and disaster mental health counseling emerges as one of the most challenging, yet misunderstood, areas in counselor education and professional practice. The search for personal meaning in one's chronic illness, disability, or traumatic experience is thought to be an existential and spiritual pursuit (Stebnicki, 2016b). Possessing the awareness, knowledge, and skills of integrating spirituality into a therapeutic environment is essential for working from both multicultural counseling and holistic perspectives in finding meaning in a multitude of critical events (Association for Spiritual, Ethical, and Religious Values [ASERVIC], 2016; Corey & Corey, 2016; Meyers & Sweeney, 2008; Miller, 2003; Shannonhouse, Myers, & Sweeney, 2016; Stebnicki, 2016b; Stebnicki & Cubero, 2008). This chapter explores the implications of infusing the client's spirituality into counseling practice with the intention to bring some level of meaning to extraordinary stressful and traumatic events. Guidelines for mental health counselors, counselor educators, and clinical supervisors are offered for integrating spirituality into disaster mental health services.

## SPIRITUALITY: IN SEARCH OF A DEFINITION

Mental health counselors work with clients who have both religious and spiritual concerns and oftentimes bring these issues into the therapeutic setting (Francis, 2016). However, the nature of a person's spiritual health presents a conceptual and empirical dilemma to both researchers and practitioners in the mental health field because the literature lacks a

*Developed from Stebnicki (2006), in *Rehabilitation Research, Policy & Education, 20*(2), © Springer Publishing Company.

precise, comprehensive definition of spirituality. Primarily this is because: (a) the conceptual boundaries between religion and spirituality are sometimes difficult to discern, (b) spiritual variables in counseling are difficult to measure, and (c) the literature on both secular and religious counseling lacks guidelines for training counselors about the degree to which they should intervene to promote a person's spiritual growth. Thus, integrating spirituality into theory, practice, and a counselor training curriculum is a difficult task.

Vaughan (1991) suggests that spirituality is not the special property of any group or religion. Spirituality exists in the hearts of all persons, races, creeds, and cultures. Spirituality is a subjective experience for persons, while religiosity involves subscribing to a set of beliefs, doctrines, and rituals that are institutional or based on a church or religious organization (Shafranske & Malony, 1990; Spilka, Hood, & Gorsuch, 1985; Vaughan, 1991). Myers, Sweeney, and Witmer (2000) suggest that religion is part of the individual's spiritual belief system because, for many, religion is an expression of their spirituality. In contrast to religiosity, spirituality describes the relationship between the person and a transcendent being or higher power. It is described as the courage to look within and to trust a deep sense of belonging, wholeness, connectedness, and openness to the infinite (Shafranske & Gorsuch, 1984). Spirituality, then, is not an entity on its own; rather, a person's spiritual being is interwoven within the individual's physical body and emotional psyche (Ellison & Smith, 1991), and is present in all human beings as a way to find and construct a personal meaning about life and its existence (Myers et al., 2000).

Csordas (1990) pointed out that because we have no universal language for spirituality, discussions rely on the language of the client's emotions. As a consequence, the client's spirituality becomes paradoxical in nature because a person's spiritual being cannot be observed (Hayes, 1984). While the person has a basic conceptual understanding of religious practices, a connection with the spiritual self is difficult to express or communicate with others. The American Counseling Association's (ACA) division of ASERVIC (2016) defines spirituality ". . . as a capacity and tendency that is innate and unique to all persons. This spiritual tendency moves the individual toward knowledge, love, meaning, peace, hope, transcendence, connectedness, compassion, wellness, and wholeness" (p. 5).

Besides the conceptual and operational definitions of spirituality, not all researchers and practitioners agree that incorporating spirituality into counseling sessions is essential. Many individuals who consider themselves as atheistic and secular humanists believe that spirituality may actually be harmful to clients in a therapeutic context. Within the context of this belief system, *spirituality* is defined as some positive belief that the individual has, which is unusual, special, or has higher meaning and purpose in life. Ellis (2000), for example, views spirituality as a list of desirable characteristics that are profoundly meaningful, purposive, and spirited goals and values that clients try and achieve. However, he considers this as "quasispiritual" and does not favor most spiritual values because ". . . they are contradicted by social reality, are superoptimistic, and can easily lead to disillusionment by those who first strongly believe them" (p. 279).

Although spirituality and religiosity continue to lack clarity in definition and application, many earlier researchers (Bergin, 1988; Worthington, 1988) and psychotherapists (Assagioli, 1965; Jung, 1937/1973) contended that spirituality is a natural part of being human. Nevertheless, spirituality can create meaning and purpose in one's life and can be a vital therapeutic resource (Frankl, 1959; Hinterkopf, 1998; Tillich, 1952). A major assumption underlying the client's disability and spiritual experience is that all perceptions by the counselor must be based on an understanding of the client's socio-cultural background (Stebnicki, Rubin, Rollins, & Turner, 1999). Counselor educators and clinical supervisors who introduce spiritual aspects of counseling within the supervisor–supervisee session may want to operationally define their concept of spirituality for supervisees. However, counselor supervisees working within the spiritual realm with clients have the potential for opening another channel of increased health and wellness for individuals with chronic illnesses and disabilities.

## INTEGRATING SPIRITUALITY IN COUNSELOR EDUCATION AND SUPERVISION

Spirituality in mental health counseling has emerged as a unique topic of interest within the counselor education and supervision literature. Understanding the client's spiritual issues is typically addressed within the context of multicultural counseling. However, spirituality is considered an "orientation to the profession and ethical practice" within the counseling profession itself. In fact, the Council for Accreditation of Counseling and Related Educational Programs (CACREP, 2016) cite under Standard 2.g that counselors understand "the impact of spiritual beliefs on clients and counselors worldviews" (p. 9). There are other sections of the standards that relate to the counselor's knowledge and awareness of spiritual practices facilitated in therapeutic engagements such as one would see in substance abuse treatment settings (i.e., Alcoholics Anonymous, Narcotics Anonymous, Celebrate Recovery).

Truly, spirituality is an important part of the clinical supervision process because cultural rapport can build a strong working alliance between clients and counselors (Bernard & Goodyear, 2009). It appears to interconnect well with understanding the cultural aspects of clients (Berkel, Constantine, & Olson, 2007). Although a majority of counselor educators agreed that facilitating spiritual interventions plays an important role during counseling sessions (Green, Benshoff, & Harris-Forbes, 2001; Polanski, 2003), it is suggested that there may be some avoidance of spiritual matters within the client–counselor sessions (Gubi, 2007). Typically, mental health counselors who integrate issues of spirituality within their therapy sessions typically do so well after they complete their graduate training program. The perception is that dealing with the client's spirituality in a session is a specialty area of clinical practice that should only be dealt with in faith-based settings (Stebnicki, 2006). The integration of the client's issues of spirituality and spiritual identity is also dependent on the mental health practitioner's level of interest, motivation, and advanced training in spiritual practices. This typically occurs developmentally after the mental health professional graduates and becomes fully licensed.

Despite the reluctance that spirituality should not be addressed in the session (Gubi, 2007), competent and skilled counselors understand the cultural significance of their clients' spiritual concerns because spiritual practices are common to almost all cultures

(Stebnicki, 2016b). Overall, it is critical that mental health counselors know how to evaluate, assess, and address their clients' spiritual values, beliefs, and concerns, particularly as they relate to the client's trauma experience. Thus, it is recommended that, first and foremost, the integration of spirituality into counseling practice begins early on with counselor education, training, and supervision offering opportunities to graduate students so they can enhance their skills under competent and skilled clinical supervisors.

Despite the current literature emphasizing the importance of integrating issues of spirituality in counseling practice (Bava, Burchard, Ichihashi, Irani, & Zunker, 2002; Francis, 2016; Johnson & Hayes, 2003; Miller, 2003; Stebnicki, 2016b), there is little evidence supporting the integration, evaluation, and effectiveness of incorporating spiritual practices within counseling sessions (Aldridge, 1993; Boswell, Knight, Hamer, & McChesney, 2001; Ganje-Fling & McCarthy, 1991; Lukoff, Lu, & Turner, 1992; Vaughan, 1991; Worthington, Dupont, Berry, & Duncan, 1988). Vash and Crewe (2004) list a number of reasons why spiritual matters have long been neglected in counselor education and training programs, including: (a) the medical model is primarily a secular discipline, (b) counselors and psychologists have not been trained in how to evaluate or deal with spiritual concerns during intake interviews and therapy sessions, (c) the influence of behaviorism has led to an increased emphasis on observable phenomena that relies primarily on empirical methods of research, and (d) even though counselors and psychologists deal with subject experiences of their clients, issues that are not related to the client's spirituality tend to be more acceptable during therapy sessions.

Ethical and competent practice in mental health counseling begins with skilled and competent clinical supervision. Seasoned counselor educators and clinical supervisors must clarify for supervisees the distinction between religious and spiritual issues that may arise during client–counselor sessions. Skilled and competent clinical supervisors challenge supervisees to monitor their own strong faith-based belief system, so it does not intermingle negatively with their clients' worldview of religion and spirituality (Bishop, Avila-Juarbe, & Thumme, 2003).

The research makes a clear distinction between religiosity and spirituality. Religiosity generally involves factors such as religious affiliation, religious participation, religious rituals and practices, religious commitment, and interpretation of religious values into spiritual beliefs, whereas spirituality belongs to all cultures and has both an individual and a cultural-specific and within-group interpretation. Spirituality is integrated into the individual's consciousness, emotions, and overall health and well-being. Overall, it is essential that preprofessional mental health counselors be offered opportunities to integrate the client's spiritual issues within the therapeutic environment.

Foundationally, the client's experience of disaster and trauma many times has a spiritual significance that should be processed with an objective, skilled, and competent mental health practitioner. Some authors (Pargament & Zinnbauer, 2000; Shafranske & Malony, 1996) have suggested that counselors have an ethical obligation to explore the spiritual aspects of their clients' lives because it is consistent with facilitating counseling approaches within a multicultural framework. Myers and Williard (2003) advocate that it is essential that counselor educators incorporate spiritual issues within a wellness orientation to prepare counselors to meet the spiritual and religious needs of their clients. Spiritual connectedness is a cultural attribute and can be a form of social support that empowers individuals with chronic illnesses and disabilities to cope with their environment (Harley, Stebnicki, & Rollins, 2000).

## Spirituality and Wellness

Empirical analyses of spiritual theory, technique, and effectiveness are limited. Thus, it is not surprising that counselor educators and clinical supervisors have not kept pace with preparing mental health counselors to address their clients' spiritual needs and assess their spiritual values, beliefs, and practices. Interestingly, the counseling literature is replete with studies on facilitating "holistic approaches" (e.g., medical, physical, emotional, psychological, psychosocial) with clients. Most research that relates to integrating spirituality in counseling is found in the literature on substance use disorders. In fact, there appears to be a special emphasis on "step programs" such as Alcoholics Anonymous and support groups that have a spiritual focus on recovery (i.e., faith-based approaches such as Celebrate Recovery; Benshoff & Janikowski, 1999; Carroll, 1999; Goodwin, 2002; Green et al., 2001). Even though spirituality has been documented as a foundational treatment approach in the alcohol and substance abuse recovery process, integrating the spiritual dimension as it relates to trauma survivors is rarely discussed.

Clearly, the foundations of mental health counseling are rooted in the counseling theories of human growth and development. The development of one's spirituality, faith, morality, beliefs, and values is also a developmental process that helps define spirituality for the individual (Worthington, 1989). Within the past 20 years, integrating spirituality into counseling and psychotherapy has been explored by a limited number of researchers. This has resulted in other research paradigms that have developed the theories of wellness, optimal functioning as a person, and human potential. This pivotal shift in delineating theories of spiritual practice has been communicated in theories of wellness that suggest all individuals can benefit from counseling, not just those with chronic and persistent mental health conditions (Shannonhouse et al., 2016).

The shift to wellness models began with Meyers and her colleagues' foundational work in the Wheel of Wellness (WoW; Myers et al., 2000). The WoW is a theoretical model that combines empirical research from 17 specific areas of health, longevity, and quality of life. This model suggests that there are five life tasks central to healthy human functioning: (a) work, (b) friendship (c) love, (d) self, and (e) spirituality. Although there are 17 categories of wellness in the WoW model, spirituality is hypothesized to be the most essential aspect of wellness and healthy human functioning (Myers et al., 2000). This particular model is useful in counselor education and supervision because it incorporates the core of medical, physical, mental, cognitive, behavioral, psychological, social, emotional, behavioral, vocational/occupational, and spiritual functioning.

## SPIRITUALITY AND PEOPLE WITH CHRONIC ILLNESSES AND DISABILITIES

Spirituality and disability have been recognized by Leal-Idrogo (1997) and Maki and Murray (1997) as an important aspect of the graduate counseling curriculum, particularly in the specialty area of clinical rehabilitation counseling. However, integrating spirituality in the counselor education curriculum requires that students be provided with opportunities for clinical practice. Additionally, preprofessional counselors must have a clinical supervisor who possesses an understanding of the significance that spirituality has on developing meaning in the client's extraordinary and traumatic experiences.

Clearly, the search for personal meaning in one's chronic illness, disability, or traumatic experience is an existential and spiritual pursuit. For example, many persons with chronic illnesses and disabilities particularly become attuned to spiritual matters when faced with loss, aging, and pain (Vash & Crewe, 2004). In many cultures, the most significant and meaningful questions are related to where we came from before birth and where we will transcend to at the time of our death (Pedersen, 2000). Spirituality within the multicultural-centered perspective enhances other cultural attributes such as race, ethnicity, gender, disability, and sexual orientation (Stebnicki et al., 1999), and it is vital for understanding the holistic needs of the individual. For quite some time, researchers and educators have advocated exploring disability and trauma experiences from a metaphysical or spiritual perspective because of the power that spiritual practices offer persons to cope with adversity (Chang, Noonan, & Tennstedt, 1998; Goodwin, 1986; Lane, 1992; McCarthy, 1995; Stebnicki, 2016a; Vash, 1994; Walker & Walker, 1995). The importance of integrating spiritual practices as they apply to the clinical rehabilitation counseling process was recognized early on in the classic work of George Wright (1980), who states:

> For those who have faith in a spiritual power, the fact of irreparable disablement may be accepted as God's will and from the same source comes strength to adapt. There is no question about the potential for positive adjustment through this mysterious force of faith. Thus, it can be an invaluable resource in rehabilitation and in adjustment to a handicap. (p. 261)

### Historical Perspective

In the early literature on spirituality in ancient Judaism and Greek society, a person's soul or spirit was considered to be the essence of the personality (McNeill, 1951). In the absence of a medical or physical disability, the physical appearance of the body reflected a perfect spirit and soul. Any abnormalities—medical, physical, or mental—were perceived as deficient, deformed, or deviant. For example, epilepsy was once believed to be caused by the possession of "evil spirits" in our mortal bodies. Indeed, persons with any medical, physical, or mental disabilities were perceived as spiritually inferior and possessed by demonic spirits. Recent studies that have examined the Christian Church's response to persons with disabilities have found that persons with mental or physical disabilities are often devalued by some church members (Lane, 1992, 1995). In contrast to the Church's worldview on disability, the early literature in psychotherapy and psychoanalytic theory drew parallels between religion and spirituality by viewing disability as both neurosis and psychosis (Lukoff et al., 1992). Although some contemporary psychoanalytic circles have revised this position (Laor, 1989), Freud (1966) viewed religion itself as a "universal obsessional neurosis" and spirituality as regression, escapism, and a projection upon the world of a primitive infantile state.

Over the course of history, four ontological concepts or ways of understanding the meaning of life with a chronic illness and disability have emerged (Arokiasamy, Rubin, & Roessler, 1987). These concepts serve to clarify our understanding of chronic illness and disability and to direct intervention and practice. Explanations are described in terms of (a) divine gifts, punishment or demonic possession that is best dealt with through prayer and ritual, (b) physical disease best dealt with through medical intervention, (c) natural causes to be treated with psychosocial intervention, and (d) social barriers and prejudice to be amended through political means. Hershenson (1992) suggests that the person's understanding and meaning of a disability may be based on faith (e.g., supernatural causes), logic (e.g., medical and natural causes), or power (e.g., society as a cause of negative impact of disability). Accordingly, there is no single explanation as to the role and meaning that spirituality plays in regard to personal coping and adjustment to disability.

Historically, rehabilitation counselors have included the concept of working with the "whole person" probably more so than any other counseling disciplines and human service professionals (Goodwin, 1986). Marceline Jaques (1970), an early rehabilitation educator, reportedly was the first rehabilitation professional to relate the theoretical concept of holism specifically to the field of rehabilitation counseling. Implicit in the holistic approach to adjustment to chronic illness and disability is the challenge of integrating treatment modalities that incorporate spiritual elements (Byrd, 1997). Successful coping, adaptation, and adjustment are not just a physical or medical rehabilitation process. In the face of adversity, the individual's mental, physical, and spiritual health can make the difference between perceiving the self as a "victim" or "survivor." Yet, despite a resurgence of religious and spiritual values in the United States, the interrelationship between body, mind, and spirit is a neglected area in rehabilitation counselor training programs (McCarthy, 1995).

Although the effectiveness of achieving spiritual well-being has been well documented in other counseling fields such as social work and psychology (Chandler, Miner-Holden, & Kolander, 1992; Ellison & Smith, 1991; McKee, 1988), it still struggles for credibility among rehabilitation counselor educators and practitioners (McCarthy, 1995). Some counselor educators who have introduced spirituality into counselor training programs have faced ridicule from their colleagues (Miller, 2003), and many educators say the topic is irrelevant in the mental health field (Cheston, 1991). Some counselors avoid spiritual issues altogether because of their perceived lack of training in this area (Presley, 1992). Others believe that dealing with clients' spiritual issues is an area for the clergy or religious institutions to deal with (Chandler et al., 1992).

## Meaning of Chronic Illness and Disability

The meaning of chronic illness and disability and how people perceive their bodies can be a powerful determinant of spiritual health and growth. Wright (1983), in her discussion of the manner in which persons with disabilities are perceived, asserts ". . . the context in which a disability appears exerts a major influence on how the individual is perceived" (p. 52). She further notes that while context is important, the perceiver interprets the context in terms of his or her own internal dynamics. Consequently, the way in which counselors interact and perceive persons with chronic illnesses and disabilities is an interplay of both external (e.g., worldview) and internal (e.g., intrapersonal awareness) forces. Such forces impact personal adjustment to disability and suggest that their sociocultural background influences the manner in which counselors form a working alliance with clients and the way in which they interact with family members and other support systems (Stebnicki et al., 1999).

Spiritual health is an especially important issue for women with physical disabilities who are seeking a sense of "self." Nosek and Hughes (2001) suggest that seeking a sense of self is a spiritual journey. These authors note that women with physical disabilities report significantly lower levels of self-esteem than women without physical disabilities, because of social isolation, social comparisons, lack of employment opportunities, and dissatisfaction with personal relationships with others. They further note that a ". . . sense of self in connection to others is a fundamental determinant of self-esteem, and that self-efficacy, when perceived as a power drawn from a divine source, is an important mechanism used to transcend the challenges to both that often accompany disability" (p. 23).

It is critical that mental health counselors, counselor educators, and clinical supervisors become sensitive to issues of spiritual health and understand the challenges that chronic illness and disability present for the individual. Understanding individuals' disability, in connection with their spiritual values, ultimately influences the way in which professional counselors understand and relate to the clients they serve.

Overall, addressing issues related to spiritual and religious concerns in counselor education and supervision is important for competent and ethical practice and has been recognized as the essential feature in enhancing the individual's mental health and wellness (Johnson & Hayes, 2003; Lukoff et al., 1992). In order for research, theory, and practice to advance in counselor education and supervision, it is essential that counselor educators and supervisors learn how to evaluate and integrate relevant spiritual issues within the counseling curriculum and in counselor supervisee's clinical experiences.

## INTEGRATING SPIRITUAL ISSUES IN COUNSELOR TRAINING AND SUPERVISION

Although articles, books, and Internet sites dedicated to spiritual issues proliferate in psychology and counseling, spirituality within the counselor education and supervision curriculum emerges as one of the most challenging, yet misunderstood, areas of the counselor training program. It is incumbent upon counselor educators and supervisors to explore opportunities for infusing spirituality into the core content of the curriculum and graduate supervisees' clinical experiences. The primary purpose for doing so is to prepare competent mental health counselors to work intentionally within a multicultural context and empower clients with other resources for increased coping and adjustment to disaster and traumatic experiences.

Spirituality does play a prominent role in the lives of individuals from many different cultural and ethnic backgrounds. To work effectively with the individual's spiritual identity and worldview, it has been suggested throughout the literature that counselor educators and supervisors need to intentionally inquire about the client's spiritual health during the supervision session (Bishop et al., 2003; Cashwell & Young, 2004; Polanski, 2003). It is recognized that incorporating spirituality in the curriculum is difficult because of the: (a) lack of the instructor's and student's personal spiritual awareness and cultural sensitivity toward the topic, (b) deficiencies in the instructor's and students' training and experience in dealing with clients'/consumers' spiritual values and needs, (c) inability of counselors to recognize the unique sociocultural attributes of their clients/consumers, (d) lack of opportunity to work with clients'/consumers' spiritual needs due to the program or setting that may limit the focus of client/consumer services and counselor training provided, and (e) ambiguous and existential nature of enhancing spiritual growth and development. Overall, incorporating spiritual theory and practice into the curriculum can be complicated by philosophical differences, definitional variances, and the lack of a unifying framework in the literature itself. Additionally, some counselor educators and supervisors risk being stereotyped or ostracized by other colleagues for their spiritual or religious perspectives (Miller, 2003).

## RECOMMENDATIONS FOR COUNSELOR EDUCATORS AND SUPERVISORS

There are currently a good number of textbooks, materials, training seminars, and other specialty training methods available for counselor educators, clinical supervisors, and mental health practitioners to increase the awareness, knowledge, and skills in working with clients' spiritual concerns. There are professional organizations and professional codes of ethics that help guide the practice of spiritual work. The following recommendations are based on the assumption that counselor educators and supervisors recognize that: (a) mental health counselors should generally understand and work with culturally salient and relevant attributes of their clients; (b) the individual's spiritual identity and worldview are important cultural attributes and addressing spiritual questions can facilitate a deeper awareness and understanding about the person's chronic illness, disability, and exposure to disaster and traumatic events; and (c) a curriculum that integrates spiritual awareness, knowledge, and skills in counselor education is important and essential in training competent and ethical mental health practitioners to work with disaster and trauma survivors.

Accordingly, the recommendations that follow are offered as strategies for incorporating spiritual issues within counselor education and clinical supervision. Viewing the client's spiritual beliefs, identity, and self-perception from the sociocultural framework may assist clinical supervisors and their supervisees to conceptualize infusing theory and practice in client services.

There are multiple areas for clinical supervisors to consider such as: (a) administering spiritual assessments during intake interviews; (b) countertransference issues and ethical guidelines for counselors; (c) self-exploration of the counselor's own spiritual/religious identity; (d) the facilitation of specific supervision strategies that are helpful during supervisees' clinical experiences; (e) the supervisee's knowledge of different Eastern, Western, and indigenous religious and spiritual practices; and (f) specific treatment issues and referral sources related to spirituality. These are all critical issues to consider prior to infusing spiritual issues in supervisees' education and clinical experiences.

1. *Integrating spirituality in course content:* Spirituality should be defined in a way that is inclusive of any spiritual or religious orientation. Graduate students in counselor education and training are already immersed in the awareness, knowledge, and skills of working with persons with diverse cultural backgrounds. Thus, the client's spiritual issues should be viewed within a multicultural context. The counselor education program has a number of different options for integrating spiritual concepts into the curriculum and the supervisee's clinical experiences. These options include separate or integrated course work in orientation to the profession, multicultural counseling, psychosocial aspects of chronic illness and disability, counseling theories, human growth and development course work, and/or special topic seminars on spirituality. Once the supervisee has some awareness and knowledge of counseling issues related to spirituality, supervisees should be encouraged to integrate this awareness and knowledge of spiritual issues within their clinical experiences. This should first begin with counseling prepracticum and/or practicum experiences prior to the supervisees' internship placement. Faculty who do not have the knowledge and skills to work in this area may consult some of the resources in the References for some commonly used resources for infusing spiritual theory and technique into counseling. There are also a number of professional counseling associations that provide training and development opportunities for counselor educators and supervisors such as the ACA's divisions of the Association for Multicultural Counseling and Development (AMCD) and the ASERVIC, as well as the National Rehabilitation Association's (NRA) National Association for Multicultural Rehabilitation Concerns (NAMRC). Counselor educators interested in developing syllabi addressing sociocultural–spiritual issues should refer to recommendation #4 that provides sample course content areas and learning objectives.

2. *Facilitating an openness and awareness of integrating the spiritual dimension:* Counselor supervisors can use the supervisory session as an opportunity to discuss any specific definitional, philosophical, and spiritual/religious values and/or beliefs that may hinder the supervisee's ability to discuss spiritual issues with his or her client. Counselor supervisors should be aware of the potential for any negative and unhealthy supervisee countertransference. Accordingly, counselor supervisors

should create a supportive environment that allows supervisees to explore, understand, and articulate a personal meaning of their own spiritual or religious practices and be aware of how their values may potentially impact the counselor–client relationship. From an ethical perspective, supervisees should be reminded that they are not providing counseling services with a particular spiritual or religious orientation (i.e., Christian counseling). Rather, after a comprehensive intake interview, supervisees should know when it is appropriate to refer their clients for religious or other types of spiritual counseling. Some of the following brief questions may be asked during the intake interview, which may also act as helpful probes for supervisors to discuss with their supervisees:

▶ Tell me about your spiritual/religious beliefs.

▶ Do you practice any particular rituals, observe any religious holidays, or find any other types of spiritual practices comforting?

▶ What role, meaning, or purpose does your spiritual/religious belief play in your life?

▶ Are there any particular beliefs that cause any anxiety or confusion for you?

▶ What do you believe your higher power or God has to teach you?

3. *Assessing spiritual well-being:* Integrating issues of spirituality during mental health counseling sessions relating to trauma and disaster can be an opportunity for clients to explore the meaning and purpose of their lives as they relate to issues of adjustment and overall well-being. Myers and Willard (2003) recommend that supervisees should be presented with assessment and intervention techniques during their clinical experiences that are consistent with the philosophy of spiritual and holistic wellness. Spirituality should be defined in a way that is inclusive of any spiritual or religious orientation. However, it is important for supervisees to know their clients'/consumers' values and beliefs so they can use the appropriate terminology, concepts, and language during the interview. Polanski (2003) provides sample questions to initiate an exploration of the client's spirituality such as:

▶ What in your life do you hold sacred or spiritual?

▶ Is there a particular poem, song, or passage from scripture that speaks to your life?

▶ I wonder what kind of spiritual growth you see yourself making as a result of your situation?

▶ If you thought of your situation as a map given to you by your higher power, where do you see this leading you?

Cashwell and Young (2005) offer the following sample questions that may be useful for exploring the individual's religious/spiritual beliefs:

▶ What are some of your earliest memories of religion, church, synagogue, or perhaps the absence of religion?

▶ What, if any, were your early images of God or your higher power?

▶ What are your earliest memories of nonordinary reality, a higher power, some mystery in the universe, or other meaningful spiritual or transpersonal experiences?

▶ What resistance or barriers exist that prevent you from connecting with sources of spirituality?

▶ Where are you at now on your spiritual journey?

If in fact the body, mind, and spirit comprise the whole person, then we should be able to demonstrate a positive relationship between the person's spiritual and psychological health using subjective measures of psychological, physiological, and spiritual well-being. Despite complex interacting variables, measuring the effects of spiritual practices on the person's spiritual well-being, the Spiritual Well-Being Scale (SWBS; Ellison, 1983; Paloutzian & Ellison, 1982) is considered the most extensively researched measure of subjective spiritual well-being (Ellison & Smith, 1991; Ledbetter, Smith, Vosler-Hunter, & Fischer, 1991; Watson, Morris, & Hood, 1990). The SWBS consists of 20 items evenly divided to comprise two subscales of religious well-being (RWB) and existential well-being (EWB). This self-report instrument has been used in a variety of settings, including colleges, universities, seminaries, hospitals, ski clubs, mental health clinics, and prisons. There are a number of studies that have shown a positive correlation between the SWBS and increased psychological health among persons with chronic medical illness and life-threatening disabilities (see Baldwin, 1995; Campbell, 1988; Carson, 1990; Carson, Soeken, Shanty, & Toms, 1990; Granstrom, 1987; Heintzman, 1999; Kaczorowski, 1989; Kohlbry, 1986; Richter, 2002; Riley et al., 1998). Overall, spiritual assessments can be used within the context of a comprehensive intake interview that is culturally sensitive and can help clients explore their religious and spiritual beliefs at a level at which they feel most comfortable. Further, counselor educators and supervisors should provide opportunities for supervisees to administer and interpret formal and informal spiritual assessments for the purpose of developing appropriate counseling goals and interventions that facilitate increased health and wellness.

4. *Developing course/clinical content and learning objectives.* There are several resources available for counselor educators that propose specific course objectives for integrating spiritual aspects of counseling within foundation content areas of the counselor education curriculum (see ASERVIC, 2016; Cashwell & Young, 2004; Miller, 2003). The following domains are typically observed within the learning objectives for coursework and clinical experiences that infuse spirituality into the course content areas: (a) an introduction and orientation to the definitions and philosophies of specific religious and spiritual belief systems and worldviews, (b) an understanding of wellness concepts and human spiritual development across the life span, (c) assessing the impact that religion and spirituality has on the individual's life, (d) working with individuals who possess characteristics of

spiritual problems within a mental health diagnostic framework (i.e., *Diagnostic and Statistical Manual of Mental Disorders* [5th ed.; *DSM-5;* American Psychiatric Association, 2013]), (e) developing an understanding of one's own spiritual belief system and how countertransference can hinder a helping session, and (f) ethical issues related to the counselor–client relationship.

A combination of lectures, discussions, debates, readings, personal reaction papers, personal theory papers, videotape models, live demonstrations, guest presenters, case studies, and oral presentations can be used to facilitate student knowledge, understanding, and practice of integrating spiritual practices into counseling settings. Hence, the following learning objectives are proposed for counselor educators and supervisors:

a.  Students will be able to explain the differences and similarities between religious and spiritual practices and beliefs within a sociocultural context.

b.  Students will explore their own religious and spiritual beliefs for the purpose of increasing their sensitivity, values, and understanding of a diversity of spiritual beliefs.

c.  Students will learn how to perform a spiritual assessment for purposes of evaluating the impact that spirituality has on their clients' chronic illnesses, disabilities, and overall well-being, as well as clarifying the level of need to address spiritual issues in counseling.

d.  Students will apply counseling strategies and techniques that will demonstrate a high degree of sensitivity and acceptance of a variety of spiritual expressions by their clients/consumers.

e.  Students will explore, define, and learn how to apply ethical guidelines while integrating spirituality practices during client/consumer services.

## Summary of Recommendations

As the research suggests, there is evidence that spiritual and/or religious issues are an important part of coping with, and adjusting to, chronic illness, disability, or an extraordinary stressful and traumatic event. Because each of these issues is associated with specific emotions and experiences, each requires different supervision techniques and approaches (e.g., role-playing, audio- or videotaped supervision, case study presentation). Thus, developing the supervisee's mental health counseling skills, especially working with the client's spiritual values, beliefs, and identity, can become quite challenging for both the supervisor and the supervisee.

The supervisory relationship is pivotal in developing supervisee skills within a sociocultural–spiritual context. Paramount to this relationship is the communication dynamics between the client/consumer, supervisee, and supervisor, referred to by Bernard and Goodyear (2009) as the triad process. This process occurs frequently within the supervisory relationship and emerges unconsciously as the supervisee can be observed taking on the attitudes, beliefs, feelings, and behaviors of his or her client while relating specific client issues to his or her supervisor. A specific example might be a supervisee who presents his or her client's feelings of loss in spiritual identity. In such a case, the supervisee may display parallel emotions of hopelessness or existential despair. Consequently, the supervisor must be aware of the meta-transference that takes place within the supervisory session because it can cause conflict in the supervisor–supervisee relationship. Several strategies are recommended that include open, honest, and direct communication with the supervisee about issues of countertransference, role-playing to gain a clearer perspective of client/consumer issues, audio/videotape review to rationally deal with some of the client's/consumer's and supervisee's abstract information, and other techniques where the clinical supervisor changes roles from the counselor educator/ supervisor to the therapist.

After the supervisor–supervisee relationship is firmly established, supervisors can begin the supervisory session by incorporating the following activities with their supervisees: (a) assess any spiritual and/or religious concerns of the supervisee in terms of the supervisee's neglect or bias of his or her client's/consumer's spiritual and/or religious issues; (b) encourage the supervisee to gain knowledge of his or her client's/consumer's spiritual/religious background so he or she may communicate better, especially within the context of his or her client's spiritual-cultural norms; (c) explore the impact that the client's/consumer's religious/spiritual values and beliefs might have within the context of a sociopolitical environment that may be prejudiced or discriminatory; (d) seek consultation from traditional healers or religious or spiritual practitioners; (e) encourage continuing education and training to become more competent with sociocultural–spiritual type assessments, treatment issues, and appropriate external resources.

## INTEGRATING SPIRITUAL APPROACHES IN COUNSELING PRACTICE

Despite a lack of guidelines offered in the literature related to integrating spirituality in mental health counseling, there appears to be increased interest in addressing spiritual issues for trauma survivors and those who have acquired chronic illnesses and disabilities (Burke & Carruth, 2012; Stebnicki, 2001; Stebnicki, 2006). Moodley and West's (2005) edited work is just one example of a growing number of professional texts that delineate the integration of indigenous approaches in traditional counseling and psychotherapy. There is also a growing body of literature in the fields of psychology and health-related sciences that suggests a person's spiritual health has a major influence on the body's immune system and may affect the ability to combat chronic illness and life-threatening disability (Aldridge, 1993; Cousins, 1979; Goleman, 2003; Kelsey, 1981; Peck, 1993; Roud, 1990; Schwartz, 1994; Siegel, 1990; Simonton, 1978; Walsh, 1999; Weil, 1995). This is an emerging area of interest to counseling professionals, primarily because allopathic models of Western medicine and psychotherapy often do not integrate complementary or holistic forms of therapy that promote an optimal level of health and healing (Bliss, 1985; Chandler et al., 1992; Frame, 2002; Goodwin, 1986; McKee, 1988; Trieschmann, 1995). Many persons are dissatisfied with the ineffectiveness of the "medical model" of treatment, primarily because of the: (a) heavy reliance on pharmaceutical products, (b) philosophy of treating the "disease" while ignoring the psychosocial aspects of the person, and (c) lack of control consumers have in choosing alternative treatment options (Astin, 1998; Weil, 1995).

It is believed by many of the earlier theorists and psychotherapists (Assagioli, 1971; Frankl, 1967; Jung, 1916, 1933; Maslow, 1971) that dealing with spiritual issues in counseling is not only powerful in facilitating personal growth, but is necessary in order to understand and work with the whole person. Discussing spiritual values and beliefs with persons receiving counseling services is perceived by some to be the most influential factor in healing negative patterns of behaviors and personal beliefs, and increasing awareness of the meaning and purpose of chronic illness and disability (Krippner & Welch, 1992; Peck, 1993; Siegel, 1990). Accordingly, understanding or making sense of a chronic illness, disability, or traumatic experience essentially is a search for the meaning, which is a spiritual pursuit (Byrd & Byrd, 1993; Garfield, 1979; Goodwin, 1986; Lane, 1992; Vash, 1994). Overall, mental health counselors who are competent in facilitating spiritual growth during the counseling session may assist clients in gaining a deeper understanding and meaning of their trauma or disaster experience.

Because spirituality relates to the person's unique cultural values and beliefs, it ultimately relates to how he or she perceives his or her overall spiritual health and wellness. Aldridge (1993) contends that people usually do not speak with their physicians about spiritual matters. This is primarily because physicians do not perceive spirituality to be connected with the patient–physician relationship. It is suspected that physicians are not the only professional group that avoids dealing with spiritual and metaphysical matters.

## CONCLUDING REMARKS

The search for personal meaning in one's chronic illness, disability, or traumatic experience is thought to be an existential and spiritual pursuit. Openness to infusing issues of spirituality into counselor education, clinical supervision, and clinical practice is essential for practicing within a multicultural counseling framework. The impact that trauma and disability have on the individual and family members is enormous. Thus, integrating spirituality into the clients' practices within therapeutic engagements assists in increasing coping and resiliency skills. I have offered strategies for counselor educators and clinical supervisors to implement across the curriculum and clinical practice. Advancing the theories and practice of spiritual integration, particularly for clients with chronic medical/physical/mental illnesses and disabilities, is essential for healing trauma.

## REFERENCES

Aldridge, D. (1993). Is there evidence for spiritual healing? *Advances, 9*(4), 4–21.

American Psychiatric Association. (2013). *Diagnostic and statistical manual of mental disorders* (5th ed.). Arlington, VA: American Psychiatric Publishing.

Arokiasamy, C. V., Rubin, S. E., & Roessler, R. T. (1987). Sociological aspects of disability. In S. E. Rubin & R. T. Roessler (Eds.), *Foundations of the vocational rehabilitation process* (3rd ed.). Austin, TX: Pro-Ed.

Assagioli, R. (1965). *Psychosynthesis: A manual of principles and techniques.* New York, NY: Viking Press.

Assagioli, R. (1971). *Psychosynthesis.* New York, NY: Viking Press.

Association for Spiritual, Ethical, and Religious Values in Counseling. (2016). Home page. Retrieved from http://www.aservic.org/resources/aservic-white-paper-2

Astin, J. A. (1998). Why patients use alternative medicine: Results of a national study. *Journal of the American Medical Association, 279,* 1548–1554.

Baldwin, L. C. (1995). *Spirituality, health, and occupational therapy.* Conference abstracts and resources (pp. 165–166). American Occupational Therapy Association, Bethesda, MD.

Bava, S., Burchard, C., Ichihashi, K., Irani, A., & Zunker, C. (2002). Conversing and constructing spirituality in a postmodern training context. *Journal of Family Psychotherapy, 13,* 237–258.

Benshoff, J. J., & Janikowski, T. P. (1999). *The rehabilitation model of substance abuse counseling.* Pacific Heights, CA: Brooks/Cole.

Bergin, A. E. (1988). Three contributions of a spiritual perspective to counseling, psychotherapy, and behavior change. *Counseling and Values, 33,* 21–31.

Bergin, A. E., Stinchfield, R. D., Gaskin, T. A., Masters, K. S., & Sullivan, C. E. (1988). Religious lifestyles and mental health: An exploratory study. *Journal of Counseling Psychology, 35*(1), 91–98.

Berkel, L. A., Constantine, M. G., & Olson, E. A. (2007). Supervisor multicultural competence: Addressing religious and spiritual issues with counseling students in supervision. *The Clinical Supervisor, 26*(1), 3–15.

Bernard, J. M., & Goodyear, R. K. (2009). *Fundamentals of clinical supervision* (4th ed.). Boston, MA: Pearson, Allyn & Bacon.

Bishop, D. R., Avila-Juarbe, E., & Thumme, B. (2003). Recognizing spirituality as an important factor in counselor supervision. *Counseling and Values, 48*(1), 34–46.

Bliss, S. (1985). *The new holistic health handbook: Living well in a new age.* Lexington, MA: The Stephen Greene Press.

Boswell, B. B., Knight, S., Hamer, M., & McChesney, J. (2001). Disability and spirituality: A reciprocal relationship with implications for the rehabilitation process. *Journal of Rehabilitation, 67*(4), 20–25.

Burke, P. A., & Carruth, B. (2012). Addiction and psychological trauma: Implications for counseling strategies. In L. L. Levers (Ed.), *Trauma counseling: Theories and interventions* (pp. 214–248). New York, NY: Springer Publishing.

Byrd, E. K. (1997). Concepts related to inclusion of the spiritual component in services to persons with disability and chronic illness. *Journal of Applied Rehabilitation Counseling, 28*(4), 26–29.

Byrd, E. K., & Byrd, P. D. (1993). A listing of biblical references to healing that may be useful as bibliotherapy to the empowerment of rehabilitation clients. *Journal of Rehabilitation, 59*(3), 46–50.

Campbell, C. D. (1988). Coping with hemodialysis: Cognitive appraisals, coping behaviors, spiritual well-being, assertiveness, and family adaptability and cohesion as correlates of adjustment (Doctoral dissertation, Western Conservative Baptist Seminary, 1983). *Dissertation Abstracts International, 49,* 538B.

Carroll, J. J. (1999). Compatibility of Adlerian theory and practice with the philosophy and practice of Alcoholics Anonymous. *Journal of Addictions and Offender Counseling, 19*, 50–61.

Carson, V. B. (1990). *The relationships of spiritual well-being, selected demographic variables, health indicators, and AIDS related activities to hardiness in persons who were serum positive for the human immune deficient virus or were diagnosed with acquired immune deficient syndrome* (Unpublished doctoral dissertation). Baltimore, MD: University of Maryland, School of Nursing.

Carson, V. B., Soeken, K. L., Shanty, J., & Toms, L. (1990). Hope and spiritual well-being: Essentials for living with AIDS. *Perspectives in Psychiatric Care, 26*(2), 28–34.

Cashwell, C. S., & Young, J. S. (2004). Spirituality in counselor training: A content analysis of syllabi from introductory spirituality courses. *Counseling and Values, 48*(2), 96–109.

Cashwell, C. S., & Young, J. S. (2005). *Integrating spirituality and religion into counseling: A guide to competent practice*. Alexandria, VA: American Counseling Association.

Chandler, C. K., Miner-Holden, J., & Kolander, C. A. (1992). Counseling for spiritual wellness: Theory and practice. *Journal of Counseling & Development, 71*, 168–175.

Chang, B., Noonan, A. E., & Tennstedt, S. L. (1998). The role of religion/spirituality in coping with caregivers for disabled elders. *Gerontologist, 38*, 463–470.

Cheston, S. E. (1991). A case presentation paradigm: A model for efficient use of small group or individual counselor supervision. *The Clinical Supervisor, 9*(2), 149–159.

Corey, M. S., & Corey, G. (2016). *Becoming a helper*. Belmont, CA: Brooks/Cole.

Council for Accreditation of Counseling and Related Educational Programs. (2016). CACREP standards. Retrieved from http://www.cacrep.org/for-programs/2016-cacrep-standards

Cousins, N. (1979). *Anatomy of an illness*. New York, NY: W. W. Norton.

Csordas, T. J. (1990). The psychotherapy analogy and charismatic healing. *Psychotherapy, 27*(1), 79–90.

Ellis, A. (2000). Spiritual goals and spirited values in psychotherapy. *Journal of Individual Psychology, 56*(3), 277–284.

Ellison, C. W. (1983). Spiritual well-being: Conceptualization and measurement. *Journal of Psychology and Theology, 11*, 330–340.

Ellison, C. W., & Smith, J. (1991). Toward an integrative measure of health and well-being. *Journal of Psychology and Theology, 19*(1), 35–48.

Frame, M. W. (2002). *Spiritual issues in counseling and psychotherapy*. New York, NY: Wadsworth.

Francis, P. C. (2016). Religion and spirituality in counseling. In I. Marini & M. A. Stebnicki (Eds.), *The professional counselors' desk reference* (2nd ed., pp. 559–570). New York, NY: Springer Publishing.

Frankl, V. (1959). *Man's search for meaning*. New York, NY: Pocket Books.

Frankl, V. (1967). *The doctor and the soul: From psychotherapy to logotherapy*. New York, NY: Bantam Books.

Freud, S. (1966). Obsessive actions and religious practices. In J. Strachey (Ed. & Trans.), *The standard edition of the complete psychological works of Sigmund Freud* (Vol. 1). London, United Kingdom: Hogarth. (Original work published 1923.)

Ganje-Fling, M. A., & McCarthy, P. R. (1991). A comparative analysis of spiritual direction and psychotherapy. *Journal of Psychology and Theology, 19*(1), 103–117.

Garfield, C. A. (1979). *Stress and survival: The emotional realities of life-threatening illness.* St. Louis, MO: C. V. Mosby.

Goleman, D. (2003). *Healing emotions: Conversations with the Dalai Lama on mindfulness, emotions, and health.* Boston, MA: Shambhala.

Goodwin, L. B. (2002). *The button therapy book: A practical psychological self-help book & holistic cognitive counseling manual for mental health professionals.* Victoria, BC, Canada: Trafford.

Goodwin, L. R., Jr. (1986). A holistic perspective for the provision of rehabilitation counseling services. *Journal of Applied Rehabilitation Counseling, 17*(2), 29–36.

Granstrom, S. L. (1987, November). *A comparative study of loneliness, Buberian religiosity and spiritual well-being in cancer patients.* Paper presented at the Conference of the National Hospice Organization.

Green, R. L., Benshoff, J. J., & Harris-Forbes, J. A. (2001). Religious and spiritual beliefs and practices of persons with chronic pain. *Journal of Rehabilitation, 67*(3), 55–60.

Gubi, P. M. (2007). Exploring the supervision experience of some mainstream counsellors who integrate prayer in counseling. *Counseling and Psychotherapy Research, 7,* 114–121.

Harley, D. A., Stebnicki, M. A., & Rollins, C. W. (2000). Applying empowerment evaluation as a tool for self-improvement and community development with culturally diverse populations. *Journal of Community Development Society, 31*(2), 348–364.

Hayes, S. C. (1984). Making sense of spirituality. *Behaviorism,12*(2), 99–110.

Heintzman, P. (1999). Spiritual wellness: Theoretical links with leisure. *Journal of Leisurability, 26*(2), 21–32.

Hershenson, D. B. (1992). Conceptions of disability: Implications for rehabilitation. *Rehabilitation Counseling Bulletin, 35*(3), 154–160.

Hinterkopf, E. (1998). *Integrating spirituality in counseling: A manual for using the experiential focusing method.* Alexandria, VA: American Counseling Association.

Jaques, M. E. (1970). *Rehabilitation counseling: Scope and services.* Boston, MA: Houghton Mifflin.

Johnson, C. V., & Hayes, J. A. (2003). Troubled spirits: Prevalence and predictors of religious and spiritual concerns among university students and counseling center clients. *Journal of Counseling Psychology, 50*(4), 409–419.

Jung, C. G. (1916). *Psychology of the unconscious.* New York, NY: Dodd, Mead.

Jung, C. G. (1933). *Modern man in search of a soul.* New York, NY: Harcourt Brace.

Jung, C. G. (1973). Psychology and religion: East and west. In W. McGuire & R. F. C. Hull (Eds. & Trans.), *The collected works of C. G. Jung* (Vol. 11, pp. 5–105). Princeton NJ: Princeton University Press. (Original work published 1937.)

Kaczorowski, J. M. (1989). Spiritual well-being and anxiety in adults diagnosed with cancer. *The Hospice Journal, 5*(3–4), 105–116.

Kelsey, M. (1981). *Transcend: A guide to the spiritual quest.* New York, NY: Crossroad.

Kohlbry, P. W. (1986). *The relationship between spiritual well-being and hope/hopelessness in chronically ill clients* (Unpublished master's thesis). Marquette University, College of Nursing, Milwaukee, WI.

Krippner, S., & Welch, P. (1992). *Spiritual dimensions of healing.* New York, NY: Irvington Publishers.

Lane, N. J. (1992). A spirituality of being: Women with disabilities. *Journal of Applied Rehabilitation Counseling, 23*(4), 53–58.

Lane, N. J. (1995). A theology of anger when living with disability. *Rehabilitation Education, 9*(2), 97–111.

Laor, N. (1989). Psychoanalytic neutrality toward religious experience. *Psychoanalytic Study of the Child, 44,* 211–230.

Leal-Idrogo, A. (1997). Multicultural rehabilitation counseling. *Rehabilitation Education, 11*(3), 231–240.

Ledbetter, M. F., Smith, L. A., Vosler-Hunter, W. L., & Fischer, J. D. (1991). An evaluation of the research and clinical usefulness of the spiritual well-being scale. *Journal of Psychology and Theology, 19*(1), 49–55.

Lukoff, D., Lu, F., & Turner, R. (1992). Toward a more culturally sensitive *DSM-IV:* Psychoreligious and psychospiritual problems. *Journal of Nervous and Mental Disease, 180*(11), 673–682.

Maki, D. R., & Murray, G. C. (1997). Practicum and internship. *Rehabilitation Education, 11*(3), 241–250.

Maslow, A. (1971). *Further reaches of human nature.* New York, NY: Viking Press.

McCarthy, H. (1995). Understanding and reversing rehabilitation counseling's neglect of spirituality. *Rehabilitation Education, 9*(2), 187–199.

McKee, J. (1988). Holistic health and the critique of Western medicine. *Social Science & Medicine, 26*(8), 775–784.

McNeill, J. T. (1951). *A history of the cure of souls.* San Francisco, CA: Harper & Row.

Meyers, J. E., & Sweeney, T. J. (2008). Wellness counseling: The evidence base for practice. *Journal of Counseling & Development, 86,* 482–493.

Miller, G. (2003). *Incorporating spirituality in counseling and psychotherapy: Theory and technique.* Hoboken, NJ: Wiley.

Moodley, R., & West, W. (Eds.). (2005). *Integrating traditional healing practices into counseling and psychotherapy.* Thousand Oaks, CA: Sage Publications.

Myers, J. E., Sweeney, T. J., & Witmer, J. M. (2000). The wheel of wellness, counseling for wellness: A holistic model for treatment planning. *Journal of Counseling & Development, 78,* 251–266.

Myers, J. E., & Williard, K. (2003). Integrating spirituality into counselor preparation: A developmental wellness approach. *Counseling and Values, 47*(2), 142–155.

Nosek, M. A., & Hughes, R. B. (2001). Psychospiritual aspects of sense of self in women with physical disabilities. *Journal of Rehabilitation, 67*(1), 20–25.

Paloutzian, R. F., & Ellison, C. W. (1982). Loneliness, spiritual well-being, and the quality of life. In L. A. Peplau & D. Perlman (Eds.), *Loneliness: A sourcebook of current theory, research, and therapy.* New York, NY: Wiley.

Pargament, K. L., & Zinnbauer, B. J. (2000). Working with the sacred: Four approaches to religious and spiritual issues in counseling. *Journal of Counseling & Development, 78,* 162–171.

Peck, M. S. (1993). *Further along the road less traveled: The unending journey toward spiritual growth.* New York, NY: Simon & Schuster.

Pedersen, P. (2000). *A handbook for developing multicultural awareness* (3rd ed.). Alexandria, VA: American Counseling Association.

Polanski, P. J. (2003). Spirituality and supervision. *Counseling and Values, 47*(2), 131–141.

Presley, D. B. (1992). Three approaches to religious issues in counseling. *Journal of Psychology and Theology, 20*(1), 39–46.

Richter, R. J. (2002). Correlation of psychological well-being and Christian spiritual well-being at a small Christian liberal arts college in the urban Midwest. *CHARIS, 2*(1), 39–46.

Riley, B. B., Perna, R., Tate, D. G., Forchheimer, M., Anderson, C., & Luera, G. (1998). Types of spiritual well-being among persons with chronic illness: Their relation to various forms of quality of life. *Archives of Physical Medicine and Rehabilitation, 79*(3), 258–264.

Roud, P. C. (1990). *Making miracles: An exploration into the dynamics of self-healing.* New York, NY: Warner Communications.

Schwartz, C. E. (1994). Introduction: Old methodological challenges and new mind-body links in psychoneuroimmunology. *Advances: The Journal of Mind-Body Health, 10*(4), 4–7.

Shafranske, E. P., & Gorsuch, R. L. (1984). Factors associated with the perception of spirituality in psychotherapy. *Journal of Transpersonal Psychology, 16*, 231–241.

Shafranske, E. P., & Malony, H. N. (1990). Clinical psychologists' religious and spiritual orientations and their practice of psychotherapy. *Psychotherapy, 27*, 72–78.

Shafranske, E. P., & Malony, H. N. (1996). Religion and the clinical practice of psychology: The case for inclusion. In E. P. Shafranske (Ed.), *Religion and the clinical practice of psychology.* Washington, DC: American Psychological Association.

Shannonhouse, L. R., Myers, J. E., & Sweeney, T. J. (2016). Counseling for wellness. In I. Marini & M. A. Stebnicki (Eds.), *The professional counselors' desk reference* (2nd ed., pp. 617–623). New York, NY: Springer Publishing.

Siegel, B. S. (1990). *Peace, love, and healing.* New York, NY: Harper & Row.

Simonton, O. C. (1978). *Getting well again.* New York, NY: Bantam Books.

Spilka, B., Hood, R. W., & Gorsuch, R. L. (1985). *The psychology of religion: An empirical approach.* Englewood Cliffs, NJ: Prentice-Hall.

Stebnicki, M. A. (2001). The psychosocial impact on survivors of extraordinary stressful and traumatic events: Principles and practices in critical incident response for rehabilitation counselors. *New Directions in Rehabilitation, 12*(6), 57–72.

Stebnicki, M. A. (2006). Integrating spirituality in rehabilitation counselor supervision. *Rehabilitation Education, 20*(2), 115–132.

Stebnicki, M. A. (2016a). From empathy fatigue to empathy resilience. In I. Marini & M. A. Stebnicki (Eds.), *The professional counselors' desk reference* (2nd ed., pp. 533–545). New York, NY: Springer Publishing.

Stebnicki, M. A. (2016b). Integrative approaches in counseling and psychotherapy. In I. Marini & M. A. Stebnicki (Eds.), *The professional counselors' desk reference* (2nd ed., pp. 593–604). New York, NY: Springer Publishing.

Stebnicki, M. A., & Cubero, C. (2008). A content analysis of multicultural counseling syllabi from rehabilitation counseling programs. *Rehabilitation Education, 22*(2), 89–99.

Stebnicki, M. A., Rubin, S. E., Rollins, C. W., & Turner, T. (1999). A holistic approach to multicultural rehabilitation counseling. *Journal of Applied Rehabilitation Counseling, 30*(2), 3–6.

Tillich, P. (1952). *The courage to be.* New Haven, MA: Yale University Press.

Trieschmann, R. B. (1995). The energy model: A new approach to rehabilitation. *Rehabilitation Education, 9*(2), 217–227.

Vash, C. L. (1994). *Personality and adversity: Psychospiritual aspects of rehabilitation.* New York, NY: Springer Publishing.

Vash, C. L., & Crewe, N. M. (2004). *Psychology and disability* (2nd ed.). New York, NY: Springer Publishing.

Vaughan, F. (1991). Spiritual issues in psychotherapy. *Journal of Transpersonal Psychology, 23*(2), 105–119.

Walker, M. L., & Walker, R. B. (1995). Mindfulness in rehabilitation practice, education, and research. *Rehabilitation Education, 9*(2), 201–204.

Walsh, R. (1999). *Essential spirituality: The 7 central practices to awaken heart and mind.* New York, NY: Wiley.

Watson, P. J., Morris, R. J., & Hood, R. W. (1990). Intrinsicness, self-actualization, and the ideological surround. *Journal of Psychology and Theology, 18*, 40–53.

Weil, A. (1995). *Spontaneous healing.* New York, NY: Ballantine.

Worthington, E. L., Jr. (1988). Understanding the values of religious clients: A model and its application to counseling. *Journal of Counseling Psychology, 35*(2), 166–174.

Worthington, E. L. (1989). Religious faith across the life span: Implications for counseling and research. *The Counseling Psychologist, 17*(4), 555–612.

Worthington, E. L., Jr., Dupont, P. D., Berry, J. T., & Duncan, L. A. (1988). Christian therapists' and clients' perceptions of religious psychotherapy in private and agency settings. *Journal of Psychology and Theology, 16*(3), 282–293.

Wright, B. A. (1983). *Physical disability: A psychosocial approach* (2nd ed.). New York, NY: Harper & Row.

Wright, G. N. (1980). *Total rehabilitation.* Boston, MA: Little, Brown.

# CHAPTER 10

# Medical Aspects of Disaster and Trauma

*Mark A. Stebnicki and Irmo Marini*

There are significant mental health challenges for individuals who have acquired a medical–physical disability during a disaster or trauma experience. Regardless of how far one is from the epicenter of person-made or natural disasters, most individuals are affected by various mental and physical health conditions in the aftermath. Depending on the severity of the physical injury, many persons acquire lifelong chronic and disabling health conditions. This chapter discusses some of the more major prevalent medical conditions that are acquired from exposure to person-made and natural disasters. These conditions include traumatic brain injury (TBI), blast wounds, amputation, spinal cord injury (SCI), and musculoskeletal and chronic pain conditions. There are other related conditions that may develop as secondary complications of acute trauma injury (e.g., cardiovascular disease, chronic obstructive pulmonary disease [COPD], hearing and vision loss). However, the intent is to describe and discuss the major health conditions that are most prevalent and have the greatest challenges for individuals who have acquired an acute medical–physical injury during extraordinary stressful and traumatic events.

The central issue in this chapter should highlight the fact that acquired medical–physical disability, as a direct result of trauma and disaster (e.g., mass shooting, hurricane, earthquake), has a pervasive effect on the individual, which imposes chronic and persistent mental health conditions. The combination of medical–physical and mental health injuries has both short- and long-term effects on the individual. Therefore, mental health counselors want to familiarize themselves with the residual functional capacity and medical aspects of each of the medical–physical conditions presented in this chapter. Ultimately, mental health providers can facilitate and coordinate services to assist their clients in achieving optimal medical and psychosocial well-being.

The medical aspects of chronic illness and disability are critical to address clinically during a disaster mental health response. For instance, stress researchers report that one of the hallmarks of the stress response, particularly in traumatic stress, is the complex physiological changes that occur in the mind–body from a systemic level. It places the individual at risk for chronic illness and disability (Lazarus, 1999; Sapolsky, 1998; Tomko, 2012; Wachen et al., 2013; Weil, 1995). Overall, the impact of acute traumatic injury and permanent disability has profound implications for the individual medically, physically, and psychologically, and affects the overall psychosocial functioning, hindering one's level of independence in all life areas (Livneh & Antonak, 2005; Marini & Stebnicki, 2012).

## FREQUENTLY REPORTED HEALTH SYMPTOMS IN EXPOSURE TO TRAUMA

Regardless of your exposure to trauma as a civilian (Baker & Cormier, 2015; Levers, 2012) or military veteran (Lehavot, Der-Martirosian, Simpson, Shipherd, & Washington, 2013; Wachen et al., 2013), there are specific health-related conditions noted among women and men who screen positive for posttraumatic stress disorder (PTSD) during visits to their health care providers. It is reported that as a result of acquired PTSD, these individuals have significantly more frequent visits to their medical health care providers and report poorer physical health outcomes in the following areas:

- *Cardiovascular:* chest pain
- *Dermatological:* skin disorders (rashes, eczema, psoriasis, unexpected hair loss, scalp problems)
- *Gastrointestinal:* frequent diarrhea, recurrent abdominal pain, recurrent nausea
- *Genitourinary:* sexual difficulties or discomfort, loss of bowel and bladder control
- *Musculoskeletal:* loss of strength, joint and muscle pain, joint stiffness
- *Neurological:* recurrent migraines, numbness, difficulty speaking, tinnitus, eye and vision problems
- *Pulmonary:* wheezing, coughing, shortness of breath, frequent coughing

These medical–physical conditions all relate to one known etiology: exposure to high levels of stress and trauma. As a consequence of posttraumatic stress symptoms, the individual is at high risk for *complex PTSD*, a construct originally discussed by Herman (1992). Basically, in complex PTSD, individuals exposed to traumatic stressors typically acquire a number of other mental health conditions (i.e., depression, anxiety, and substance use disorders) and experience multiple other losses related to their physical, mental, and functional capacities. This results in complex healing and somatization of their medical–physical condition many times, which can be disabling for the person. Consequently, the combination of symptoms related to one's mental and physical health requires focus on the medical–physical and mental health and psychosocial issues imposed by the trauma.

# TRAUMATIC BRAIN INJURY

TBI is known as the signature injury of Operation Enduring Freedom (Afghanistan, 2001), Operation Iraqi Freedom (Iraq, 2003), and Operation New Dawn (Afghanistan, 2001). Because of the current conflicts, a significant amount of research has been developed related to TBI, which can be helpful in understanding civilian trauma-related TBI. For instance, all brain injuries acquired during extraordinary stressful and traumatic events, whether in civilian or military life, have one common factor: They are traumatic by nature, which creates a host of mental health conditions. TBI is typically a co-occurring condition associated with posttraumatic stress symptoms, depression, suicide ideation/attempts, anxiety, and substance use disorders (Stebnicki, 2016).

Clearly, exposure to combat stress increases the risk for acquired chronic and persistent mental and physical health problems throughout one's life. Complicating the issues of combat stress are the co-occurring mental and physical health conditions that limit functional capacity due to service-connected disabilities (Government Accountability Office [GAO], 2016a). About two million troops have deployed overseas since post-9/11; there has been upward of 100,000 injuries with about 6,889 fatalities at the time of this writing (Department of Defense [DoD], 2016). TBI affects 13% to 25% of combat military personnel. These injuries typically occur from mortar, rocket, artillery, small arms, roadside bombs, improvised explosive devices (IEDs), sniper attack, and blast wounds. In civilian life, the leading causes of most TBIs are falls, motor vehicle accidents (MVAs), physical assaults, and violence including gunshot wounds to the head (Falvo, 2014).

As a consequence of TBI, high rates of mental health concerns exist and include the following co-occurring conditions: posttraumatic stress (15%–60%), depression (23%), anxiety (43%), and substance use disorders (10%–34%). Of particular importance for mental health counselors is that individuals with a history of TBI and a diagnosis of PTSD have significantly higher rates of suicide attempts (Brenner et al., 2011). Studies vary on attempted suicide rates, from 3% to 15% of those who have a history of both TBI and PTSD. However, the point is that TBI complicates good mental health functioning.

TBI is often diagnosed in civilian populations in war-torn countries as a result of exposure to blasts. In the United States, TBI can occur as a result of person-made disasters. For instance, the homemade bombs at the Boston City Marathon that took place April 15, 2013, killed three individuals and injured 264. Many who attended this event and were closest to the epicenter sustained not only musculoskeletal injuries and amputations, but also TBIs. In regard to natural disasters, flying debris and persons propelled against immovable objects often result in a TBI. This can occur as a closed head or open head injury and ranges from mild to moderate to severe.

## Residual Functional Capacity of TBI

The residual functional capacity of individuals who acquire a TBI depends on the severity of the injury and which part of the brain was injured (Falvo, 2014). Injuries to the left side of the brain impact primarily the person's receptive cognitive processing skills.

This is because the left brain is responsible for (a) spoken and written language, (b) technical and scientific skills, (c) number skills, and (d) analytical thinking. The right brain is typically responsible for (a) artistic awareness and imagination, (b) intuition, (c) apprehension of three-dimensional objects and figures, and (d) characteristics that are unique to our personality and behavior. Current research in neurological and neuropsychological conditions suggests that the right- and left-side hemispheres of the brain are networked and work in coordination with sensory-motor tasks. Interestingly, the right side of the brain controls the left side of the body and left side of the brain controls the right side of the body. Thus, depending on the severity of the TBI, injury to the right brain may result in left side hemiparesis and injury to the left brain results in right side hemiparesis. Overall, Falvo (2014) notes some functional limitations that have long-term implications for individuals with TBI:

- ▶ Persons with Wernicke's aphasia (receptive aphasia) may have normal speech and grammar but may lack the ability to comprehend and process information.

- ▶ Persons with Broca's aphasia (expressive aphasia) may comprehend the spoken word and be able to read, but will have communication problems in regards to speech and articulation, as well as difficulties putting words and sentences together.

- ▶ Motor coordination and balance problems may be present, depending on the location and severity of the injury.

- ▶ Depth perception, ability to judge distances, and interpretation of visual stimuli may be affected.

- ▶ Difficulties may exist with activities of daily living (ADLs) such as eating, swallowing, bowel and bladder function, cooking, cleaning, and bathing safely.

- ▶ Cognitive problems of memory, concentration, and attention may develop.

- ▶ Concept formation, judgment, reasoning, and insight may be affected.

- ▶ Other signs include lack of self-awareness, proneness to irritability, anger outbursts, labile emotions, and depression.

Mild TBI (referred to sometimes as postconcussive syndrome) accounts for about 85% of all TBIs. As a consequence, individuals may experience the following symptoms:

- ▶ An altered state of consciousness for up to 30 minutes
- ▶ Reduced concentration and focus, as well as short-term memory loss
- ▶ Diminished ability to learn new tasks
- ▶ Persistent headaches, vertigo, and tinnitus
- ▶ Sleep disturbance, depression, irritability, and anger

# BLAST WOUNDS

Blast wounds are slightly different than the open or closed brain injury but can result in the same functional limitations. Blast injuries are sustained as the result of a high-intensity detonation or explosion. Regardless of how close or far one is from a blast, it can be a serious injury with long-term complications and all the conditions associated with TBI.

Blast injuries are divided into three areas: primary (changes in atmospheric pressure caused by a blast wave), secondary (blast injuries occurring as a result of objects accelerated by energy of the explosion striking the victim), and tertiary (injury as a result of the victim's body being thrown by the blast; Warden, 2006; Wightman & Gladish, 2001). All blast injuries involve high-explosive detonations where the person is exposed to some level of inhalations of dust, smoke, carbon monoxide, chemicals, and burns from hot gases or fires, and in some cases has a penetrating wound or has been thrown against a hard surface. Regardless of whether an individual has an open or closed head injury, the nature of such experiences results in complex TBI (i.e., posttraumatic stress symptoms, musculoskeletal injury, and decrease in cognitive abilities) and co-occurring medical conditions (i.e., COPD, loss of hearing, vision).

Professional mental health counselors must be mindful of the long-term medical, psychological, and vocational implications that result in TBIs. Facilitating and consulting with the appropriate supports and resources from competent professionals who specialize in neurorehabilitation are critical.

# CHRONIC TRAUMATIC ENCEPHALOPATHY

Chronic traumatic encephalopathy (CTE) is now being recognized in the neurosciences as a very serious condition that can affect the service member's neurocognitive functioning long after separation from the service. CTE results from repeated blows to the head; it is often seen in National Football League (NFL) and National Hockey League (NHL) players, professional boxers, military personnel, and those civilian populations that live in war-torn countries that have been exposed to physical violence such as torture. Neurocognitive researchers have shown significant neurodegenerative changes within certain structures of the brain where abnormal brain tissue develops. These neurodegenerative changes can occur months, years, or even decades after the person's last concussion. As a consequence, there are signs of reduced cognitive functioning such as memory loss, confusion, impaired judgment, poor concentration and focus, paranoia, low impulse control, major depression, aggression, and eventually dementia.

Current treatment protocols among members of the armed forces and professional and nonprofessional athletes, such as those in public school sports programs, require a more detailed, mandatory neurological and neuropsychological assessment after returning from deployment if the service member has had three critical incidents related to blasts, concussions, and mild TBI.

## TRAUMATIC AMPUTATION

Traumatic amputation refers to the severance of a body part due to an acute trauma incident, most typically as a result of an IED explosion, MVA, or other injuries sustained during armed conflict. In some cases, amputation is necessary when the individual has severe frostbite. The first priority in either battlefield or civilian emergency medicine is to save the upper or lower extremities. In some situations, reimplantation surgery may be attempted so as to reattach the severed limb. Even though reimplantation studies show that less than 50% actually have functional use or sensation of the affected limb, quality of life and psychosocial adjustment improve as a result of the individual's preserved body image (Brown & Wu, 2003). In civilian populations where severe type 1 diabetes is diagnosed, it is sometimes necessary for the vascular surgeon to remove lower extremity body parts (e.g., legs, feet, toes). Although most amputations in the diabetic patient are planned surgical procedures and do not result in acute traumatic injury, the loss of a body part itself can be quite traumatic for most individuals, requiring some degree of psychosocial adjustment to their newly acquired disability.

Complications may develop after amputation surgery, which include edema, skin ulceration, contractures, bone spurs, and scoliosis. Phantom sensation and phantom limb pain are a common occurrence among many disabled veterans. This is experienced by some individuals as chronic and severe pain in a body part that is no longer present. Phantom pain diminishes over time. However, some can be incapacitated by the severity of this atypical chronic pain condition (Knotkova, Crucian, Tronnier, & Rasche, 2012).

Prosthetic devices are commonly fabricated as a substitute for the missing body part. These artificial limbs increase independence and functioning for the individual and can be used for cosmetic purposes. The results of higher independent functioning also increase the person's body image, self-esteem, and vocational capacity for performing jobs more safely, and improves overall psychosocial adjustment.

## MUSCUOLOSKELETAL CONDITIONS

There are a number of research studies in medicine and psychology that suggest trauma and depression are part of the known etiology of some specific musculoskeletal conditions such as chronic low back pain, neck pain, and fibromyalgia (Antai-Otong, 2005; Miquel, 2009; Robinson et al., 2004). The intention of this section is not to discuss all musculoskeletal conditions (e.g., bone fractures, carpel tunnel syndrome, torn tendons, osteoarthritis) but rather to concentrate on the most common musculoskeletal problems seen in health care settings, particularly those conditions caused by traumatic incidents (e.g., MVAs, falls, physical assaults and violence). Chronic pain is present in almost all musculoskeletal conditions but is discussed separately, particularly since some pain conditions have an unknown etiology.

### Chronic Low Back Pain

One of the most frequently treated musculoskeletal conditions in medical practice settings is low back pain. If back pain persists beyond 6 months or longer, it is considered chronic low back pain (CLBP). CLBP is defined as pain that is located in the lumbar or sacral region of the lower back. It is experienced by the individual in erect, nonmoving (static) positions or during physical exertional activities (kinetic). CLBP can occur as the consequence of poor body mechanics such as the individual's poor posture or engaging in activities that cause a sprain or strain such as in sports injuries. There are a number of degenerative conditions that cause CLBP, such as arthritis, osteoporosis, and degenerative disk disease. A significant number of musculoskeletal CLBP conditions occur as a result of injury due to falls, MVAs, physical assault, and violence. These extraordinary stressful and traumatic events can result in a number of acute musculo-skeletal conditions including slipped disk, bulging disk, and sciatica, a chronic pain syndrome that radiates from the lower back into the hip and down the legs. Addition-ally, many of the traumatic physical injuries present with the co-occurring conditions of posttraumatic stress symptoms, depression, generalized anxiety disorders, anxiety with panic reaction, and substance use disorders. Consequently, the combination of physical, mental, psychological, and emotional trauma creates a type of complex trauma that is difficult for mental and physical health care providers to treat and makes it hard to coordinate services.

## CHRONIC PAIN CONDITIONS

The condition of chronic pain is defined as pain that persists beyond the expected period of healing or as pain that persists longer than 3 to 6 months (Cohen & Raja, 2012). Chronic pain has over 30 years of research, theory, and clinical practice by which to draw upon in regard to treatment modalities. It is one of the most difficult conditions to treat in the mental, medical, and allied health professional settings. Foundationally, pain is what the person reports in regard to his or her perception, level, intensity, and fre-quency of his or her pain experiences.

Almost everyone experiences some degree of pain at various points throughout their lives, between childbirth, childhood injuries, burning their fingers on a hot stove, or going to the dentist. However, pain that results from traumatic injuries is classified as a separate medical and psychological condition. Chronic pain is multidimensional in its diagnosis and treatment based on a number of factors. Even though chronic pain is uni-versal among all acute and chronic illnesses, disabilities, and traumatic injuries, the experience is highly individualized (Falvo, 2014).

Early pain researchers such as Fordyce (1982) classified pain reactions as *pacers* and *recliners*. Pacers react to pain by maintaining their daily activities, frequently changing positions to reduce their levels of pain. Recliners are more likely to require physical reha-bilitation services because they have higher levels of frequency and intensity while in a resting position. Stiller (1975) classifies pain in three different groups: (a) *pain reducers*—those who attempt to minimize and downplay their experience of pain, (b) *pain augmentors*—those who magnify their experiences of pain, and (c) *moderators*—those who neither magnify nor minimize their experiences of pain. Turk, Meichenbaum, and Genest (1983) have developed four categories of pain that vary along dimensions of inten-sity, quality, duration, and meaning of their pain. These are (a) *acute pain*—pain that has a sudden onset, (b) *chronic periodic pain*—pain that is acute but with intermittent periods, (c) *chronic intractable benign pain*—pain that is present most of the time where the intensity varies, and (d) *chronic progressive pain*—pain that is typically present in malignancies.

Many pain experts today suggest that the condition of chronic pain is influenced by the person's physical, psychological, spiritual, cultural, and social experiences (Milks, 2012). The individual's home and work environments also influence how the person responds to pain. For instance, after an acute physical injury has healed and has reached maximum medical improvement, a physician may release the patient to return to work full time. If the individual's pain persists into a more chronic condition, many times the medical model of disability perceives the patient's pain condition as "psychological" in nature and the person may be viewed as malingering with his or her illness. There are many factors involved with malingering and somatoform disorders. Following this example, professional providers must look at motivating influences that cause the individual to avoid work or job-seeking activities (i.e., pending legal issues concerning their disability). The home environment may include family members who can reward or positively reinforce the individual's chronic pain condition by allowing him or her to recline and stay inactive. Some family members and cultures do not recognize the intensity of their family member's chronic pain condition. In other words, there may be little tolerance for reclining because the family is dependent on the injured family member to work and bring home money for the family to survive. Thus, understanding family relationships, work environment, medical restrictions, residual functional/physical capacity, mental health issues, and other factors that influence the person's level and intensity of chronic pain assist in treatment planning with the intention to reduce and decrease the person's chronic pain experience.

The research is clear that there are a significant number of mental health-related conditions and symptoms that are co-occurring with chronic pain conditions (Winterowd & Sims, 2016). A variety of symptoms such as negative thoughts and feelings toward self and others, as well as feelings of depression, anxiety, irritability, anger, out-of-control stress and panic reactions, and even posttraumatic stress symptoms, all make chronic pain a complex condition to treat both medically and physically.

Complicating chronic pain conditions are the use, overuse, and abuse of pharmaceutical products prescribed by the medical community to reduce the severity of pain and discomfort. Goodwin (2016) suggests that the use of medications to treat physiological symptoms related to chronic conditions can develop into substance use disorders. Many of the medications prescribed by physicians to treat pain (i.e., opioid analgesics) and co-occurring mental health issues (i.e., alprazolam for treating anxiety, selective serotonin reuptake inhibitors (SSRIs) and benzodiazepines for treating depression) can be highly addictive in nature.

Overall, in the management of chronic pain there are multiple approaches that range from medications such as acetaminophen or nonsteroidal anti-inflammatory drugs (NSAIDs) to corticosteroids and opioid analgesics. Medical technology may be used such as a transcutaneous electrical nerve stimulation (TENS) unit; this is a small battery-operated electronic device placed over the painful area that stimulates nerve fibers to help block pain receptors. Invasive interventions include a nerve block, a surgical procedure whereby the neurologist, physiatrist, or anesthesiologist injects a local anesthetic into the affected area to block or reduce the sensation of pain. Acupuncture is a commonly used procedure based on Chinese medicine that uses fine needles inserted into selected energy vortexes or trigger points with the intention to block pain. Physical therapy may also be helpful with some individuals to decrease pain levels through exercise, and proper body mechanics may be used to increase range of motion, flexion, and extension and to reduce the sensation of pain. Commonly used mental health approaches include stress reduction, regulated breathing, meditation, visualization, relaxation therapies, and cognitive behavioral therapy, as well as biofeedback used in conjunction with talk therapies.

## Assessment of Chronic Pain

The following facilitative questions may be useful to the mental health practitioner to assess the areas of the person's life that are most affected by chronic pain. Based on the person's response, evidence-based treatment or integrative medicine approaches may be facilitated with the goal of decreasing or managing the person's chronic pain condition.

1. What is the location of your pain?
2. How frequently do you experience pain?
3. Describe your pain (i.e., dull, aching, sharp, burning, throbbing).
4. How long does your pain last?
5. If you were to rate your pain on a scale of 1 to 10, with 1 being a pin prick and 10 so severe that you would have to go into an emergency room/hospital, how would you rate this?
6. What activities do you do that tend to cause the onset of pain?
7. What do you do to alleviate the pain?
8. What activities do you engage in that aggravates your pain?
9. What kinds of activities are you able to perform when your pain is present?
10. What activities do you avoid?
11. How does your pain change your daily activities (work, home, school, hobbies, socially, emotionally)?
12. How does your pain affect your relationships with others (family, friends, partner, and so forth)?
13. Are you involved in any litigation related to your pain?

During the initial interview, it may be helpful to receive the input from family members and take a comprehensive history of behavior and personality traits that may predispose the individual for chronic and persistent thoughts, feelings, actions, and experiences that promote increased levels of pain. Overall, chronic pain conditions, particularly as they relate to extraordinary and traumatic experiences, require a treatment team approach coordinating multiple modalities to reach optimal mental and physical well-being.

## SPINAL CORD INJURY

The onset of a traumatic SCI is a physically paralyzing and functionally limiting condition that can disrupt one's independence, family and social life, and employability. There are a number of individualized circumstances within and outside of an individual's control that may or may not assist him or her in maintaining optimal health and quality of life (Marini & Brown, 2016). Specifically, factors such as one's age at onset, premorbid health conditions, injury severity, ethnicity/race, socioeconomic status, education, motivation, support system, and marital status are all key factors supported in the literature regarding outcomes for SCI (Blackwell, Krause, Winkler, & Steins, 2001; Krause & Saunders, 2012).

There are approximately 12,000 new cases of SCI reported annually and an estimated 238,000 to 332,000 persons living with SCI in the United States as of 2013 (National Spinal Cord Injury Statistical Center [NSCISC], 2013). Although over half of all SCIs are between 16 and 30 years of age, the average age of onset has increased from 28.7 years in the mid-1970s to 42 years of age in 2010. Males account for approximately 80% of all injuries that occur from MVAs (36%), falls (28.5%), violence (14.3%), other causes (11%), and sports injuries (9%; NSCISC, 2013). Men engaging in higher risk activities have been cited for a proportionally large percentage of occurrences.

### Spinal Cord Anatomy and Consequence of Injury

At a basic rudimentary level of understanding, our spinal cord essentially acts as a conduit relaying motor messages via billions of nerve cells interconnected from the brain to activate/control our muscles and extremities, while conveying sensory information back to the parietal lobe in the brain. The severity of an injury largely depends on the location on the spinal cord where the neurological lesion occurs. A cervical (C) or neck lesion SCI (damaging the C1–C8 nerve roots) often results in tetraplegia (formerly termed quadriplegia), whereby all four extremities sustain some (incomplete injury) or all (complete injury) functional loss of motor and sensory ability. Each level of a cervical injury carries significant meaning to functional independence. For example, an individual with a C2–C3 SCI typically can only move his or her head, neck, and shoulders, and is ventilator dependent. Such an injury also requires the use of a power wheelchair controlled by head, sip and puff, or voice control technology. Conversely, someone with a C6 SCI has additional musculature of the biceps and wrist extensors that enable the individual to push a manual wheelchair, drive with vehicle modifications, and eat/brush/write/shave with assistive devices (Blackwell et al., 2001). The majority of individuals with cervical injuries require varying levels of caregiving and homemaking assistance, generally ranging from 10 to 24 hours per day (Consortium for Spinal Cord Medicine [CSCM], 1999). Caregiving assistance often includes assistance with dressing, showering, bowel and bladder care, cooking, cleaning, and shopping, which are generally considered ADLs.

Neurologically, aside from a cervical injury affecting all four limbs to some degree, individuals may sustain a thoracic, lumbar, or sacral level lesion SCI termed *paraplegia* that affects the motor and sensory ability sequentially down the spine, impairing some degree of chest, lower back, and lower extremity function. Most persons with paraplegia are able to function almost totally independently on their own in carrying out their ADLs. However, higher level thoracic injuries often require several hours a day of home health care or attendant care assistance (Blackwell et al., 2001; CSCM, 1999). In the vast majority of SCI cases, individuals also lose bowel and bladder functions (neurogenic bowel and bladder); in these situations, catheterization or some other form of urinary collection is required and a suppository or enema is needed for feces evacuation. Relatedly, women with SCI may still have children, although they are typically monitored closely and may be hospitalized earlier by their OB/GYN as they near term for edema or autonomic dysreflexia (for those with T6 or higher injuries). Males often can obtain an erection by direct stimulation, and may maintain an erection with common erectile dysfunction medications and/or assistive devices.

Finally, the secondary complications of SCI should be noted so counselors can be aware of the medical conditions that sometimes disrupt their functional independence or maintaining their daily lives. These conditions once again are exacerbated or more frequent in prevalence depending on the individual's diet, lifestyle, self-care diligence, premorbid disabilities such as obesity or type 2 diabetes, and access to health care (Krause & Saunders, 2012). Common complications include pressure sores, urinary tract infection, respiratory dysfunction such as pneumonia or atelectasis, autonomic dysreflexia, repetitive motion injuries generally involving the shoulders and wrists, osteoporosis, musculoskeletal changes such as atrophy and contractures, chronic pain, and others (Ysasi, Kerwin, Marini, McDaniels, & Antol, 2016).

## Psychological Implications of SCI

How successfully someone adapts or adjusts to SCI is based on a number of individual and environmental factors that are inextricably connected. Specifically, no matter how psychologically strong or mentally prepared an individual is to deal with extreme adversity, if he or she lives in an inaccessible environment with few financial resources, no social support, or no access to assistive technology, then such an individual faces numerous obstacles to his or her physical and mental well-being as well as quality of life (Marini, 2012). For those individuals living in a war-torn or Third World country where daily life is a simple struggle for food, warmth, and safety, persons with SCI would not survive long. Similarly, during the days and weeks following a natural disaster, persons with SCI who are not immediately tended to would not survive, either. Unfortunately, to this day, agencies such as the Federal Emergency Management Agency (FEMA), the Red Cross, and related agencies are ill prepared to house and care for the needs of persons with SCI.

The immediate or acute stage of traumatic SCI generally is one of chaos and shock for the individual and his or her family. Although numerous researchers cite a variety of theories regarding the adjustment or response to disability (Livneh & Antonak, 2005; Marini, 2012), some describe the common stages of adjustment as: (a) initial onset involving shock and anxiety; (b) defense mobilization involving bargaining with God or some higher power for recovery and denial of one's prognosis; (c) initial realization—grief and possibly depression as well as internalized anger or self-blame; (d) retaliation or externalized anger onto others; and (e) final adjustment or reintegration, where the individual mentally and emotionally comes to terms with his or her prognosis and seeks to discover a new disabled self-identity. This grief and loss of self typically lasts months and perhaps years. Varying rates of clinical depression, sometimes cited up to 40% in some studies, can occur, and suicide risk is highest in the first year following injury (Craig, Hancock, & Dickson, 1994; DeVivo, Black, Richards, & Stover, 1991).

Counselors who work with this population should understand that successful adaptation to SCI involves more than just intrinsic motivation, although this is one of many factors. Family and caregiver support is perhaps the most important factor in healthy recovery. Such support is critical in assisting (when needed) with ADLs, emotional support, and socialization into the community. The support of family and friends is also a key factor in enhancing one's self-esteem following SCI (Li & Moore, 1998). In the same vein, this is one disability where the family needs must be given almost equal attention. The ripple effect of the loved one with SCI's needs of caregiver stress, potential financial costs for uncovered medical expenses, role reversal, role strain, potential drop-off of social support and isolation postinjury, and real or perceived societal barriers all require family involvement and/or family counseling (Blanes, Carmagnani, & Ferreira, 2007; Boschen, Tonack, & Gargaro, 2005).

Mental health practitioners would also benefit from knowing the hundreds of assistive devices available in the market to assist persons with SCI to become more independent. There are various websites (see Disability Products, 2016; Disabled World, 2016; Spin Life, 2016) that assist individuals in acquiring driving, transferring, and various sports and exercise equipment; ADLs; voice recognition environmental control units; and devices that interface with computers. Many of the same devices/equipment allow persons with SCI to successfully become employed and attend school. Those with SCI pursuing a postsecondary education have a much greater statistical likelihood of becoming employed than individuals with high school or less education. Unfortunately, over 50% of all persons with SCI remain chronically unemployed for a variety of reasons, including lack of education, ongoing disruptive medical complications, poor family support, lack of transportation, and lack of caregiver assistance (Blackwell et al., 2001).

Overall, over half of all persons with SCI require some level of caregiving support in the home to accomplish ADLs, and this factor alone is critical in the overall picture for greater independence, better health outcomes, and improved quality of life. The injured individual and the family often go through a grieving period of many months while struggling to adapt to family role changes, adjusted finances, uncertain health complications, and caregiver strain. Establishing caregiver support, transportation, and diligent health monitoring; obtaining needed assistive technology; and establishing relevant community supports are all imperative in the successful rehabilitation of persons with SCI.

## CONCLUDING REMARKS

The medical aspects of chronic illness and disability are critical to address during disaster mental health response. Stress researchers report that one of the hallmarks of the stress response, particularly in traumatic stress, is the complex physiological changes that occur in the mind–body from a systemic level. It places the individual at risk for chronic illnesses and disabilities. The combination of medical–physical and mental health injury has both short- and long-term effects on the individual and family members. Therefore, mental health counselors want to familiarize themselves with the residual functional capacity and medical aspects of each of the medical–physical conditions that commonly co-occur in exposure to traumatic events. Ultimately, in disaster recovery complex trauma presents itself as both a mental health and medical–physical health condition.

## REFERENCES

Antai-Otong, D. (2005). Depression and fibromyalgia syndrome (FMS): Pharmacologic considerations. *Perspectives in Psychiatric Care, 41*(3), 146–148.

Baker, L. R., & Cormier, L. A. (2015). *Disasters and vulnerable populations: Evidence-based practice for the helping professions.* New York, NY: Springer Publishing.

Blackwell, T. L., Krause, J. S., Winkler, T., & Steins, S. A. (2001). *Spinal cord injury desk reference.* New York, NY: Demos Medical Publishing.

Blanes, L., Carmagnani, M. I., & Ferreira, L. M. (2007). Health-related quality of life of primary caregivers of persons with paraplegia. *Spinal Cord, 45,* 399–403.

Boschen, K., Tonack, M., & Gargaro, J. (2005). The impact of being a support provider to a person living in the community with a spinal cord injury. *Rehabilitation Psychology, 50,* 397–407.

Brenner, L. A., Betthauser, L. M., Homaifar, B. Y., Villarreal, E., Harwood, J. E. F., Staves, P. J., & Huggins, J. A. (2011). Posttraumatic stress disorder, traumatic brain injury, suicide attempt history among veterans receiving mental health services. *Suicide and Life-Threatening Behavior, 41*(4), 416–423.

Brown, R. E., & Wu, T. Y. (2003). Use of "spare parts" in mutilated upper extremity injuries. *Hand Clinics, 19*(1), 73–87.

Cohen, S. P., & Raja, S. N. (2012). Pain. In L. Goldman & A. I. Schafer (Eds.), *Goldman's Cecil medicine* (24th ed., pp. 133–140). Philadelphia, PA: Elsevier Saunders.

Consortium for Spinal Cord Medicine (CSCM). (1999). *Outcomes following traumatic spinal cord injury: Clinical practice guidelines for health-care professionals.* Washington, DC: Paralyzed Veterans of America.

Craig, A. R., Hancock, K. M., & Dickson, H. G. (1994). A longitudinal investigation into anxiety and depression in the first two years following spinal cord injury. *Paraplegia, 32,* 675–679.

Department of Defense (DoD). (2016). U.S. casualty status: Fatalities as of October 2016. Retrieved from http://www.defense.gov/casualty.pdf

DeVivo, M. J., Black, K. L., Richards, S., & Stover, S. L. (1991). Suicide following spinal cord injury. *Paraplegia, 29,* 620–627.

Disability Products. (2016). Home page. Retrieved from http://www.disabilityproducts.com

Disabled World. (2016). Disability news and information. Retrieved from http://www.disabled-world.com

Falvo, D. R. (2014). *Medical and psychosocial aspects of chronic illness and disability* (5th ed.). Burlington, MA: Jones & Bartlett.

Fordyce, W. E. (1982). Forward. In J. Barber (Ed.), *Psychological approaches to the management of pain* (pp. v–x). New York, NY: Brunner/Mazel.

Goodwin, L. R., Jr. (2016). Treatment for substance use disorders. In I. Marini & M. A. Stebnicki (Eds.), *The professional counselor's desk reference* (2nd ed., pp. 457–468). New York, NY: Springer Publishing.

Government Accountability Office. (2016). Human capital: Additional actions needed to enhance DoD's efforts to address mental health care stigma. Retrieved from http://www.gao.gov/assets/680/676633 .pdf

Herman, J. (1992). *Trauma and recovery: The aftermath of violence: From domestic abuse to political terror.* New York, NY: Perseus Books Group.

Knotkova, H., Crucian, R. A., Tronnier, V. M., & Rasche, D. (2012). Current and future options for the management of phantom limb pain. *Journal of Pain Research, 5,* 39–49.

Krause, J. S., & Saunders, L. L. (2012). Socioeconomic and behavioral risk factors for mortality: Do risk factors observed after spinal cord injury parallel those from the general U.S. population? *Spinal Cord, 50*(8), 609–613.

Lazarus, R. S. (1999). *Stress and emotions: A new synthesis.* New York, NY: Springer Publishing.

Lehavot, K., Der-Martirosian, C., Simpson, T. L., Shipherd, J. C., & Washington, D. L. (2013). The role of military social support in understanding the relationship between PTSD, physical health, and healthcare utilization in women veterans. *Journal of Traumatic Stress, 26,* 773–775.

Levers, L. L. (2012). *Trauma counseling: Theories and interventions.* New York, NY: Springer Publishing.

Li, L., & Moore, D. (1998). Acceptance of disability and its correlates. *Journal of Social Psychology, 138*(1), 13–25.

Livneh, H., & Antonak, R. F. (2005). Psychological adaptation to chronic illness and disability: A primer for counselors. *Journal of Counseling & Development, 83,* 12–20. http://dx.doi.org/10.1002/j.1556–6678.2005.tb00575.x

Marini, I. (2012). Theories of adjustment and adaptation to disability. In I. Marini, N. Glover-Graf, & M. J. Millington (Eds.), *Psychosocial aspects of disability: Insider perspectives in counseling strategies,* (pp. 133–166). New York, NY: Springer Publishing.

Marini, I., & Brown, A. D. (2016). Family care and spinal cord injury. In M. J. Millington and I. Marini (Eds.), *Families in rehabilitation counseling: A community-based approach* (pp. 193–212). New York, NY: Springer Publishing.

Marini, I., & Stebnicki, M. A. (2012). *The psychological and social impact of illness and disability* (6th ed.). New York, NY: Springer Publishing.

Milks, J. W. (2012). Pain. In E. T. Bope & R. D. Kellerman (Eds.), *Conn's current therapy 2012* (pp. 24–31). Philadelphia, PA: Elsevier Saunders.

Miquel, F. (2009). Depression and fibromyalgia: Two distinct disorders with a "hard life" in common. *European Psychiatry, 24,* 661–671.

National Spinal Cord Injury Statistical Center. (2013). Spinal cord injury facts and figures at a glance. Retrieved from https://www.nscisc.uab.edu/PublicDocuments/fact_figures_docs/Facts%202013.pdf

Robinson, R. L., Birnbaum, H. G., Morely, M. A., Sisitsky, T., Greenberg, P. E., & Wolf, W. (2004). Depression and fibromyalgia: Treatment and cost when diagnosing separately or concurrently. *Journal of Rheumatology, 31*(8), 1621–1629.

Sapolsky, R. M. (1998). *Why zebras don't get ulcers: An updated guide to stress, stress-related diseases, and coping.* New York, NY: W. H. Freeman.

Spin Life. (2016). Home page. Retrieved from http://www.spinlife.com

Stebnicki, M. A. (2016). Military counseling. In I. Marini & M. A. Stebnicki (Eds.), *The professional counselor's desk reference* (2nd ed., pp. 499–506). New York, NY: Springer Publishing.

Stiller, R. (1975). *Pain: Why it hurts, where it hurts, when it hurts.* Nashville, TN: Thomas Nelson.

Tomko, J. R. (2012). Neurobiological effects of trauma and psychopharmacology. In L. L. Lopez Levers (Ed.), *Trauma counseling: Theories and interventions* (pp. 59–76). New York, NY: Springer Publishing.

Turk, D. C., Meichenbaum, D., & Genest, M. (1983). *Pain and behavioral medicine.* New York, NY: Guilford Press.

Wachen, S. J., Shipherd, J. C., Suvak, M., Vogt, D., King, L. A., & King, D. W. (2013). Posttraumatic stress symptomatology as a mediator of the relationship between warzone exposure and physical health symptoms in men and women. *Journal of Traumatic Stress, 26,* 319–328.

Warden, D. (2006). Military TBI during the Iraq and Afghanistan wars. *Journal of Head Trauma Rehabilitation, 21*(5), 398–402.

Weil, A. (1995). *Spontaneous healing: How to discover and enhance your body's natural ability to maintain and heal itself.* New York, NY: Fawcett.

Wightman, J. M., & Gladish, S. L. (2001). Explosions and blast injuries. *Annals of Emergency Medicine, 37*(6), 664–678.

Winterowd, C., & Sims, W. F. (2016). Counseling persons with chronic pain. In I. Marini & M. A. Stebnicki (Eds.), *The professional counselor's desk reference* (2nd ed., pp. 565–570). New York, NY: Springer Publishing.

Ysasi, N. A., Kerwin, S., Marini, I., McDaniels, B., & Antol, D. L. (2016). A comprehensive literature review of secondary complications of spinal cord injury. *Journal of Life Care Planning, 14*(1), 25–58.

# CHAPTER 11

# Psychosocial Adjustment Issues in Disaster Mental Health Counseling

Typical persons in the United States spend nearly 12 years of their lives—particularly in their older years—in a state of limited daily functioning because of chronic medical, physical, or psychological conditions (Eisenberg, Glueckauf, & Zaretsky, 1999). Because of the onset of chronic illnesses and disabilities (CIDs), most individuals have significantly higher levels of chronic and persistent stress in their lives (Falvo, 2014). Exposure to extraordinary stressful and traumatic events complicates healing, particularly those persons who have preexisting CIDs. It also profoundly affects the lives of persons who have acquired their disabilities through a disaster incident or critical event. Ultimately, CIDs place most trauma survivors in a high-risk category for dealing with the long-term medical and mental health effects of their disability across multiple life areas (Levers, 2012; Livneh & Antonak, 2005; Marini & Stebnicki, 2012). This chapter offers: (a) an overview of the dynamic process of psychosocial adjustment and adaptation to CID, (b) key variables in coping and resiliency with such chronic and persistent mental and physical health conditions, and (c) recommended treatment interventions to assist mental health counselors in helping others adjust in postdisaster recovery and the rehabilitation process.

The majority of professional counselors (with the exception of rehabilitation counselors) do not have training in working with the psychosocial adjustment issues found in persons with CIDs (Smart, 2016). Most professional counselors who have completed training in traditional counselor education and psychology programs received training in the biomedical model, as opposed to the biopsychosocial model, of disability. They lack training in critical biopsychosocial counseling issues related to disability culture and stigma, disability rights legislation, independent living, job accommodation, and overall psychosocial adjustment issues. This is a significant point because of the combination of medical, physical, and mental health conditions that present in the aftermath of natural, person-made, and biological disasters.

Statistically, the U.S. Census Bureau in 2010 estimated that there are more than 56.7 million Americans with acquired CIDs (U.S. Census Bureau, 2010). The WHO (2016) reports that about one billion persons live with a disability worldwide. Many of these disabilities are caused by motor vehicle accidents; falls causing catastrophic injury; acts of physical, sexual, and intimate partner violence; and war. The medical/physical injuries acquired are of a very serious nature and typically include traumatic brain injury, traumatic amputation, spinal cord injury, musculoskeletal injuries, and chronic pain conditions.

Mental health counselors could benefit greatly from having awareness, knowledge, and skills in working with the unique medical/physical injuries that accompany post-traumatic stress and other mental health conditions. Additionally, having the awareness, knowledge, and skills of working with the cultural attributes of persons with mental and physical disabilities is a therapeutic advantage while integrating services with this vulnerable population.

## PSYCHOSOCIAL ADJUSTMENT AND ADAPTATION TO CID

Psychosocial adjustment, adaptation, and response to CID is a complex interaction that requires a holistic combination of treating the medical, physical, psychological, spiritual, emotional, social, and vocational aspects of the person. The prolonged course of medical and mental health treatment, often uncertain prognosis of different conditions, constant and intense psychosocial stressors, and associated impact on family members all combine to create a profound effect on the lives of persons with disabilities (Falvo, 2014; Marini & Stebnicki, 2012). Indeed, the combination of mental, emotional, psychological, medical, and physical stress complicates adjustment and adaptation to trauma survivors who have acquired permanent and lifelong disabilities.

Psychosocial adjustment to healing trauma has both medical–physical and mental health challenges for trauma survivors. For example, as a result of trauma-based lifesaving medical advances, there are more active duty and military veterans who have survived traumatic injuries than ever before (Jackson, Thoman, Suris, & North, 2012; Pincus, House, Christenson, & Adler, 2014). Regardless if you are at the epicenter of a critical incident as a civilian or combat service member, physical trauma is almost always accompanied by posttraumatic stress-related symptoms and mental health conditions (i.e., depression, anxiety, substance use disorder [SUD]; Livneh & Antonak, 2005; Stebnicki, 2016b). Overall, disaster mental health counselors should be aware of the complex mental and physical trauma adjustment issues involved with healing from natural, person-made, and/or biological disasters. Indeed, such critical events place survivors with chronic and persistent mental and physical health conditions in a higher risk category.

## PSYCHOSOCIAL STAGE MODELS OF DISABILITY

There are a number of stage models offered in the literature regarding psychosocial adaptation to disability, trauma, crisis, grief, and loss (Antonak & Livneh, 1991; Garfield, 1979; Kubler-Ross, 1969; Livneh, 2001; Mitchell & Everly, 1996; Shontz, 1975; Young, 1998). These models emphasize that the (a) prolonged course of treatment, (b) often uncertain prognosis, (c) constant intense psychological–emotional stressors, (d) limited daily functioning, and (e) psychological impact on family and friends all combine to create complications in adjustment and adaptation to extraordinary stressful and traumatic events.

Stage models of psychosocial adjustment and adaptation also make it clear that: (a) there is no universal experience or response to chronic illness, trauma, or disability; (b) a state of final adjustment (sometimes referred to as resolution, acceptance, assimilation, or reintegration) is not always achieved by the individual; and (c) based on the available clinical and empirical evidence, psychological recovery does not follow an orderly sequence of reaction phases. Thus, individuals may experience phases of adjustment on a continuum and may regress to an earlier phase, skip one or more phases, or overlap with other phases (Livneh & Antonak, 2005). Overall, it is suggested that each stage of adjustment requires different coping patterns, may be both maladaptive and adaptive, and has a variety of emotional triggers that hinder the survivor's ability to adapt to his or her experience of trauma, loss, or disability.

The overall intent and purpose of stage models of disability are to assist mental health practitioners with a conceptual clinical perspective of how the individual perceives the consequences of his or her CID and where he or she is at in terms of adjustment, response, and adaptation. It can also assist mental health practitioners in treatment planning and deciding what course of action needs to be facilitated through the rehabilitation process.

Livneh and Antonak (2005) offer the following stage model based on over 25 years of research. This model provides a comprehensive overview of the psychosocial reaction and experiences of a typical person with a CID. Using this model as a guide should assist mental health counselors in conceptually understanding personal adjustment issues and the rehabilitation process for persons with CIDs. Livneh and Antonak (2005) remind us that it is important to recognize first that there are several common assumptions related to all stage models of adaptation. These include the following:

- ▶ Adaptation is a dynamic and individualized process whereby the person's premorbid or preinjury level of functioning may determine how well he or she deals with the loss and grief associated with his or her illness or disability.

- ▶ The adaptation process is not a linear progression; rather, the individual may regress to an earlier phase or skip one or more phases altogether.

- ▶ The duration of each phase of adaptation depends on factors such as age of onset, premorbid personality, prior experience with crisis situations, nature and severity of the illness or disability, extent of social support, and human and financial resources available to the person.

- ▶ Successful transition through the phases of adaptation should produce increased psychological growth and maturity as observed by the person's coping mechanisms.

- ▶ Not all individuals reach the theoretical end point of adaptation and adjustment.

A brief description of the reactions and experiences within each stage of Livneh and Antonak's psychosocial adaptation model is as follows:

*Shock/initial impact:* This is generally perceived as the individual's initial or emergency reaction to the onset of a sudden and severe physical injury or psychological trauma. It is a reaction resulting from the impact of an overwhelming extraordinary stressful event during exposure to combat and is characterized by psychic numbness, depersonalization, cognitive disorganization, and often dramatic loss of communication abilities.

*Anxiety:* This is viewed as a panic reaction typically experienced upon the initial sensing of the magnitude of the physically or psychologically traumatic event. Typical reactions to anxiety are signified by confused thinking, cognitive overload, numerous physiological responses, and purposeless hyperactivity.

*Denial:* This is observed as the painful realization of the extent, duration, and future implications of the chronic illness or disability. It involves the individual reacting resistively, defensively, or minimizing the chronicity of his or her disabling condition. Denial often includes an irrational and unrealistic expectancy of recovery by developing a distorted picture of reality.

*Depression:* This is a reaction often observed among most persons with an acquired mental, emotional, or physical disabling condition. Symptomatology varies depending on the disability and is based on the impact and perceived loss associated with the individual's physical, social, emotional, vocational, and economic functioning. Depending on the person's predisability personality, past reactions to stressors, and other biological and neurochemical attributes, the person often feels helpless, hopeless, isolated, or self-depreciated.

*Anger/hostility:* This represents self-directed anger, resentment, bitterness, and is often associated with feelings of self-blame. Feelings of self-guilt and survivor guilt, as well as self-harm and suicidal ideation, are often observed. This reaction is most evident in persons who realize their impairment is chronic. This is also viewed as the person's attempt to retaliate against other family members or health care professionals. This phase is characterized by aggressive verbal and physical threatening behaviors, antagonistic and overly critical responses to others, and passive–aggressive behaviors.

*Acknowledgment:* This is regarded as the first indication that the individual has cognitively reconciled with or accepted the permanency of his or her chronic or disabling condition. The future implications that result in major life changes are also realized. Persons in this phase attempt to gain a new sense of acceptance and self-concept. They reappraise their life values, and actively seek new meanings and goals that lead them to the final theoretical stage of "adjustment."

*Adjustment/integration and growth:* This is theoretically conceptualized as the final phase of the adaptation process. This involves multiple factors that support the person's total awareness and meaning (affectively and cognitively) of the functional limitations or barriers imposed by the chronic or disabling condition. Persons can be observed reintegrating into their new life situation by fully assimilating and successfully adapting to the environment around them. Individuals who reach this phase reestablish a positive self-worth, realizing the existence of their residual functioning and newly discovered potentials, while actively pursuing and implementing social, vocational, and other goals.

Overall, there are a plethora of personal, social, and emotional supports; person–environment interactions; coping strategies; searches for meaning; and other internal–external resources that influence the outcome of one's overall psychosocial health and well-being during the adjustment process (Livneh, 2001).

## PSYCHOSOCIAL STRESSORS ASSOCIATED WITH CID

Falvo (2014) suggests that the degree of psychosocial stress associated with medical–physical health is often related to the degree of threat it represents to the individual. Potential threats include the following:

- ▶ Threats to one's life and physical well-being
- ▶ Threats to body integrity and comfort as a result of the illness or disability itself, diagnostic procedures, or treatment
- ▶ Threats to independence, privacy, autonomy, and control
- ▶ Threats to self-concept and fulfillment of customary roles
- ▶ Threats to the goals and future plans
- ▶ Threats to relationships with family, friends, and colleagues
- ▶ Threats to economic well-being

Clinical studies demonstrate how persons who are in a constant state of hyperarousal due to high and intense levels of stress exposure have developed significant health problems (Kabat-Zinn, 1990; Sapolsky, 1998; Wachen et al., 2013; Weil, 1995). For some, chronic stress and anxiety can become a persistent pattern involving one's physical, mental, emotional, and cognitive health. Once the emotional brain maps extraordinary stressful and traumatic incidents, this becomes an intense experience that can lead to high levels of chronic stress. Additionally, exposure to traumatic stress can increase oxidative stress, inflammation in brain and nervous system tissue, and the release of multiple stress hormones in the bloodstream creating an enduring neurological pattern, resulting in multiple mental and physical health conditions (Prasad & Bondy, 2015). When CID is acquired during trauma (e.g., traumatic brain injury [TBI], amputation, spinal cord injury) this places the individual in a whole other risk category for multiple mental health conditions (i.e., major depression, anxiety disorders, SUDs, chronic pain conditions).

Overall, as Sapolsky (1998) elucidates, the study of stress and disease is complex because each person turns on his or her stress mechanism differently. Furthermore, we each attribute personal meaning toward how we experience specific stressors, respond differently to stress based on how we perceive or anticipate its intensity, and form a unique pattern response to daily and traumatic stressors.

## COPING STRATEGIES

Coping strategies and stress appraisal have been studied for decades by classical theorists and stress researchers (e.g., Frankl, 1963; Kabat-Zinn, 1990; Lazarus, 1999; Lazarus &

Folkman, 1984; Selye, 1950). The literature specific to how persons with CID cope is also quite vast. Coping has been viewed as a psychological strategy to decrease, modify, or diffuse the impact of stress-related life events (Livneh & Antonak, 2005). The defining characteristics of coping include variables such as how the person: (a) exhibits and experiences coping as a state or traits, (b) controls or manipulates his or her coping strategies, (c) organizes his or her coping style on a range of internal–external characteristics, and (d) responds from an affective, cognitive, and/or behavioral style of coping.

Falvo (2014) describes *coping strategies* as a subconscious mechanism to deal and cope with stress. The intent is for the person to reduce his or her levels of stress and anxiety. Coping styles are particularly relevant for persons coping with CIDs. This is because in psychosocial adjustment to disability, there is a strong need for the person to bring balance, normalcy, productivity, and a certain quality of life back for optimal functioning. There are many coping strategies mentioned in the literature. However, the more common ones associated with persons who have acquired CIDs are as follows:

*Denial:* Extraordinary stressful and traumatic events can be extremely overwhelming for the individual. This can be experienced by the person medically, physically, cognitively, mentally, psychologically, socially, emotionally, and spiritually. As a result of this overwhelming experience, the individual may deny the stark reality of his or her newly acquired disabling condition that many times leaves the person in a dependent state of functioning. Denial can be expressed both consciously and unconsciously, as well as in healthy and unhealthy ways. For example, an individual who may have acquired a spinal cord injury (i.e., C-5 level quadriplegic) may verbalize, "I need to walk again so I can get back to my job as a carpenter." The conscious expression of "the need to work again" is healthy. However, if the person has acquired a permanent condition to the degree where ambulation is not possible, particularly engaging in the physical-exertional levels required to do carpentry, then the individual does not have a realistic grasp of his or her permanently disabling condition, requiring lifelong medical treatment and rehabilitation. Thus, denying the reality of the need for medical treatment and rehabilitation therapy, as well as the existence of one's diminished mental, physical, and cognitive functional capacity, is quite normal and expected. It is a way for the person to cope with the overwhelming odds of his or her predisability functioning. However, if these unconscious or conscious thoughts and expressions persist past a few days or weeks, it is likely the person is in unhealthy denial. This ultimately hinders his or her ability to progress to the point of maximum medical improvement or psychosocial functioning.

*Regression:* Psychosocial response, adaptation, and adjustment to CID as described earlier in this chapter make the assumption that the person develops from one stage of adjustment to another. Once the individual theoretically completes one developmental stage, this produces enhanced psychosocial functioning. The individual then has the confidence, functional ability, self-concept, and mental and emotional balance to achieve other necessary tasks and behaviors, which theoretically moves this person along to optimal functional capacity. However, in *regression* the individual reverts or defaults to an earlier stage of psychosocial adjustment, which signals that he or she did not grow psychologically or emotionally from previous challenges of having a newly acquired CID. Reverting to early stages of dependency is quite normal and even expected with some serious injuries. However, if the person remains in a state of dependency for days, weeks, or months, it is difficult to reach optimal levels of mental and physical well-being. Some individuals intentionally (consciously) or unintentionally (unconsciously) choose *not* to take responsibility for their overall mental/physical health and well-being. This may be seen by others in their environment as poor psychosocial adjustment, exhibiting low or no motivation for daily activities, and/or dependency on others.

*Compensation:* A natural artifact of having reduced physical, mental, or cognitive capacity is to feel, think, or behave in a different manner. Thus, problem-solving with a newly acquired disability becomes a challenge with every daily task. It is quite natural to attempt daily tasks using modifications or accommodations in different environments to deal with the experience of disability. Compensation as a coping strategy is used by persons with CID to counterbalance functional incapacity in one area of life by becoming stronger or more proficient in another area. Persons who use compensation that is directed toward positive goals and outcomes are generally considered resilient because they are trying out new behaviors or challenges not attempted prior to their disabling conditions. For instance, a person with a T-5 spinal cord injury (paraplegic) who has achieved some level of positive psychosocial adjustment and stability decides that he or she would like to join a wheelchair basketball team. This hypothetical person, predisability, was a highly successful business executive who traveled internationally. Even though this person has never played basketball before (predisability), this person is viewed as compensating for his or her disability by trying out an adaptive recreational sport such as wheelchair basketball. Thus, in compensation, when the individual loses functional capacity in one area of life, he or she may try to excel in other areas. At times, persons with disabilities may be seen by others as "overcompensating" for their disabilities, which has negative attributes. For instance, if this same person with a T-5 spinal cord injury wants to try out sky diving, scuba diving, and surfing besides wheelchair basketball, others in the environment may sense that the person has become overinvolved as a way of proving to self and others that physical capacity has not limited his or her ability to function. The concept of overcompensation is not without controversy because most of the time we use our own personal values, philosophy, and beliefs about how others should live their lives. The primary consideration while viewing compensation and overcompensation as a coping strategy is whether the activities or behaviors derive positive benefits to the persons with a disability or if there is harm to self and others.

*Rationalization:* Most individuals have the ability to rationalize, justify, explain, or defend their reasoning for choosing everything from an intimate partner to a particular occupation. It is part of being human. Rationalization as a coping strategy allows the individual to find socially acceptable reasons for his or her behavior. It also serves as a way to provide justification for not accomplishing a task or feeling motivated to achieve therapeutic goals. For most individuals, rationalizing feelings, emotions, thoughts, and behaviors is a personality state or trait and a normal way of being. A primary consideration for assessing the use of rationalization as a coping strategy is to look at the positive and negative effects it has on the person's mental and physical health. In many instances, rationalization serves as an avoidance mechanism or an irrational reaction to something that most others deem healthy.

*Diversion of feelings:* Many individuals with acquired CID feel a range of emotions related to their chronic and persistent disabling condition. Mood and affect can range from a sense of irritability and anger to hostility. Diverting negative emotions and behaviors to others in the external environment (e.g., spouse, family members, health care providers) is unhealthy. Diverting feelings and behaviors internally can be self-destructive and equally unhealthy. Emotional energy that is redirected toward something more positive or has beneficial coping strategies that allow the person to grow psychologically and emotionally should be seen as healthy. Ultimately, the person chooses his or her feelings and actions. A natural artifact of acquired mental and physical trauma is to find a healthy balance of feelings, thoughts, and actions that leads toward optimal levels of psychosocial adjustment and overall well-being.

## CID: A LOSS AND GRIEF RESPONSE

Many individuals who experience permanent medical illness and disabling conditions experience a complex level of psychosocial adjustment related to their residual functional capacity. There are many factors involved in the mental and physical rehabilitation process. Choosing goals with your client and family members in this therapeutic process requires some knowledge related to: (a) stability, (b) progressive nature, (c) episodic nature, (d) degenerative nature, and (e) periods of exacerbation and remission of the individual's CID. It also requires an understanding that loss can be experienced by the individual in the following ways:

- ▶ Loss over the control of one's life and overall independence
- ▶ Loss of a sense of fairness and justice
- ▶ Loss of emotional and mental security
- ▶ Loss of mental capacity to make decisions independently
- ▶ Loss of physical capacity, body image, and ability for sexual or intimate relationships
- ▶ Loss of career identity, vocational opportunities, and ability to progress academically

## FOUNDATIONS OF PSYCHOSOCIAL DISASTER MENTAL HEALTH COUNSELING

The focus of disaster mental health counseling has changed since 2001 because of the: (a) nature, severity, and frequency with which critical incidents have occurred both in the United States and globally (e.g., natural disasters and war); (b) research on the long-term impact of critical incidents, which leads to chronic and persistent mental and physical conditions (e.g., posttraumatic stress disorder [PTSD], suicide completions, SUDs); (c) shift toward critical incidence that creates mass violence and mass causalities (e.g., school shootings, shootings in malls and movie theaters, bombings at sporting events such as the Boston Marathon); (d) negative mental and physical health effects of those serving as primary and secondary responders (e.g., paramedics, police, health care providers, counselors); and (e) emphasis on violence prevention because of the research suggesting that immediate and brief interventions decrease the negative long-term symptoms associated with posttraumatic stress symptoms (e.g., mental health and substance prevention programs, active shooter exercises, recognition of mental health symptoms at work and school). Accordingly, disaster mental health counselors should have the awareness, knowledge, and skills to work with the whole person in disaster recovery, recognizing the effects on mental and physical health of those at the epicenter of the disaster. The following are foundational psychosocial elements that mental health counselors should integrate while facilitating clinical interventions with individuals, groups, families, and communities by extraordinary stressful and traumatic events:

*Recognize the person as a survivor:* Viewing persons as "victims" of traumatic events discounts their survival skills and negatively reinforces the stereotype of being help-less, hopeless, dependent, and defenseless. Although the person may be a victim of violence or a natural disaster, mental health counselors can facilitate interventions that empower individuals to view themselves as "survivors" of such critical inci-dents. The search for meaning begins with the realization that being a survivor has many therapeutic advantages in coping, resiliency, and psychosocial adjustment. The experience of maintaining the "victim role" leads to feelings and thoughts of help-lessness, hopelessness, and dependence.

*Accept that the stressors accompanying traumatic events are real and legitimate:* Persons involved in extraordinary stressful and traumatic events are typically physiologically and psychologically affected and require some short-term therapeutic interventions. Many persons at the epicenter of disaster feel like they are "going crazy" or are "emo-tionally weak" or that "it will always feel this way . . . recovery is not possible." The physiological and psychological effects associated with trauma are a normal response to an abnormal event. Research indicates that generally between 30% and 60% of those individuals most affected by trauma require long-term mental and physical health services. Most trauma survivors do not have somatoform disorders. Rather, most experience the clinical presentation of posttraumatic stress, major depression, anxiety and substance use disorders, and suicide ideation. The research generally agrees that there are at least 30% to 40% of trauma survivors who heal on their own with family and other natural supports.

*Preexisting mental and physical conditions produce a synergistic reaction of a more intense nature:* Researchers have identified that persons with CIDs are among the most vulnerable populations during times of disasters (Baker & Cormier, 2015). It is important to recognize that when trauma strikes, persons with preexisting mental or physical health conditions are most affected. Preexisting mental and physical health can predict posttrauma recovery. The combination and synergistic effects of preexisting conditions (i.e., major depressive, anxiety, and substance use disorders, as well as cardiovascular conditions) may intensify the person's response to an extraordinary stressful or traumatic event. Exposure to extreme stressors or critical incidents may be "trigger events" for those who are under treatment for a current mental or physical health condition. Trauma can exacerbate current medical and mental health conditions, often causing some persons to relapse.

*Empathy fatigue is a natural response to working with persons at intense levels of service:* Empathy fatigue results from a state of psychological, emotional, mental, physical, spiritual, and occupational exhaustion that occurs as the counselor's own wounds are continually revisited by the client's life stories of chronic illness, disability, trauma, grief, and loss (Stebnicki, 2016a). It is of paramount importance that disaster mental health counselors recognize the symptoms of empathy fatigue and the negative shift that occurs within the professional counselor's mind, body, and spirit.

*Interventions should be person-centered as opposed to treating a diagnostic category:* Diagnostic categories and mental health symptoms abound in clinical settings. The old adage "if the only tool you have is a hammer then everything looks like a nail" applies also to mental health professionals who are training to diagnose and treat mental health conditions. Diagnostic categories can be dehumanizing to trauma survivors because it places emphasis on their "mental health conditions" as opposed to having a normal reaction to an abnormal experience. Thus, any treatment efforts must consider the unique individual, sociocultural, and environmental characteristics focusing on symptom relief of the person's acute stress.

*Cultivating rapport is essential with all clients:* Mental health professionals must view trauma survivors in relation to their unique individual, sociocultural, and environmental characteristics. Trauma survivors acquire mental health issues from a variety of sources. Many times the environment itself causes the trauma (e.g., intimate sexual violence, brutal governments in war-torn countries, civil unrest due to civil rights violations). Thus, there may be a general distrust of mental health professionals. Cultivating a genuine and trusting rapport with the use of compassion and empathy is important in gaining a working alliance with the trauma survivor.

*Empowering survivors with natural support systems:* Family, friends, coworkers, faith-based organizations, nonprofit agencies, and other support groups can be pivotal in coping, recovery, and psychosocial adaptation to disaster. Natural support systems by definition are positive influences in the person's life and are readily available to clients in their natural environments: home, school, work, community, spiritual–religious institutions, clubs, and nonprofit organizations. Natural supports change and evolve over time; the natural supports that one utilized last year at this time may not exist because individuals change geographic locations, jobs, schools, and friends. Natural support systems promote independence, responsibility, and psychological, social, and emotional growth for the trauma survivor. Mostly, natural supports can be an extension of the therapeutic environment. Thus, it is critical that mental health professionals know how to cultivate and have individuals and groups tap into natural support system resources. Ultimately, the real therapy takes place before and after a 45-minute therapy session.

*Individuals heal at different rates:* An individual's ability to cope, bounce back, cultivate resiliency, and display hardiness and overall adjustment psychosocially to the grief and loss experienced during a critical incident can vary significantly. Many times psychosocial adjustment to trauma and disability does not fit neatly into a theoretical stage model of adaptation or adjustment. Victor Frankl (1963) sums up this point by suggesting that it is not necessarily the nature of the trauma itself that most affects one's ability to cope psychologically with its consequences, but rather the person's own attitude and perception toward the trauma. Placing expectations and conditions upon trauma survivors for meeting goals, moving along, and coming out of a depressive state requires the mental health professional to view the person qualitatively as a unique individual who comprises many attributes and characteristics. As a society, we particularly place an overemphasis on when persons "should be done grieving" or be "moving along with their grief." As seasoned mental health professionals can attest, each individual heals at his or her own rate, some relapse and regress, and healing is a journey—not the destination.

## CONCLUDING REMARKS

Disaster mental health and crisis response is not a new phenomenon in the counseling and mental health field. In the early 1970s, the psychology and counseling literature was replete with brief and immediate interventions for clients who were in crisis (see Aguilera & Messick, 1974; Lester & Brockopp, 1973; Specter & Claiborn, 1973). Because of increasing trends in violence against groups of people (e.g., minority groups, school children, work-related violence, immigrants, refugees, asylum seekers) and naturally occurring disasters (e.g., hurricanes, floods, earthquakes), there is a need for trained and qualified crisis responders who can intervene with persons who are directly and indirectly affected by the aftermath of extraordinary stressful and traumatic events. Such events require a different understanding and a unique set of strategies to facilitate brief and immediate psychosocial adjustment interventions.

## REFERENCES

Aguilera, D. C., & Messick, J. M. (1974). *Crisis intervention: Theory and methodology* (2nd ed.). St. Louis, MO: C. V. Mosby.

Antonak, R. F., & Livneh, H. (1991). A hierarchy of reactions to disability. *International Journal of Rehabilitation Research, 14*, 13–24.

Baker, L. R., & Cormier, L. A. (2015). *Disasters and vulnerable populations: Evidence-based practice for the helping professions.* New York, NY: Springer Publishing.

Eisenberg, M. G., Glueckauf, R. L., & Zaretsky, H. H. (1999). *Medical aspects of disability: A handbook for the rehabilitation professionals.* New York, NY: Springer Publishing.

Falvo, D. R. (2014). *Medical and psychosocial aspects of chronic illness and disability* (5th ed.). Burlington, MA: Jones & Bartlett.

Frankl, V. E. (1963). *Man's search for meaning.* New York, NY: Pocket Books.

Garfield, C. A. (1979). *Stress and survival: The emotional realities of life-threatening illness.* St. Louis, MO: C. V. Mosby.

Jackson, J., Thoman, L., Suris, A. M., & North, C. (2012). Working with trauma-related mental health problems among combat veterans of the Afghanistan and Iraq conflicts. In I. Marini & M. A. Stebnicki (Eds.), *The psychological and social impact of illness and disability* (6th ed., pp. 307–330). New York, NY: Springer Publishing.

Kabat-Zinn, J. (1990). *Full catastrophe living: Using the wisdom of your body and mind to face stress, pain, and illness.* New York, NY: Dell Publishing.

Kubler-Ross, E. (1969). *On death and dying.* New York, NY: Macmillan.

Lazarus, R. S. (1999). *Stress and emotion: A new synthesis.* New York, NY: Springer Publishing.

Lazarus, R. S., & Folkman, S. (1984). *Stress, appraisal, and coping.* New York, NY: Springer Publishing.

Lester, D., & Brockopp, G. W. (1973). *Crisis intervention and counseling by telephone.* Springfield, IL: Charles C. Thomas.

Levers, L. L. (2012). *Trauma counseling: Theories and interventions.* New York, NY: Springer Publishing.

Livneh, H. (2001). Psychosocial adaptation to chronic illness and disability. *Rehabilitation Counseling Bulletin, 44*(3), 151–160. http://dx.doi.org/10.1177/003435520104400305

Livneh, H., & Antonak, R. F. (2005). Psychological adaptation to chronic illness and disability: A primer for counselors. *Journal of Counseling & Development, 83,* 12–20. http://dx.doi.org/10.1002/j.1556-6678.2005.tb00575.x

Marini, I., & Stebnicki, M. A. (2012). *The psychological and social impact of illness and disability* (6th ed.). New York, NY: Springer Publishing.

Mitchell, J. T, & Everly, G. S. (1996). *Critical incident stress debriefing: An operations manual for the prevention of traumatic stress among emergency services and disaster workers* (2nd ed.). Ellicott City, MD: Chevron Publishing.

Pincus, S. H., House, R., Christenson, J., & Adler, L. E. (2014). The emotional cycle of deployment: Military family perspective. Retrieved from http://www.military.com/spouse/military-deployment/dealing-with-deployment/emotional-cycle-of-deployment-military-family.html

Prasad, K. N., & Bondy, S. C. (2015). Common biochemical defects linkage between post-traumatic stress disorders, mild traumatic brain injury (TBI) and penetrating TBI. *Brain Research, 1599,* 103–114.

Sapolsky, R. M. (1998). *Why zebras don't get ulcers: An updated guide to stress, stress-related diseases, and coping.* New York, NY: W. H. Freeman.

Selye, H. (1950). Stress and the general adaptation syndrome. *British Medical Journal, 1,* 1383. http://dx.doi.org/10.1136/bmj.1.4667.1383

Shontz, F. C. (1975). *The psychological aspects of physical illness and disability.* New York, NY: MacMillan.

Smart, J. (2016). Counseling individuals with disabilities. In I. Marini & M. A. Stebnicki (Eds.), *The professional counselor's desk reference* (2nd ed., pp. 417–421). New York, NY: Springer Publishing.

Specter, G. A., & Claiborn, W. L. (1973). *Crisis intervention: A topical series in community-clinical psychology.* New York, NY: Behavioral Publications.

Stebnicki, M. A. (2016a). From empathy fatigue to empathy resiliency. In I. Marini & M. A. Stebnicki (Eds.), *The professional counselor's desk reference* (2nd ed., pp. 533–545). New York, NY: Springer Publishing.

Stebnicki, M. A. (2016b). Military counseling. In I. Marini & M. A. Stebnicki (Eds.), *The professional counselor's desk reference* (2nd ed., pp. 499–506). New York, NY: Springer Publishing.

U.S. Census Bureau. (2010). Nearly 1 in 5 people have a disability in the U.S., Census Bureau reports. Retrieved from https://www.census.gov/newsroom/releases/archives/miscellaneous/cb12-134.html

Wachen, J. S., Shipherd, J. C., Suvak, M., Vogt, D., King, L. A., & King, D. W. (2013). Posttraumatic stress symptomatology as a mediator of the relationship between warzone exposure and physical health symptoms in men and women. *Journal of Traumatic Stress, 26,* 319–328.

Weil, A. (1995). *Spontaneous healing.* New York, NY: Ballantine.

World Health Organization. (2016). Injury-related disability and rehabilitation. Retrieved from http://www.who.int/violence_injury_prevention/disability/en

Young, M. A. (1998). *The community crisis response team training manual* (2nd ed.). Washington, DC: National Organization for Victim Assistance.

# CHAPTER 12

# Career Transition in Disaster Mental Health

## VOCATIONAL AND OCCUPATIONAL IMPACT OF DISASTER

For many Americans, education, jobs, and careers take up a majority of one's waking hours (Szymanski & Parker, 2010). Current research in occupational choice suggests that work positively affects the mental health of individuals because it provides structure and life satisfaction, and improves the social, psychological, and physical health of those engaged in work activities (Arnold, Turner, Barling, Kelloway, & McKee, 2007; Fabian, 2016). One unmistakable difference between Americans and natural-born citizens of countries at the epicenter of war or natural disaster is the amount of opportunities that Americans have for the pursuit of education, jobs, and careers. In the case of immigrants, refugees, or asylum seekers, where the life and safety of the family depend on frequent geographic relocations, the psychological stress of trauma exposure, and the fight for basic survival, return to school and work is not even an immediate consideration (Stebnicki, 2015). Thus, in many noncapitalistic and socialistic cultures where there are few if any opportunities for education, jobs, or careers, the focus may be on food, shelter, clothing, and minimal government resources to sustain the family. Regardless of what country you are from, education and work activities are important to one's emotional and physical well-being. At least in the United States, education and vocational pursuits beyond high school are of critical importance and a pathway to sustainable careers.

Traditional disaster mental health counseling focuses on the survivor's medical and psychological health (Stebnicki, 2016). Psychological first aid and other stress debriefing approaches are essential within the hours and days of many natural disasters and other person-made tragedies. In the immediate aftermath of a disaster and trauma, first responders work to triage persons with the most severe medical and psychological conditions. Others on a crisis management team assist in arranging temporary structures that provide basic food, shelter, and clothing. Although one's medical and psychological health is of critical importance in disaster recovery, getting back to balance requires working with the holistic needs of disaster survivors. For school-age children and adolescents, this would include going back to school in the days and weeks that follow a disaster. For those who have jobs and careers, return to work may be essential to maintain financial stability in the family. Certainly, return to work and/or school is particularly complicated for individuals with severe chronic medical, physical, and psychological health conditions.

The intent of this chapter is to offer mental health counselors the knowledge and skills to assist disaster and trauma survivors in the return-to-work and/or school process. Skilled and competent counselors are mindful of multiple resources that facilitate the survivor's experience of "getting back to normal" by helping the survivor: (a) search for predisaster resiliency traits that can carry them through the "new normal" using career counseling approaches, (b) understand the residual physical, mental, emotional, and vocational capacities that would assist them in the return-to-work/return-to-school process, and (c) engage in career exploration and transferable skills analysis that would assist the person/client with new job and educational opportunities. The assumption is made in this chapter that the trauma or disaster survivor: (a) is willing and motivated, and has the mental and physical capacity to engage in work activities and (b) has some degree of medical, physical, cognitive, and psychological stability. Overall, skilled and competent professionals make attempts to work with the holistic needs of individuals by facilitating postdisaster recovery strategies that assist the person/client to transition into the "new normal" way of life.

## VOCATIONAL AND CAREER TRANSITION AFTER TRAUMA

Why is vocational, career, and educational transition so difficult after exposure to trauma and disaster? For obvious reasons, individuals may lack the medical, physical, or mental health capacity for returning to work or school. Assuming that the individual has reached optimal medical and psychological functioning and has attained some level of stability, multiple resources (e.g., family, friends) and supports (e.g., financial) that existed pretrauma/disaster may be depleted in the recovery process. Exposure to traumatic stress also has the long-term effects of decreased ability to concentrate, focus, be productive, and perform essential job tasks (Stebnicki, 2012). Indeed, with the presence of posttraumatic stress symptoms there is a productivity cost to employers and a psychological consequence to employees. This can lead to extended absences, termination, and separation from work activities.

Other factors in returning to work after trauma and disaster include the reality of today's world of work that is characterized by company takeovers, mergers, downsizing, and an increase in workplace violence. Trauma and disaster exposure, whether acquired at work (e.g., workplace violence) or outside the work environment, has a financial cost to employers. The cost to businesses is somewhere between $3 and $5 billion per year. These costs are related to lower employee productivity, increased absenteeism, time spent in visits to health care practitioners, and overall higher employee turnover (Peterson & Gonzalez, 2005).

Employers, companies, and organizations many times are reliant on health care practitioners' (i.e., physicians, physical therapists, mental health counseling) ability to assist in the return-to-work process (Shrey & Lacerte, 1995). They generally do well preparing workers for health and wellness opportunities (e.g., health club/fitness programs) or through employee assistance programs for short-term brief mental health interventions (e.g., divorce, grief, loss, substance abuse). Many midlevel managers and top executives regularly attend educational seminars and training that assist in fulfilling leadership roles, as well as organizational and managerial skills. At a minimum, companies across a variety of industries (e.g., retail store chains, service or fast food industry, sales) provide basic skills training programs to their employees. Many companies want employees who are good problem solvers, flexible and adaptable to new work processes (i.e., computer software programs), and perform multiple jobs proficiently and effectively (Bissonnette, 1994).

Despite intensive organizational training and development programs, most employers do little to train their employees and managers on how to deal with the psychological/emotional stress of work, especially after trauma exposure within the worker community such as an incidence of workplace violence (Peterson & Gonzalez, 2005). It is typically the responsibility of the employee to seek mental health assistance. Thus, mental health practitioners are called upon to facilitate new meaning and approaches that help bring employees back to balance in the aftermath of trauma or disaster. It is of paramount importance that mental health counselors not just treat the "mental health condition" or "diagnosis." Rather, skilled and competent mental health professionals utilize strategies that bring meaning to their clients' lives whether it is a job, relationship, or their psychological and emotional well-being. If career transition is necessary, then mental health professionals should be available to assist in utilizing some of the approaches offered in this chapter.

## MENTAL AND PHYSICAL CHALLENGES IN RETURN TO WORK

Assuming that trauma exposure and disaster have depleted the individual's mental and physical resources and have resulted in unemployment, then why is it difficult for survivors to independently prepare for, seek, and maintain employment? The truth is that career development is difficult for almost everyone and it takes a skilled and competent professional counselor to assist in navigating career exploration and job seeking. It is especially difficult for the person with chronic medical, physical, and psychological health conditions who has a decreased capacity for personal resiliency and coping skills (Department of Labor [DOL], 2016; Stebnicki, 2012).

The use of mental–physical functional capacity evaluations is paramount in finding the right job match for persons with acquired mental health, as well as psychiatric, neuro-cognitive, and medical–physical conditions that limit job efficiency and productivity (Marini, 2016). These individuals in particular have multiple challenges that may require the use of pharmaceutical products, medical equipment, assistive technology, or on-the-job accommodations so the employee can perform work safely and productively. At the very minimum, mental health professionals can employ career counseling strategies for career exploration and find transferable skills to other careers and occupations.

Competent and high functioning professional counselors can offer more than mental health counseling in disaster recovery after medical and mental health stabilization.

At some point in the therapy session, mental health professionals may need to ask questions such as—*What are some next steps you thought about in your return to work/ school? Would you be open to engaging in some career exploration activities? Given your current situation (e.g., unemployed, disabled), what are some current career/academic obstacles or challenges you see for yourself during the next year or so?* Such questions can be daunting for clients if they have not achieved some level of mental or physical stability. Thus, it is essential that mental health professionals are skilled and competent in assessing the client's work readiness at the very minimum. If mental health professionals do not have the training or background to perform vocational assessment, assist in career exploration and work readiness strategies, and analyze occupations consistent with the client's functional mental and physical capacity for good job matches, then they may want to consider special training.

Mental health counselors have traditionally worked independently of other professional counselors (e.g., career counselors, school counselors, substance abuse counselors) and have minimally engaged in the coordination of client services. Despite these gaps in services for clients in the aftermath and recovery process, counseling strategies that assist in the functional capacity for the return to school or work process have therapeutic value (Sligar & Thomas, 2016).

## WORK READINESS AND FUNCTIONAL CAPACITY EVALUATIONS

If mental health counselors truly want to work with the holistic needs of trauma and disaster survivors and assist them in getting back to their normal work and school routines, they first and foremost want to assess their clients' mental and physical capacity for work. The structured and formal physical capacity assessments are typically performed by medical practitioners, particularly in cases where a chronic illness or disability has been acquired, which may ultimately hinder the person's ability to return to work (Cooke, 2009; Marini, 2016). Despite the structured medical–physical capacity assessments, there are many other functional assessments that mental health counselors can perform in order to assess the client's residual psychological and mental capacity for his or her return to work. Several functional capacity evaluations are offered in the next sections that help mental health professionals determine the physical, mental, and emotional capacities of their clients' ability for work. It is critical that mental health counselors address the vocational implication of the individual's mental and emotional health in the return-to-work process.

### Assessment of Work Readiness

The following guidelines are offered as an assessment checklist for work readiness:

▶ What degree of medical, physical, functional, psychological, emotional, and vocational stability does the client exhibit?

▶ Does the client have a chronic and persistent medical/physical or mental health condition that is progressive, episodic, or stable in nature?

▶ What resources and supports does the client have to assist him or her in getting back to balance medically/physically, psychologically, or emotionally?

▶ How would you describe your client's coping, hardiness, and resiliency skills?

▶ Is your client motivated to return to school and/or work?

## Assessment of Cognitive Behavioral Stress Capacity

The following functional capacity assessments are typical items in 10 separate categories that are addressed in the assessment of the client's cognitive, behavioral, and stress capacity as it relates to his or her work readiness.

1. Describe the client's ability to perform the following cognitive activities:

    ▶ Remember simple instructions on a short-term basis?

    ▶ Able to read and write?

    ▶ Able to organize, plan, and initiate an activity?

    ▶ Able to concentrate and stay focused long enough to complete a task?

2. Describe how the client typically interacts with coworkers or supervisors:

    ▶ Impulsive (says things he or she did not really mean to say)?

    ▶ Feels irritable working around others?

    ▶ Feels awkward in social situations (such as coffee breaks or lunchtime)?

    ▶ Feels frustration or anger?

    ▶ Feels nervous?

    ▶ Feels depressed?

3. How would you characterize your client's quality or productivity of work? Do you feel the client has difficulties with completing work tasks with sufficient:

    ▶ Accuracy?

    ▶ Speed?

    ▶ Quality?

4. Does the client feel excessive amounts of fatigue at the end of the day?

5. Does the client get headaches on a regular basis (not on occasion)?

6. Does the client have difficulty sleeping at night? Difficulties getting up in the morning?

7. Describe how your clients experience stress (mental or physical). How do they relieve stress?

8. Are there any things that your client enjoys doing outside of work life? Hobbies? Special interests? Social visits?

9. Describe how your client spends a typical day.

10. Describe work activities that your client perceives that he or she cannot do or would have difficulty doing.

## Physical Residual Functional Capacity Assessment Questionnaire

To assist mental health professionals in the assessment of the client's work readiness, the following assessment of physical residual functional capacity is offered.

### Exertional Limitations

1. What is the maximum amount of weight that you can lift and/or carry?

2. What is the amount of weight that you can lift and/or carry on a frequent daily basis?

3. For what period of time are you able to stand without having to sit down?

4. How far can you walk?

5. For what period of time are you able to sit at one time without having to stand up?

6. How much weight can you push or pull?

7. How well are you able to climb on such objects as stairs or a ladder?

Rate the following items in the Postural Limitations section using the traditional worker traits scale: N = none or never; O = occasional; F = frequent; C = constant.

### Postural Limitations

8. Are you able to do any of the following physical activities?

Climb stairs?

Balance (on an object such as a ladder or scaffold)?

Bend forward/backward?

Stoop?

Kneel?

Crawl?

Crouch?

### Handling/Manipulative Limitations

9. Are you able to do any of the following tasks that involve your arms and hands?

Reaching overhead and sideways?

Handling large objects?

Fingering or utilizing fine motor manipulative skills?

## Visual Limitations

10. How good is your vision for any of the following?

    Reading or seeing objects close to you?

    Seeing objects at a distance?

    Seeing objects that are in your peripheral vision?

## Hearing Limitations

11. Do you have any problems with your hearing?

## Environmental Limitations

12. Do you have any problems when you are around any of the following environmental conditions?

    Extreme cold?

    Extreme heat?

    Wetness/humidity?

    Dust, odors, fumes?

## CAREER RESILIENCY

Mental health professionals who work in disaster recovery have many opportunities to assist clients with stress, trauma, depression, and substance use disorders. All of these mental health conditions affect the person's return to work and school. Accordingly, mental health professionals may be in the best position to assist their clients with career counseling and development activities because they are attuned to the mental, emotional, social, and psychological health of the individual. Mental health counselors have opportunities to serve in multiple roles to assist clients in accomplishing career goals and educational opportunities. Mental health professionals can gain therapeutic leverage with their clients as they seek to understand the vocational impact of their clients' mental health conditions. Career counseling strategies can be offered to clients engaged in job seeking activities such as career exploration, resume and cover letter writing, interviewing skills, dealing with workplace stress, defining transferable skills to other occupations that are potential job matches, and other skills to seek and maintain employment. The resources and materials in this chapter help mental health counselors facilitate strategies to transform a trauma disaster victim into a survivor. As many who are at the epicenter of trauma and disaster cannot return to school or work, mental health professionals can provide multiple recovery interventions such as enriched career and vocational services.

### Career Resiliency Portfolio (CRP)

The following material is based on the commonly utilized CRP. CRPs are utilized primarily as a career counseling tool directed toward assisting clients, particularly persons with mental and physical disabilities, to identify careers, interests, and aptitudes; develop awareness of strengths and limitations; and cultivate career resiliency traits (Szymanski, 1999). CRPs can be used as a compass for navigating career direction. It is particularly useful for those who have not had opportunities for independent decision making, for acquiring traditional work experiences, and for building specific skills and competencies that would potentially transfer into multiple careers. Overall, CRPs involve career counseling strategies that can assist clients in career transition and develop job seeking skills in the multiple work settings.

A good place to begin the career counseling process is to get a better idea of what the client did prior to his or her trauma or disaster exposure. This can be done through the following steps:

1. Complete a work history form asking the person to detail his or her past occupations, job title, role and function of his or her job, work tasks, job duties, tools and materials used to do his or her job, knowledge acquired from past work, specialized training, and any other piece of information that he or she can legally share.

2. Acquire information about the highest level of grade completed; favorite subjects in school; college major, if any; practical, internship, or mentoring experiences; credentials or certifications earned before, during, and after the service; vocational, technical, or any specialized training; and any other information related to academic training and certifications.

3. Ask: What are your career/educational goals? What would you really like to do in life? Where do you see yourself working now or a few years from now?

Now that you have some basic information about your client's work history, career, and/or educational goals, try using the following sample career exploration questions as a nontraditional career exploration tool. Notice that some of the questions and information you gather are more demographic in nature. However, the open-ended questions assist counseling professionals in obtaining deeper material. Thus, the following questions may be used to collect information regarding your client's total life experiences. This would include, but is not limited to, values and beliefs regarding career, education, and work; identification of critical mental and physical capacities that may hinder employment or educational opportunities; barriers to his or her career path; or resiliency skills he or she can draw upon while in career transition.

## Sample Career Counseling Exploration Interview Questions

1. Tell me something interesting about you as a person.

2. What is your family or home life like—what was it like when you were in service or deployed?

3. Tell me some things that are unique about yourself—or unique in regard to your cultural background.

4. Do you have any special interests, hobbies, or activities that you like to do?

5. What things in life do you feel that you are most talented or gifted at doing? What things come the easiest for you?

6. What things have other people (family, friends) complemented you on in terms of what you are best at doing?

7. If you could do more of what you wanted to do in a job, what would that be like— what would that look like for you?

8. When you think back over your life, what have been some of your greatest achievements and accomplishments in life?

9. What have been some of your greatest challenges or hardships that have confronted you in your life?

10. Discuss some things that you feel would stand in the way (or that would be a barrier for you) in fulfilling your employment or career goals.

11. Do you have any specific limitations that you could share with me—ones that may interfere with employment or that may be a barrier to your career goals?

12. Do you have any special academic, educational, or job training?

13. Describe your past work experiences to me. What jobs have you held in the past? How did you perform these jobs? What were some of the special skills or knowledge that you had to have to perform your job effectively?

14. Talk about some things in your past work that you would totally like to avoid.

15. If you could have any job in the world, what would you want to be doing? What would be your dream job?

16. What are some immediate goals (short and long term) that you have at this moment?

## Career Self-Assessment

Career self-assessments can assist your client with narrowing down his or her worker traits, interests, and goals. There are three types of career assessments: (a) tested interests (use of standardized and nonstandardized assessments), (b) manifest interests (those interests that have developed through a lifetime of career development), and (c) expressed interests (verbalizing interests such as the 16 questions listed in the previous section). You can utilize some of the career self-assessment tools as found in the References section, but make sure that your client completes his or her own self-assessment. You can then help your client interpret and summarize this self-assessment information. Make sure that your client can verbalize, summarize, and identify salient features concerning his or her self-assessment. This includes some of the 16 sample career exploration questions in the previous section. Make sure that you use good facilitative skills and share what you "heard" your client say in regard to the content, feelings, emotions, or other experiences that you could share with your client. As you review his or her career self-assessment, help your client identify important items on his or her assessment such as the identification of satisfactions and dissatisfactions, likes and dislikes, preferences, and so forth. Feel free to use additional assessments if you are qualified to administer them (e.g., standardized tests that reflect aptitude, abilities, skills, personality traits, workplace stress).

## Personal Life Story or Testimonial

Guide your client to write a personal life story or testimonial that is educational, as well as work and career related. Writing engages a different part of the brain and allows the individual to communicate deeper thoughts and insight as opposed to answering questions impulsively or in free form. The personal life story or testimonial should include, at a minimum, work or professional experiences, interests, aptitudes, special skills and abilities, hobbies, key decisions, personal experiences, peak insights that prompted them to their specific educational or career paths, significant life events or adversity that helped them cultivate who they are, and lastly, where they see themselves going in life. The intention of the life story/testimonial for your client is to begin building career and personal resiliency skills. There are some items that your client could share with an employer and others that they may only share with you, the mental health professional. This material can be utilized to facilitate self-awareness and insight as to where they came from and where they are going.

## Applications, Cover Letters, and Resumes

Now that you have abundant information on your client, you can assist him or her in completing the basic job applications and develop cover letters and resumes using the multiple resources in the References section. Cover letter and resume guidelines are offered in the next section as a checklist of essential items to assist mental health professionals in creating these documents. Your client may have had few experiences in careers and career exploration. Thus, you might have to take more responsibility for facilitating such strategies. Remember that your client has an application, cover letter, and resume as the first employer contacts. It is critical that you help guide your client through this process so that he or she can present himself or herself in the most positive, competent, and skillful manner to an employer.

## Cover Letter and Resume Review Form

Effectiveness rating scale:

1 = Not effective at all

2 = Only slightly effective

3 = Moderately effective

4 = Very effective

5 = Extraordinarily effective

### Cover Letter

1. Does the first paragraph of the letter explain the reason that the job seeker is writing? What does he or she want from the person or organization/company? How did he or she become familiar or come to contact the person or organization/company?                                           Rating_____

2. Does the second paragraph highlight the person's accomplishments? Does it appear to match the elements or tasks in the job he or she is applying for?   Rating_____

3. Does the third paragraph demonstrate good closure by communicating to the employer how the applicant intends to follow-up?                    Rating_____

4. Overall, how is the readability of the cover letter? Is it direct, concise, to the point, written grammatically correct, and flow easily?          Rating_____

## Resume

At a minimum, has the student included the following items (check all that apply)?

Job Objective:____

Education/Degree(s):____

Professional Employment Experience:____

Volunteer Experience:____

Professional Affiliations/Organizations:____

Special Abilities and Projects:____

1. How effectively does the resume communicate the person's educational background?                                                              Rating_____

2. How effectively does the resume highlight the person's qualifications in regard to his or her professional experiences?                           Rating_____

3. How effectively does the resume communicate the person's volunteer experience?                                                                   Rating_____

4. How effectively does the resume demonstrate the person's professional activities?
                                                                     Rating_____

5. How effectively does the resume highlight the person's special abilities and projects?                                                           Rating_____

6. After reviewing the cover letter and resume tips found in the various class materials, comment on how well the writer considered some of these important points:

_____

_____.

## CONCLUDING REMARKS

Dealing with the disaster or trauma survivors' medical and psychological health is of critical importance in disaster recovery. However, getting back to balance requires working with the holistic needs of disaster survivors. For school-age children and adolescents, this would include going back to school in the days and weeks that follow a disaster. For those who have jobs and careers, return to work may be essential to maintain financial stability in the family. Certainly, return to work and/or school is particularly complicated for individuals with severe chronic medical, physical, and psychological health conditions. Thus, it is critical that mental health counselors have the awareness, knowledge, and skills to work with the career and educational transition needs of disaster and trauma survivors. Work and school can be therapeutic outcomes. Even though traditional mental health counseling does not deal in vocational assessment and career counseling as its primary focus, this chapter offers the primary career counseling tools to assist disaster survivors on the path to healing trauma in a holistic sense.

## REFERENCES

Arnold, K. A., Turner, N., Barling, J., Kelloway, E. K., & McKee, M. C. (2007). Transformational leadership and psychological well-being: The mediating role of meaningful work. *Journal of Occupational Health Psychology, 13*, 193–203.

Bissonnette, D. (1994). *Beyond traditional job development: The art of creating opportunity.* Santa Cruz, CA: Milt Wright & Associates.

Cooke, C. (2009). Work capacity evaluation and return to work rates. The Thirteenth National Forum on Issues in Vocational Assessment: Sponsored by Vocational Evaluation and Career Assessment Professionals. Auburn University, Auburn, Alabama.

Department of Labor. (2016). America's heroes at work: Veterans hiring toolkit. Retrieved from http://www.dol.gov/vets/ahaw

Fabian, E. S. (2016). Occupational choice and the meaning of work. In I. Marini & M. A. Stebnicki (Eds.), *The professional counselor's desk reference* (2nd ed., pp. 261–265). New York, NY: Springer Publishing.

Marini, I. (2016). Understanding mental and physical functional capacity evaluations. In I. Marini & M. A. Stebnicki (Eds.), *The professional counselor's desk reference* (2nd ed., pp. 321–327). New York, NY: Springer Publishing.

Peterson, N., & Gonzalez, R. C. (2005). *The role of work in people's lives: Applied career counseling and vocational psychology* (2nd ed.). Belmont, CA: Thomson Brooks/Cole.

Shrey, D. E., & Lacerte, M. (1995). *Principles and practices of disability management in industry.* Winter Park, FL: GR Press.

Sligar, S. R., & Thomas, S. W. (2016). What counselor should know about vocational assessment and evaluation. In I. Marini & M. A. Stebnicki (Eds.), *The professional counselor's desk reference* (2nd ed., pp. 339–350). New York, NY: Springer Publishing.

Stebnicki, M. A. (2012, April). *Psychosocial aspects of chronic illness and disability: Integral approaches for healing the mind, body, and spirit.* Presentation given at the Annual Conference of the North Carolina Rehabilitation Counselors Association (NCRCA) and the Vocational Evaluation and Work Adjustment Association (VEWAA), Pine Knoll Shores, NC.

Stebnicki, M. A. (2015, October). *The psychosocial cost of war on non-military civilian populations: A global perspective.* Presentation given at the Annual Conference of the Licensed Professional Counseling Association of North Carolina, Raleigh, NC.

Stebnicki, M. A. (2016). Disaster mental health response and stress debriefing. In I. Marini & M. A. Stebnicki (Eds.), *The professional counselor's desk reference* (2nd ed., pp. 439–447). New York, NY: Springer Publishing.

Szymanski, E. M. (1999). Disability, job stress, the changing nature of careers, and the career resiliency portfolio. *Rehabilitation Counseling Bulletin, 42*(4), 279–289.

Szymanski, E. M., & Parker, R. M. (2010). *Work and disability: Contexts, issues, and strategies for enhancing employment outcomes for people with disabilities.* Austin, TX: Pro-Ed.

# CHAPTER 13

# Interventions in Disaster Mental Health Counseling

## A NEW GENERATION OF DISASTER MENTAL HEALTH COUNSELORS

Catastrophic events have accelerated worldwide within the past 15 years. In America, the horrific terrorist attacks of Tuesday, September 11, 2001, and the devastation that took place from Hurricane Katrina that took place on August 29, 2005, left emotional, physical, spiritual, and environmental scars upon our minds, bodies, and spirits. The desolation left in the aftermath has created a sort of historical trauma among Westerners. This has prompted a consciousness shift within the mental health counseling field and other allied helping professions. Since 9/11, there have been a multitude of other catastrophic events that have required the direct and indirect interventions of mental health counselors. Indeed, medical and physical interventions by first responders are critical for survival. The psychological first aid and mental health rescue in the aftermath and recovery phase are critical in working with individuals, families, and communities that have experienced civil unrest, acts of terrorism, school shootings, workplace violence, and the unending natural events that keep the Earth out of balance, such as fires, floods, hurricanes, tornadoes, and droughts.

There are many geographic regions of the planet that are not safe places to live. In part, many areas of the United States, as well as the world, have been destabilized by human engineering and climate change; hence, they are prone to natural disasters (e.g., hurricanes, floods, tornadoes, tsunamis, earthquakes). Since World War II, person-made disasters have grown exponentially (e.g., war, civil unrest, genocide, ethnic cleansing) along with a host of biological pandemics (e.g., HIV/AIDS, Ebola, Zika viruses). Each of these catastrophic events requires a multitude of first responders to provide medical, physical, psychological, emotional, social, and psychosocial first aid.

We are all impacted by critical incidents in the United States and abroad. Critical incidents are replayed on the nightly news, and we are all affected at some level of consciousness. As a consequence, many in the United States may be experiencing the emotional, social, physical, spiritual, and occupational exhaustion that is associated with a new world at war, the daily threat of global terrorism, and natural disasters that have increased in frequency and intensity (Stebnicki, 2008, 2016; Stebnicki & Marini, 2016). The psychosocial impact of catastrophic events creates multiple mental health conditions (i.e., depression, anxiety, posttraumatic stress, and substance abuse disorders) and creates functional limitations that can become disabling for individuals, families, and communities.

It is of paramount importance that we cultivate, recruit, train, and prepare a new generation of skilled and competent mental health counselors to provide services in the specialty areas of: (a) disaster mental health response, (b) counseling approaches that focus on issues related to complex grief, death, and dying, (c) counselors who specialize in various models of critical incident response for specific incidents (i.e., school shootings, terrorism, pandemics), and (d) counselor education programs that dedicate curriculum and practical experiences for coping with stress, reducing posttraumatic stress symptoms, and cultivating resiliency skills.

This chapter offers (a) a practical approach for facilitating disaster mental health response using a variety of models, (b) specific guidelines for structuring such interventions and responding to individuals and groups, and (c) resources to assist in graduate training and professional development within this specialty area known as disaster mental health response. Additionally, three case scenarios are provided at the end of the chapter for the purpose of practicing the skills of disaster mental health and stress debriefing interventions.

A variety of mental health disaster response models and strategies exist for mental health professions to acquire the skills of clinical interventions. The intent of this chapter is not to discuss the plethora of disaster or trauma theories, models, strategies, and interventions or endorse any one particular model over another. The intent is to offer a practical approach using the structure of multiple stress debriefing models that can be facilitated in a variety of person-made and natural disasters. The interested reader is encouraged to review the reference section for additional resources.

## DISASTER MENTAL HEALTH RESPONSE MODELS: COMMONALITIES IN APPROACHES

While medical professionals, police, and rescue workers all prepare for the physical rescue in the multitude of disaster scenarios, mental health professionals are called upon to provide the mental health rescue. Today, many counselors and other human service professionals are required to have training in various models of crisis intervention and critical incident response. These include, but are not limited to (listed in alphabetical order): Acute Traumatic Stress Management (ATSM, 2016), American Red Cross (ARC, 2016), Disaster Mental Health response model, Critical Incident Stress Debriefing (CISD, 2016), Critical Incident Stress Management (CISM, 2016), National Organization for Victim Assistance (NOVA, 2016) Group Crisis response model, and Psychological First Aid (National Center for Posttraumatic Stress Disorder [NCPTSD], 2016).

There are many other crisis and disaster response models, many of which are organization specific and include protocols found in other models as cited previously.

Others have adopted their own training programs and crisis response certifications such as the Department of Homeland Security, Environmental Protection Agency, commercial airline industry, banking industry, computer and Internet cyber-security specialists, public schools and higher education, private corporations, faith-based and charity organizations, and many others whose focus is to serve a specific population or setting. There are various employee assistant programs (EAPs) that also endorse their own programs of critical incident response and stress debriefing.

Commonalities exist among the various disaster and trauma response models. Some of these common factors are delineated as follows:

1. Most models have evidence-informed (e.g., individual perceptions of helpfulness) principles, objectives, and techniques that have been facilitated in specific disaster scenarios (e.g., hurricanes, floods, school shootings) and settings (e.g., schools, businesses, governmental organizations, staging areas, homeless shelters), and with specific populations (e.g., school children, military, law enforcement).

2. Most models lack sufficient validation and evidence-based research, which supports the statistical significance of one particular model over another.

3. Some models have empirical support, suggesting that specific aspects or core principles of the model result in positive adaptation, coping, and resiliency following trauma-guided interventions (e.g., promoting a calming effect, sense of safety and security, promoting a sense of community, instilling feelings of hope for the future).

4. Most models are based on specific trauma and disaster theories and techniques that pull from a variety of counseling and psychology models, theories, and techniques.

5. Most models have been repeatedly facilitated in the aftermath and recovery phase of multiple disaster scenarios with the primary focus on short-term interventions.

6. Most models focus on interventions within the first 24, 48, or 72 hours of the trauma or disaster with goals being solution-focused, brief interventions, and do not integrate long-term psychotherapeutic interventions.

7. Some models have application across the life span with specific interventions focused on children, adolescents, and/or adults.

8. Most models are grouped in specific recommended modules, phases, or protocols that direct the use of specific interventions at specific phases of the disaster response process.

Indeed, there are similarities and differences in the various models of disaster mental health response. Mental health practitioners should be assured that there are multiple opportunities for learning disaster and trauma interventions in a wide range of critical incidents. However, object research findings suggest that, overall, there is no one evidence-based or validated mental health disaster model, protocol, or intervention that can be applied to all possible critical incident scenarios and with full attention to the associated mental health symptoms present during acute stress conditions

(Burke & Carruth, 2012; Levers, 2012; Lynch, 2012; Smith & Jankoski, 2012; Stebnicki, 2016; Vernberg et al., 2008). Despite gaps in empirical evidence, most researchers would agree that the psychological and mental health consequence of trauma and disaster reach far beyond the survivors' coping and resiliency resources (Tol et al., 2011). The consequence of limited or no intervention on survivors of trauma and disaster events has a long-term negative mental health impact (Yun, Lurie, & Hyde, 2010). Facilitating appropriate interventions for a particular population in a specific setting with competent and skilled mental health practitioners trained in specific disaster and trauma interventions is of paramount importance to begin the process of healing trauma.

## CONSIDERATIONS FOR CHOOSING DISASTER RESPONSE MODELS

The first consideration in the use of any disaster mental health response model is to consider the setting in which the critical incident occurred (e.g., schools, hospitals, workplace). As suggested earlier, there is no one model of crisis response that is superior or comprehensive enough to provide interventions in all extraordinary stressful and traumatic events, particularly when considering the diversity of cultures in the United States and worldwide in which mental health interventions may be required. Much like the research in counseling theories (e.g., Cognitive Behavioral, Humanistic, Motivational Interviewing, Gestalt), many models have evidence-based and evidence-informed assertions of effectiveness and application for the use with specific populations and settings. Accordingly, it is important to evaluate the efficacy of the intervention and its use for a particular critical incident.

One essential feature common to all interventions is the facilitation of genuineness, empathy, compassion, rapport, and connection with survivors. The quality of the working relationship is key to facilitating and reinforcing coping and resiliency skills. Essential also are culturally specific supports and resources that disaster mental health professionals can help cultivate for survivors. The ability to intently listen, attend to, and empathically respond can therapeutically empower survivors for coping resources within the first few hours, days, and weeks after a critical event.

Accordingly, the primary purpose of a disaster mental health intervention is to facilitate brief interventions in a highly dynamic and supportive environment that focuses on (a) identifying the person's behavioral, affective, somatic, interpersonal, cognitive, and spiritual capacities that increase the individual's safety and security needs; (b) creating an empathic environment and opportunity for the individual to talk about the trauma experience (when he or she is ready) for the purpose of psychological or empathy first aid; and (c) reducing acute stress and offering an environment that can cultivate seeds of hope to restore balance and normalcy by building resiliency skills.

Most practitioners and researchers would agree that disaster mental health response should not serve as a substitute for longer term therapeutic interventions. Thus, competent and skilled practitioners understand that creating a supportive, safe, empathetic, and compassionate environment is the first therapeutic step in the survivor's journey into healing the mind, body, and spirit.

## PREINTERVENTION STRUCTURE

The preintervention stage is critical in the planning and triage of individuals and/or groups. Initially, mental health professionals must assess, coordinate, and communicate with others on the disaster team. Screening and assessment should occur with concern for the trauma survivors' medical, physical, psychological, and emotional level of functioning. The nature and timing of the traumatic event (e.g., 24 hours, 48 hours, 5 days postdisaster) will determine the mental health interventions that will be required. The mental health professional should first select individuals and/or groups that may be closest to the epicenter of the critical event or those that are most at-risk psychologically. In large-scale disasters, other groups may be formed by those individuals and groups that are secondary survivors or further from the epicenter.

Begin by establishing a rapport with the individual or group in a private area if possible. Once the group or individual session is formed, the disaster mental health professional should:

1. Make sure to introduce himself or herself and others on the disaster response team and begin to establish a rapport with the survivor

2. Explain the purpose and intention of the stress debriefing or intervention

3. Ask for permission to talk with the survivor

4. Discuss issues of confidentiality and safety

5. Provide a professional statement of disclosure and emphasize the counselor's role as mental health specialist

6. Encourage personal disclosure with the survivor but only at the level where the person feels most comfortable when discussing the traumatic experience

7. Focus on interventions and educate the individual or group, and reinforce that the counselor is there for emotional/psychological support with the intention of empowering them with resources that will help build short-term coping and resiliency skills

## COMPASSION AND EMPATHY: ESTABLISHING SAFETY AND SECURITY OF THE PERSON'S WELL-BEING

Timing is critical during disaster mental health response. The immediate needs of trauma survivors may be on a physical rescue or emergency medical care, not mental health care. They may require food, water, shelter, and clothing. The assumption is that in this phase of intervention the person has been stabilized physically and functionally to some degree to be able to engage in the emotional rescue.

Competent and skilled mental health counselors provide opportunities for individuals to receive positive human contact (compassionate communication and appropriate physical touch) and to reaffirm their needs for physical and psychological safety and security. Establishing a psychological, social, and emotional environment that attends to the overall mental health and well-being of individuals and groups are of paramount importance. Mental health professionals are encouraged to use the skills of listening, attending, and empathic responding to validate the survivor's experience as they choose to verbalize at the level they feel most comfortable. This is particularly important in the preintervention phases of any disaster mental health response model.

Mental health professionals must be aware of the general behavioral, affective, somatic, interpersonal, cognitive, and spiritual responses to acute stress and trauma stress (see Table 13.1). This is critical for distinguishing between predisaster (underlying mental and physical health conditions) and postdisaster symptoms of acute stress reaction. In the aftermath of trauma, mental health professionals can anticipate a range of physical, mental, cognitive, and behavioral symptoms. For example, there is a sympathetic arousal involving all body systems, creating a sense of psychic shock, panic, anxiety, and other physiological signs, as shown in Table 13.1. Most importantly in this phase of critical incident or disaster response, the practitioner creates an environment that reinforces the survivors' safety and security needs, as well as provides hope for their future.

During this first phase of intervention, individuals and groups are extremely concerned with how they will cope with the pain, suffering, losses, and grief associated with the catastrophic events. There is a tendency to feel an overwhelming sense of hopelessness, discouragement, and mental, physical, and spiritual exhaustion. Thus, it is critical to use statements that encourage and reflect their positive traits of internal locus of control and life areas they can and cannot control. Reinforce the individual's or group's coping and resiliency skills from the past events of adversity.

## TABLE 13.1 Response to Acute and Posttraumatic Stress Symptoms

| Physical | Cognitive | Emotional | Behavioral |
|---|---|---|---|
| Fatigue | Tendency to blame others | Anxiety | Changes in normal activities |
| Insomnia | Confusion | Severe panic (rare) | Change in speech |
| Muscle tremors | Poor attention | Grief | Withdrawal from others |
| Twitches | Inability to make decisions | Survivor guilt/ self-blame | Emotional outbursts |
| Difficult or rapid breathing | Heightened or lowered alertness | Emotional numbness | Change in communication |
| Bowel and bladder problems | Poor concentration | Uncertainty | Suspiciousness |

*(continued)*

| | | | |
|---|---|---|---|
| **TABLE 13.1 Response to Acute and Posttraumatic Stress Symptoms** *(continued)* | | | |
| **Physical** | **Cognitive** | **Emotional** | **Behavioral** |
| Elevated BP | Forgetfulness | Loss of emotional control | Inability to rest |
| Rapid heartbeat | Trouble identifying known objects or people | Fear of loss/of going crazy | Substance abuse |
| Chest pain | Increased or decreased awareness of surrounding | Depression | Intensified startle reflex |
| Headaches | Poor problem solving | Lack of capacity for enjoyment | Antisocial acts |
| Visual difficulties | Loss of a sense of time, place, or person | Apprehension | Pacing |
| Nausea/vomiting | Disturbed thinking | Intense anger | Erratic movements |
| Thirst | Nightmares | Irritability | Decreased personal hygiene |
| Loss of appetite | Inescapable images | Agitation | Diminished sexual drive |
| Dizziness | Flashbacks | Helplessness | Appetite disturbance |
| Excessive sweating | Suicidal ideas | Mistrust | Prolonged silences |
| Chills | Disbelief | Feelings of worthlessness | Accident proneness |
| Weakness | Change in values | Apathy/boredom | |
| Fainting | Search for meaning | | |

## VERBALIZING, VALIDATING, AND USE OF EMPATHY

Encourage individuals to verbalize their stories related to their disaster or traumatic experiences. Allow individuals to verbalize at the level they feel most comfortable with, which may change moment-to-moment. Provide a compassionate environment where you allow or "give permission" to talk about the physical, mental, emotional, psychosocial, and spiritual thoughts and concerns they have regarding the critical incident. Never force disclosure or attempt psychotherapeutic approaches with clients who are trauma and disaster survivors. This would apply to the first few days and weeks of a particular extraordinary stressful and traumatic event. Skilled and competent mental health professionals know the difference between interventions associated with acute stress (i.e., traumatic stress symptoms experienced by the survivor within the first 30 days of a critical incident) and posttraumatic stress (i.e., chronic, persistent, and/or delayed onset of traumatic symptoms that occur continuously after 30 days of a critical incident). Thus, the primary approaches facilitated during this phase allow room for clients to tell their stories.

Disaster mental health counselors can then use the client's traumatic experiences as a therapeutic opportunity to validate and normalize the experience, which is an ordinary response to a nonordinary critical event. Reassure the client that his or her sadness, grief, sense of enormous loss, and feelings of hopelessness are a normal response to an abnormal or traumatic event. Reassure the person that he or she will not always feel this sense of overwhelming grief. The person may never forget the traumatic event; however, with time, the intensity of emotion will ease or diminish.

## Response to Acute and Posttraumatic Stress Symptoms

Table 13.1 lists symptoms related to both acute and posttraumatic stress. Generally, the person's exposure to disaster and trauma is a whole-body experience. Most react from a physiological, cognitive, emotional, and behavioral point of view. The response to disaster and trauma is a highly individualized experience that is described from different levels of the mind, body, and spirit, as explained in other chapters. The experience of traumatic stress varies with individuals based on the level of intensity, frequency, and duration. Trauma survivors may present clinically with preexisting psychological conditions (e.g., major depression, anxiety, or substance use disorder [SUD]), which may intensify the acute stress reaction. It is critical that mental health professionals focus on symptom-relief and short-term brief interventions consistent in the various models of crisis response.

Overall, Table 13.1 may be presented to trauma survivors, which for some may normalize their physical, cognitive, emotional, and behavioral responses. However, disaster mental health counselors will have to assess the trauma survivor's readiness for psychoeducational materials. Considerations would include (a) the person's ability to read and understand signs and symptoms of acute and posttraumatic stress, (b) if the person is exhibiting signs of psychic shock and numbness, and (c) if clinical judgment determines that psychoeducational materials could potentially exacerbate the person's acute stress condition.

Timing is important in the educational phase of any trauma response or stress debriefing. For some survivors, seeing the list of symptoms too early in their exposure may actually exacerbate their whole-body experience of trauma. Many times during group stress debriefings, the group members describe what they are experiencing. Thus, the mental health professional can facilitate a common awareness of what others are experiencing by shared validation. Hearing and seeing other group members disclose the clinical symptoms of acute stress (as shown in Table 13.1) sometimes is a much more powerful tool for the trauma survivor than reading psychoeducational materials.

## Verbalizing Feelings and Storytelling

The mental health professional will want to reinforce that being open and honest with one's feelings and emotions is healthy for one's overall psychological and emotional well-being. Disclosure of feelings, emotions, or the individual's story concerning the traumatic event is very individualized. The ethical and competent disaster mental health practitioner knows that he or she should never force emotions or shame individuals for not verbalizing or disclosing their trauma, especially early on in the grieving and healing process (e.g., 24, 48, or 72 hours posttrauma experience). Many trauma survivors require a period of silence as a coping response before talking to someone who may initially be a stranger or an acquaintance. Overall, it is essential that disaster mental health practitioners support trauma survivors when they are ready to disclose.

If the disaster mental health practitioner is facilitating a group stress debriefing, he or she should reemphasize and describe the focus and intention of the group as an opportunity to allow trauma survivors to cultivate their own coping and resiliency skills. When the survivor is ready, reinforce that it is healthy to "talk about it," and by putting our heads together, we may be able to see how we can get our lives "back to normal" or "back to balance again." Facilitators may use the following questions during this phase of disaster response:

- ▶ Where were you when this incident occurred?
- ▶ Try and remember back to this event. What were some of the things that you saw, heard, felt, smelled, and experienced?
- ▶ What other memories stood out for you?
- ▶ Since the time of this incident, how have you been affected? Can you describe how this event has significantly impacted your life right now?
- ▶ How did your family and friends react to this incident?
- ▶ Are there any particular family members or friends who are more of a support than others?

Mental health counselors should use the skills of attending, listening, empathic reflection, paraphrasing, clarifying, and summarizing to facilitate individual or group interventions. Educate the survivors on the mental, physical, cognitive, spiritual, and other things they may experience during this particular time of their lives. Using Table 13.1 may again help normalize for some what they are experiencing as they read through the list of symptoms.

Despite the fact that the individual may have experienced an extraordinary stressful and traumatic event, he or she may feel and respond in the role as a "victim." The primary point here is that it is essential that mental health counselors reinforce the idea that the role of the *victim* is a normal response to an abnormal event. However, the person who perceives himself or herself as a *survivor* is empowered with awareness of his or her experience. This awareness will eventually bring meaning to his or her trauma experience. Clarify for the person that he or she may have a certain degree of negative thoughts, feelings, emotions, and experiences; however, "it will not always feel this intense . . . as time goes on they may never forget what just happened . . . but the intensity won't always be present."

## PREDICTION, PREPARATION, AND MAKING MEANING OF THE CRITICAL INCIDENT

Timing is critical during disaster mental health response. During this phase, the immediate needs of trauma survivors may continue to be related to medical stabilization with emotional support and human contact. However, the assumption is that trauma survivors have already engaged in the two previous phases where they felt some level of safety and security and have verbalized at the level they felt most comfortable. Thus, the readiness of trauma survivors to look toward the future is highly individualized. Overall, in this phase of intervention the trauma survivor should feel somewhat comfortable with the process.

Mental health counselors should encourage the person to try and think about how he or she can get back to normal again and how to reconnect with his or her life (e.g., job, school, friends, family, regular routines). As a disaster mental health responder, you may feel the need to provide all the answers. However, the most effective strategies are those that (a) educate the person about psychosocial reactions to trauma, loss, and grief; and (b) facilitate meaning of the critical event and brainstorm ideas for healing, support, and building capacity for coping and resiliency. Mental health practitioners may ask the following questions:

- ▶ What have you discovered about yourself in this experience?
- ▶ What keeps you going through this painful time right now?
- ▶ Have you made any sense of this painful experience?
- ▶ After all that you have been through, what do you expect to face in the next few days, weeks, or months?
- ▶ What are some things that help you to continue on after all that you have been through?
- ▶ How do you think that your family, friends, or community will continue to be affected?
- ▶ What other concerns do you have right at this time?

▶ What are some things (coping strategies) that you can do (today) to help you prepare for getting back to normal again at (school, work, home, and parenting)?

▶ Are there any specific things that you could share with others that might help them through this event, to help them cope right now?

▶ If I came in contact with you a few weeks or months from now, what might I notice would be different about you? What would you be feeling or thinking?

Significant life-stressors and challenges lie ahead for many trauma survivors at this point in the process. The critical event may have taken away some sense of meaning, purpose, and hope for their future. They may have feelings such that life for them will never get back to normal again. However, the skilled and competent mental health professional facilitates approaches that help the survivor begin a path of healing and allow the person to heal at his or her own pace.

Finding meaning in an extraordinary stressful or traumatic event may not occur for days, weeks, months, or even years after the critical event. These may be long-term goals for the trauma survivor. Many will need to work through some of the complex loss and grief (e.g., survivor guilt, disability adjustment, loss of a child). From an existential perspective, meaning occurs at different levels of consciousness for the survivor. Over time, some of the physical, emotional, and psychological traumatic symptoms may begin to lessen, dissipate, or scar-over as the survivor attempts to integrate the traumatic experience into some existential or spiritual meaning. Accordingly, the professional must make a holistic assessment of the individual and then facilitate appropriate interventions at the survivor's level of understanding and perception toward the critical incident.

## CORE MESSAGES AND FACILITATIVE RESPONSES OF WHAT TO COMMUNICATE TO CHILDREN, ADOLESCENTS, AND ADULTS

There are a host of vulnerable populations that may be more affected than others during critical incidents (i.e., older adults with medical/physical problems, persons with a preexisting psychiatric disability, minority groups). The seasoned disaster mental health or trauma specialist knows how to communicate words of comfort, compassion, and empathy that are culturally sensitive. Mental health professionals may not be prepared to intervene in every environmental setting, disaster scenario, or cultural group. However, it is essential that the counselor gather information prior to convening an individual or group stress debriefing. For example, it is important to anticipate any cultural differences (e.g., racial/ethnic identity, gender, rural versus urban settings, physical disability) so that interventions can be facilitated in a culturally responsive manner such as described in other chapters in *Disaster Mental Health Counseling*.

One population that is particularly affected by extraordinary stressful and traumatic events is composed of children and adolescents. Typically, mental health counselors who specialize in children and adolescents understand the unique developmental, cognitive, social, and emotional aspects of psychosocial adjustment to disaster and trauma. The following section offers some guidelines and facilitative responses that may be helpful early on in disaster mental health response with dealing with children, adolescents, and adults.

## Children and Adolescents

▶ Assure the child/adolescent that feeling frightened, sad, or confused is very normal given what he or she has been through. It is healthy to express emotions. It will help the individual get better, much like if he or she is feeling sick or injured (i.e., flu, colds, healing a broken bone). Emotions will heal too just like broken bones or a cut.

▶ Explain to the child/adolescent that part of what he or she is feeling emotionally and physically will actually help him or her feel better and more balanced. Say to the child, "You are not a weak person. Most kids and even adults feel the same way you do after an experience like yours." It especially helps heal emotions when kids can verbalize their feelings.

▶ Reinforce that it is important for the child/adolescent to accept help and support for a while until he or she feels better and less sad. We are not totally independent in our lives. Everyone needs help from others at some point in his or her life.

▶ Reassure the child/adolescent that right now, it may take a lot of effort and focus to get back to normal daily routines (i.e., school, homework, sports, other activities). Allow children/adolescents to transition at their own pace back to normal routines. The more they practice trying to get back to normal routines, the easier it will become.

▶ Explain to the child/adolescent that he or she does not have to share his or her thoughts and feelings with everyone. It is OK to share them with you (professionals) or someone else who the child/adolescent trusts.

▶ Say to the child/adolescent: "You have been through something very few others have. It is normal to feel sad. Crying over something sad and terrible is not the same as acting like a baby."

▶ Say to the child/adolescent: "People's hearts can hurt the same way a broken bone does. Hurting is just part of healing, and broken hearts do heal, just like broken bones."

## Facilitative Responses for Adults

▶ I'm sorry this has happened to you. I can't imagine what you are going through right now.

▶ I'm glad you're safe right now; let's think of some ways that you can feel even more safe.

▶ It is hard to forget or stop the pain because this is something too painful to forget.

- ▶ What you are feeling right now is very normal. What you have been through is very abnormal.

- ▶ Feeling sad only means that you are a human being.

- ▶ Your feelings may change from day to day. You may have many different feelings all at the same time. It may feel confusing to you at times because of all that you have been through.

- ▶ You may never completely forget or be able to erase what happened. As time goes on, you will feel less frightened or sad, and things will begin to feel normal again.

- ▶ You will feel happy again. If you get upset again, that's OK. This is just your heart telling you how much you miss him or her right now. It's OK to remember.

## SUICIDE RISK AND LETHALITY

Suicide represents a self-inflicted, unexpected, traumatic, and violent death that commonly co-occurs with homicide and exposure to trauma and violence (Malinga-Musamba & Maundeni, 2012). Suicide has traditionally been separated into three categories: suicide ideation or thoughts of suicide, suicide attempts, and suicide completions. In disaster mental health response, it is critical that mental health practitioners know how to assess disaster and trauma survivors in all categories of suicide. The Behavioral, Affect, Somatic, Interpersonal, Cognitive, and Spiritual (BASICS) model as well as other material offered in this chapter will assist mental health professionals to evaluate all levels of lethality and guidelines for actions to take on behalf of this high-risk population of trauma survivors.

The Centers for Disease Control and Prevention (CDC) reports that suicide was the tenth leading cause of death among Americans in 2013 (CDC, 2015). Among 10- to 13-year-olds, suicide is the third leading cause of death. In fact, adults 18 to 25 years of age have the highest rates of suicide ideation at 7.4%. Overall, about 4% of adults 26 to 49 years of age have a suicide completion. Men are four times more likely than women to attempt suicide. Suicide among men is the seventh leading cause of death. Fifty-seven percent of men who commit suicide do so by use of firearms, whereas 35% of women use poisoning as the most common form.

It has been well documented in the grief counseling literature that grieving a loss due to suicide has a more complex mourning process than loss of life that results in a natural disaster (e.g., flood, hurricane, fire; Rando, 1984; Worden, 2009). Both events are traumatic and each person's perceptions toward trauma and disaster are different. However, one of the primary differences is that self-inflicted suicide has an attributable cause (the person) that is stigmatized by society as a whole. Rarely do families want to talk to friends and neighbors about their loved one's act of suicide.

Even though many individuals with suicide ideation have a diagnosable mental health condition (i.e., major depressive disorder, SUD), most family members, coworkers, and peers do not recognize the warning signs. Accordingly, there appears to be a lot of self-blame among family members, close friends, and coworkers for not being attuned to the deceased person's serious mental health condition that led up to taking one's life. In naturally occurring disasters, many individuals rationalize, justify, or bring meaning to the event as an unexplained phenomenon that perhaps has a divine cause or could not be controlled or avoided. Thus, survivors have no one to blame as the perpetrator. However, in acts of suicide or homicide there is an identifiable person(s) involved. The stigma associated with suicide is particularly painful, shameful, and wounding for the person who may have had a failed suicide attempt. Family members are affected enormously by such events.

## SUICIDE AND LETHALITY ASSESSMENT

Traditional models for assessing the potential risk of suicide focus primarily on the lethality of the individual and the intended level of threat to complete an act of suicide. Despite the statistical significance of a plethora of epidemiological research that has identified at-risk populations, the fact remains that persons who have sustained extraordinary stressful and traumatic events are in the highest risk category for lethality and suicide completion. Thus, disaster mental health counselors should be well versed in the screening, assessment, and diagnosis of co-occurring mental health conditions associated with suicide lethality.

Suicide behavioral assessment must consider multiple factors such as age; current chronic medical conditions; mental, physical, and cognitive capacity; and exposure to specific types of disasters and trauma; as well as preexisting mental health conditions that predispose the individual to a higher risk of lethality. Mental health counselors who are skilled and competent in crisis response, lethality, and suicide assessment know how to utilize good clinical judgment, follow-up questions, and resources that bring the crisis to some resolution. Traditional suicide assessments typically evaluate the person's level of lethality in the following six areas:

1. Does the individual communicate an intent to harm self or others?

2. Has the individual devised a detailed plan? Are any weapons accessible? Is there a history of anger, aggression, or violence?

3. Does the individual have a history of any suicide ideation, threats, or attempts?

4. Are there any specific life stressors that the individual has experienced recently (e.g., exposure to disaster and traumatic events, loss of a loved one, chronic illness, life-threatening disability, legal issues or incarceration)?

5. Does the individual have any current mental health conditions that predisposes him or her to suicide risk and lethality (e.g., depression, anxiety, PTSD, SUDs)?

6. What type and level of support does the individual have (e.g., family, friends, support groups, others)?

In the context of establishing contact with the person who has exposure to disaster or trauma, it is important that mental health professionals recognize the person as a *survivor* rather than a *victim*. Accordingly, interventions addressing the person's level of lethality should begin with the facilitation of empathetic and compassionate connections and use of resiliency strategies as therapeutic leverage. If the individual can view himself or herself as a *survivor* of a traumatic event, then this should provide an opportunity to refocus the crisis on potential support systems and resources.

## The BASICS Model of Multimodal Assessment

**The BASICS model is based on Slaideu**'s (1990) application of **Lazarus**'s (1981) multimodal assessment and has recently been presented by **Echterling**, Presbury, and Edson-McKee (2005, p. 13) as an assessment of lethality and suicide ideation. The strength of the BASICS model, as delineated in the following, is that it offers prompts for a multimodal assessment of the survivor's resiliency traits and coping skills. The acronym (BASICS) was developed to guide crisis responders through critical areas of lethality assessment and is defined in the following holistic areas: Behavioral (what people do); Affective (how people feel); Somatic (how people respond physically); Interpersonal (how people relate to others); Cognitive (how people think); Spiritual (what people believe and value). This protocol may be helpful for disaster mental health professionals to integrate with other assessment items related to the survivor**'s suicide ideation and co-occurring mental health conditions.**

### Behavioral

Observe the person's appearance and nonverbal communication that might indicate a suicide risk (e.g., poor grooming, flat affect, detached or dissociative traits). Is the person only hinting at the possibility of hurting self or others, or is he or she openly verbalizing suicide intention? If the person openly states: *"I'm thinking of killing myself . . . ."* respond empathically to the person's pain: *"It takes a lot of courage to talk about this—I can't imagine how this must feel to you. . . . Tell me more specifically what you mean by this."* If preparations are being made by the person (gathering of the implements to inflict harm), ask directly: *"Are you planning to do anything right now to carry out your plan?"* If previous attempts have been made by the individual, this places the person in a high-risk category. State: *"You said that you've tried to kill yourself in the past. . . . I'm very concerned about your safety and would like to ask you some questions about this issue. . . ."* If the person has chosen life, then this is an opportunity to begin assessing the individual's coping resources. You might state: *"What did you tell yourself when you talked yourself out of hurting yourself?"* Or, *"How were you able to get through that terrible event without trying to kill yourself?"*

### Affective

Evaluate the individual's level/intensity of feelings of fear, rage, depression, or mood disorder that would place him or her in a high-risk category. You could state: *"I can't imagine what you are going through right now. . . . Other people that have been through what you have been through have feelings like yours (hopeless, depression, and thoughts of suicide) . . . sometimes these feelings pass. . . . I'm concerned about you. . . . What are you feeling right now?"* You could use a scaling technique: *"On a scale of 1 to 10 with 1 being no hope whatsoever and 10 feeling very hopeful . . . where are you right now? What might be different in your life right now if you felt more hopeful?"*

## Somatic

If someone has been injured and you sense he or she is in a high-risk category, you might state: *"I'm sorry this has happened to you, you've shared that you are struggling now. . . . I've had this question running through my mind, are you thinking about hurting yourself?"* Or in a less direct way: *"Now that you're dealing with this injury that threatens your life, how are you finding the will or the strength to continue on?"*

## Interpersonal

The presence of fewer supports and coping resources in the person's life places individuals in a higher risk category for suicide attempt or completion. Assess the level of support from family, friends, and/or social group by asking: *"Who are the important people in your life?. . . How can they be more involved in your situation right now?"*

## Cognitive

An occasional, vague, nondescriptive, and fleeting moment of suicide ideation is not uncommon during the time of a crisis. It is important to check the individual's thoughts about this if you feel the lethality is high. You might say directly: *"I'm sensing that you really want to end it all now."* Or, *"You suggested that you might want to end it all right now— do you have a plan or idea how you would do this?"* This is an opportunity to explore coping resources and the person's internal emotional and psychological strengths. Try to tap this energy source and state: *"It sounds like you've maybe got some ideas about an alternative possibility. . . . Tell me more about this."*

## Spiritual

A particularly troubling sign of high-risk lethality is when someone is expressing the belief system that he or she no longer matters to anyone, or life has no meaning, or that his or her death will send a signal to others (e.g., a personal cause, philosophical ideology, or indication of how much pain he or she was in). Someone who is feeling a profound sense of spiritual alienation may see suicide as his or her only choice. You might state: *"After all that's just happened to you it sounds like you're wondering if there's any point to your life right now. . . . What would need to happen for you to begin feeling better about going on with your life?"*

## DISASTER MENTAL HEALTH RESOURCES WEBSITES

The following is a list of various professional associations and organizations that specialize in disaster response. Each association and organization has its mission, purpose, endorsed training approaches, and membership that may be a valuable resource for disaster mental health counselors.

American Academy of Child and Adolescent Psychiatry (AACAP): www.aacap.org

The American Academy of Experts in Traumatic Stress (AAETS): www.aaets.org

American Counseling Association (ACA): www.counseling.org

American Psychiatric Association (APA): www.psych.org

American Psychological Association (APA): www.apa.org

American Red Cross (ARC): www.redcross.org

Centers for Disease Control and Prevention (CDC): www.cdc.gov

National Association of School Psychologists (NASP): www.nasponline.org

National Association of Social Workers (NASW): www.naswdc.org

National Institute of Mental Health (NIMH): www.nimh.nih.gov

National Mental Health Association (NMHA): www.nmha.org

Substance Abuse Mental Health Services Administration (SAMHSA): www.samhsa.gov

## DISASTER SCENARIO ROLE-PLAY EXERCISES*

The intention for the following section is to present multiple disaster scenarios for practice with crisis or critical incident teams. There are a wide range of critical incidents that could be written for inclusion in a disaster mental health training. However, the three scenarios presented offer a structure for developing other critical incidents for role-play exercises.

### Scenario 1: Critical Incident: School Bus Crash Scenario

Two nights ago, three busloads of your middle school seventh to eighth graders were returning home from a daylong field trip. As the three buses were driving back at night in a strong rainstorm, the bus in the middle slid off into a ditch, crashed, and was turned on its side. Apparently, there was a car that the bus driver was trying to avoid. Currently, we do not have much information beyond this; an investigation is pending.

The bus that crashed had about 35 riders. Two of the students, Marcus and Joy, sustained some broken bones, and Joy also suffered a moderate brain injury. They are both listed in critical condition at Dare County Hospital. Marcus has a reputation of being somewhat "obnoxious and irritating" to others. He is an average student with poor interpersonal skills and does not handle problem solving well. Marcus spends time living between his grandparents' and mother's house and is not involved in any extracurricular school activities. Joy is an academically talented student, plays on the girls' softball team, and belongs to a number of school clubs. The remaining children were treated and released with only minor injuries of cuts and bruises. The bus driver also went to the hospital and is listed in stable condition.

### Roles

*Teacher:* You have Marcus and Joy in your class as well as many of the other adolescents that were injured. You have contact with these students on a daily basis. You were riding in the bus that was following behind the bus that crashed. You didn't

---

*Adapted from Chapter 70, Stebnicki (2016), in *The Professional Counselor's Desk Reference* (2nd ed.), © Springer Publishing Company.

actually see the crash, but you heard the students on your bus scream and then you passed by the bus that was lying off in the ditch.

*Girls' softball coach:* Joy is one of the star softball players on your team and you have coached her for the last two seasons. Three of the other adolescents who sustained minor injuries are also on the team. However, you've got the Regional Tournament coming up, and you really need Joy.

*School nurse:* You really don't have much contact with Joy, but you see Marcus several times a month because he always seems to have frequent injuries during gym class. You were on the field trip and riding on the bus in front of the one that crashed. No one on your bus saw or heard anything until a few minutes later when your bus driver heard the emergency call over the radio.

*School counselor:* You see Marcus regularly to coordinate outside social services for him and his mother. Although he is not one of your favorite students, he does follow through on things.

*Mental health case worker:* You don't know Joy or any of the other youth that were injured. You see Marcus twice per month for family intervention services. You do have infrequent contact with some of the kids who were riding in the other two buses.

*School principal:* You have frequent contact with Marcus because of his behavior problems. You've got a soft spot in your heart for Marcus because you can relate with his family situation, which reminds you of your own as you were growing up between two homes while in school.

## Scenario 2: Critical Incident: Toxic Chemical Spill Scenario

One August afternoon in a rural community in your state (population about 20,000 residents), a train carrying tanker cars of chemicals derailed in the center of town. Before emergency disaster personnel knew what was contained in the tanker cars, many people within a mile or so of the accident became ill with flulike symptoms from the toxic fumes. Officials of this small rural town had to wait about 2 hours before federal officials could identify exactly what chemicals were being transported by this train. The local hospital emergency department was in chaos because of the overwhelming number of local residents being transported there for emergency medical treatment of some unknown toxin. Fortunately, there were no related deaths, only some lingering upper respiratory effects from the exposure to the chemicals.

At the time of the accident, the clients of a local day-care facility were swimming at the local public pool close to the downtown area. In all the confusion and chaos during the train derailment, one particular 4-year-old child who could not swim was left unattended for a very brief period of time (less than 1 minute). Sadly, little Leslie drowned. You have been called in to provide mental health disaster relief to this rural community 4 days after this toxic spill. Discuss and role-play the following:

1. Discuss the characteristics of such a critical incident (e.g., transportation disaster, sociocultural aspects, existing county/town infrastructure, time of day or month of event, duration or intensity of this transportation event, effects of media coverage).

2. Discuss the types of losses that individuals in this rural community have sustained.

3. Anticipate and discuss some of the familiar feelings/emotions, thoughts, or stories that you would expect to encounter after such an incident.

4. Who might be the persons most affected (emotionally, behaviorally, physically, cognitively, and spiritually) by this critical incident (e.g., populations such as elderly or disabled, children, family members, friends, firefighters, police, paramedics, rescue personnel, other surrounding support systems, day-care facility workers)?

5. What coping mechanisms and resiliency factors would you want to assess/evaluate and facilitate with this community?

### Role-Play Scenario

Discuss how you might set up or arrange your crisis intervention. Role-play one on one with a partner, with each taking different roles; if time allows, role-play Group Crisis.

▶ Town mayor

▶ Emergency service personnel (firefighters, paramedics, police)

▶ Parent with child in day-care setting

▶ Lifeguard on duty at time of drowning

▶ Director of day-care facility and day-care teachers

▶ Parent of "Little Leslie"

▶ Director of parks, pools, and recreation

▶ Create your own role

## Scenario 3: Critical Incident: Tornado Scenario

One night in March 1999, there were about 30 tornadoes that ripped through the central part of the state of Arkansas. One particular rural town (population about 5,000) was almost entirely destroyed and about the only thing left standing was the local school. You are called to the school gymnasium within 48 hours of this critical incident to do a stress debriefing with many of the towns' folk. Discuss and role-play the following:

1. Discuss the characteristics of such a critical incident (e.g., natural disaster, sociocultural aspects, existing county/town infrastructure, time of day or month of event, duration or intensity of this weather event, effects of media coverage).

2. Discuss the types of losses that individuals in this small rural community have sustained.

3. Anticipate and discuss some of the familiar feelings/emotions, thoughts, or stories that you would expect to encounter after such an incident.

4. Who might be the persons most affected (emotionally, behaviorally, physically, cognitively, and spiritually) by this critical incident (e.g., populations such as

elderly or disabled, family members, friends, firefighters, police, paramedics, rescue personnel, other surrounding support systems)?

5.  What coping mechanisms and resiliency factors would you want to assess/evaluate and facilitate with the townspeople?

## Role-Play Scenario

Discuss how you might set up or arrange your crisis intervention. Role-play one on one with a partner, with each taking different roles; if time allows, role-play Group Crisis.

► Town mayor

► Emergency service personnel (firefighters, paramedics, police)

► Parent of school-aged children

► School principal

► Schoolteacher

► Older person with roots in the community for 100-plus years

► Create your own role

## CONCLUDING REMARKS

Disaster mental health and trauma counseling is a challenging field. There is a noticeable change in the types of individuals and groups being served by professional counselors. Thus, there is an enormous need for qualified and competent mental health professionals who can provide disaster mental health relief and stress debriefing groups in a wide range of critical incidents. Client stories that have such themes as physical or sexual abuse, psychological trauma, or loss, pain, and suffering can adversely affect the mind, body, and spirit of the professional counselor. Many professionals who work this close to the epicenter are naturally predisposed to an empathy fatigue experience. Thus, it is essential that counselor self-care approaches be initiated for working at such intense levels of service.

## REFERENCES

Acute Traumatic Stress Management. (2016). Comprehensive Acute Traumatic Stress Management. Retrieved from http://www.atsm.org

American Red Cross. (2016). Red Cross mental health teams help people cope during disaster. Retrieved from http://www.redcross.org/news/article/Red-Cross-Mental-Health-Teams-Help-People-Cope-During-Disaster

Burke, P. A., & Carruth, B. (2012). Addiction and psychological trauma: Implications for counseling strategies. In L. L. Levers (Ed.), *Trauma counseling: Theories and interventions* (pp. 214–230). New York, NY: Springer Publishing.

Centers for Disease Control and Prevention. (2015). Suicide: Facts at a glance. Retrieved from http://www.cdc.gov/violenceprevention/pdf/suicide-datasheet-a.pdf

Critical Incident Stress Debriefing. (2016). Critical Incident Stress Debriefing (CISD). Retrieved from http://www.info-trauma.org/flash/medie/mitchellCriticalIncidentStressDebriefing.pdf

Critical Incident Stress Management. (2016). What is CISM? Retrieved from http://www.criticalinci dentstress.com/what_is_cism

Echterling, L. G., Presbury, J. H., & Edson-McKee, J. (2005). *Crisis intervention: Promoting resilience and resolution in troubled times*. Columbus, OH: Pearson, Merrill/Prentice-Hall.

Lazarus, A. A. (1981). *The practice of multimodal therapy*. New York, NY: McGraw-Hill.

Levers, L. L. (2012). An introduction to counseling survivors of trauma: Beginning to understand the context of trauma. In L. L. Levers (Ed.), *Trauma counseling: Theories and interventions* (pp. 1–22). New York, NY: Springer Publishing.

Lynch, M. F. (2012). Theoretical contexts of trauma counseling. In L. L. Levers (Ed.), *Trauma counseling: Theories and interventions* (pp. 47–58). New York, NY: Springer Publishing.

Malinga-Musamba, T., & Maundeni, T. (2012). Traumatic aftermath of homicide and suicide. In L. L. Levers (Ed.), *Trauma counseling: Theories and interventions* (pp. 249–263). New York, NY: Springer Publishing.

National Center for Posttraumatic Stress Disorder. (2016). Psychological first aid model. Retrieved from http://www.ptsd.va.gov/professional/manuals/psych-first-aid.asp

National Organization for Victim Assistance. (2016). 42nd Annual NOVA training event. Retrieved from http://www.trynova.org

Rando, T. (1984). *Grief, death, and dying*. Champaign, IL: Research Press.

Slaideu, K. A. (1990). *Crisis intervention: A handbook for practice and research* (2nd ed.). Boston, MA: Allyn & Bacon.

Smith, J. A., & Jankoski, J. A. (2012). Disaster behavioral health: Counselors responding to terrorism. In L. L. Levers (Ed.), *Trauma counseling: Theories and interventions* (pp. 454–470). New York, NY: Springer Publishing.

Stebnicki, M. A. (2008). *Empathy fatigue: Healing the mind, body, and spirit of professional counselors*. New York, NY: Springer Publishing

Stebnicki, M. A. (2016). From empathy fatigue to empathy resiliency. In I. Marini & M. A. Stebnicki (Eds.), *The professional counselor's desk reference* (2nd ed., pp. 533–545). New York, NY: Springer Publishing.

Stebnicki, M. A., & Marini, I. (2016). The psychosocial impact of global disasters. In I. Marini & M. A. Stebnicki (Eds.), *The professional counselor's desk reference* (2nd ed., pp. 611–615). New York, NY: Springer Publishing.

Tol, W. A., Barbui, C., Galappatti, A., Silove, D., Betancourt, T. S., Souza, R., . . . van Ommeren, M. (2011). Mental health and psychosocial support in humanitarian settings: Linking practice and research. *The Lancet, 378*(9802), 1581–1591.

Vernberg, E. M., Jacobs, A. K., Layne, C. M., Pynoos, R. S., Steinberg, A. M., Brymer, M. J., . . . Ruzek, J. I. (2008). Innovations in disaster mental health: Psychological first aid. *Professional Psychology, 39*(4), 381–388.

Worden, W. (2009). *Grief counseling and grief therapy: A handbook for the mental health practitioner*. New York, NY: Springer Publishing.

Yun, K., Lurie, N., & Hyde, P. S. (2010). Moving mental health into the disaster-preparedness spotlight. *New England Journal of Medicine, 363*(13), 1193–1195.

# CHAPTER 14

# Immigrants, Refugees, and Asylum Seekers: The Psychosocial Cost of War on Civilians

The world has been at war since the beginning of time. The majority of deaths that occur during times of war do not involve military personnel. Rather, 90% comprise civilian casualties (Wiist et al., 2014). Since World War II there have been 127 different wars fought globally with over 40 million civilian deaths (Hanson & Vogel, 2012). World War II alone was responsible for over 27.3 million civilian casualties (War Chronicle, 2016). Other examples since the 20th century include over 5.4 million civilian deaths in the Democratic Republic of Congo; two million civilian deaths related to the Khmer Rouge killing fields; two million civilian deaths in Rwanda; and 200,000 civilian deaths from the Bosnian civil war in the Balkins (Genocide Intervention Network, 2016). Our most recent conflicts, Operation Iraqi Freedom, Operation Enduring Freedom, and Operation New Dawn, have resulted in over 210,000 civilian casualties. Civilian causalities (direct and indirect) due to enemy combatants are difficult to obtain because there are no standardized reporting procedures (Physicians for Social Responsibility [PSR], 2016). PSR suggests that the U.S. military and the Department of Defense do not do an accurate accounting of civilian causalities during war time.

Global security is reportedly at one of the most capricious states seen in modern times. Some would say that we are in the midst of World War III as a result of the Islamic State of Iraq, al Qaeda, Taliban, Russia, China, and other hostile insurgencies where civilians are at the epicenter of armed conflict and the quest for power and control of land and resources. Geographic relocation to the United States and other countries is no longer for immigrant job seekers or a quest to improve one's quality of life. Rather, the journey is long, perilous, and primarily for the purpose of basic survival, just to breathe and have basic food, shelter, and clothing.

What is at stake is the safety and security of U.S. citizens and other global civilian populations' mental and physical well-being. We are confronted by simultaneous technological, person-made, and biological threats perpetrated by antigovernment groups,

terrorist networks such as the Islamic State in Iraq and Syria (ISIS), and other dark entities that have flown under the radar for decades (Joint Chiefs of Staff, Unified Combatant Commands, & Office of the Secretary of Defense, 2016).

The United States has been blessed with a democracy that respects and upholds civil
liberties for the most part. It has a strong humanitarian base of nonprofit organizations
and faith-based groups to help those in need of food, clean water, shelter, clothing, and
mental and physical health care. However, the same opportunities are not afforded to
civilians in war-torn countries where torture, rape, imprisonment, and execution are
daily threats to minority and disempowered indigenous groups. As a consequence, millions of immigrants, refugees, internally displaced persons, and asylum seekers from
war-torn countries seek to find safe havens in the United States and other nations that
value human life and civil liberties.

## DEFINITIONS

The U.S. Citizenship and Immigration Services (USCIS, 2016c) under the U.S. Department of Homeland Security delineates the complex law and path to citizenship as it
relates to immigrants, refugees, and asylum seekers. The USCIS (2016a) makes decisions based on policies and laws that were first introduced in the Immigration and
Nationality Act (INA). The INA was shaped by the McCarren-Walter bill in 1952, which
created Public Law 82–414. An extensive policy manual exists (USCIS, 2016b), which
provides full disclosure of all policies related to rights, responsibilities, and processes of
naturalization, continuous residence, individuals and groups under temporary pro-
tected status (TPS), and overall policies related to immigration. The intent of the chapter is to provide transparency to all public, private, and governmental entities. The law
itself is quite complex and is beyond the scope of this chapter to be discussed comprehensively. However, definitions are described in the following sections so as to clarify
the individuals who comprise the populations and cultures we refer to as immigrants,
refugees, and asylum seekers.

## Immigrant

The term *immigrant* is defined as a person who is a migrant from another country, either
lawfully or unlawfully, with the intent to take up permanent residence (Homeland Security, 2016). If granted legal residency, he or she is provided the status of a *permanent
resident alien*. Those who migrate from another country unlawfully are also referred to
as *immigrants,* but not in legal status and not as a *permanent resident alien*. The uni-
formed and culturally insensitive often use the term *illegal aliens* for immigrants who
have entered the United States unlawfully. There is a certain degree of stigma and stereotype associated with the term *alien* due to the dehumanizing aspects. Thus, it
becomes more humanistic and culturally appropriate to use the terms *permanent resident* and *U.S. citizen* when referring to those who immigrated lawfully to the United
States and have been granted residency or citizenship status. The term *unauthorized
immigrant* likewise reflects a greater degree of humanism as opposed to *alien*.

The Secretary of Homeland Security has the power to designate individuals and groups from foreign countries under the *TPS*, which grants foreign nationals temporary residence in the United States. This would typically be done in cases where if the person returns to his or her country of origin this would likely result in imprisonment, harm to his or her safety and welfare, and in many circumstances result in death. At the time of this writing, foreign nationals from the following countries have been granted TPS by the U.S. government: El Salvador, Guinea, Haiti, Honduras, Liberia, Nepal, Nicaragua, Sierra Leone, Somalia, South Sudan, Sudan, Syria, and Yemen.

## Refugee

The USCIS (2016c) defines a *refugee* as someone who: (a) is located outside the United States and is in need of humanitarian assistance; (b) demonstrates he or she has been persecuted due to race, religion, nationality, political opinion, or membership within a particular social group, and is not firmly resettled in another country; and (c) meets all the requirements for admission contingent on background screenings (i.e., mental, physical, criminal).

## Asylum Seeker

Each year people come to the United States seeking asylum because of threats to their safety and fear of persecution. The USCIS defines an *asylum seeker* as a person who, because of race, religion, nationality, membership in a particular social group, or political opinion, has been threatened with violence, persecution, and fear that he or she will suffer persecution. Asylum seekers are a new phenomenon to the United States and European nations for the 21st century due to the immense volume of populations seeking safety and security from war-torn countries. This sociopolitical phenomenon requires governments to seriously consider the human, moral, and ethical issues related to accepting and not accepting, screening, and adjudicating such populations of individuals. Issues related to terrorism, criminality, pandemic viruses, and other consequences are quite challenging for the mental and physical health and welfare of the civilized world today.

## PREVALENCE, INCIDENCE, AND ETIOLOGY

Worldwide there are more than 51 million refugees, asylum seekers, and internally displaced persons from war-torn countries forced to flee their homelands (United Nations High Commissioner for Refugees [UNHCR], 2016). The UNHCR's global trend report compiled by governments and nongovernmental-partnering organizations shows an enormous increase in these indigenous populations due to war and threats of safety and security. At the time of this writing, the largest number of refugees have come from Afghanistan (2.5 million), Syria (2.4 million), Somalia (over 1.1 million), Sudan (650,000), Democratic Republic of the Congo (500,000), Myanmar (480,000), Iraq (402,000), Columbia (307,000), and Vietnam (314,000). In January 2016, there were 51,000 Afghan, Syrian, and Iraqi refugees who traveled through the harsh winter conditions over the

Mediterranean Sea (Mercy Corps, 2016) to seek asylum in various other countries. All were forced out of their homelands and spread geographically across bordering countries due to war. Presently, over 1.1 million people worldwide have submitted applications for asylums with an additional 25,300 asylum seekers who are children separated or unaccompanied by their parents. The parents of these children were likely seriously injured or killed as a casualties of war.

Despite some of the hysteria among American citizens, the majority of applications for asylum are being handled by Germany and other European nations, not the United States. However, since 1975, the U.S. State Department has welcomed over three million refugees from all over the world (U.S. State Department, 2016). There are multiple governmental and nongovernmental organizations in all 50 states that have provided basic needs for these indigenous groups. Since 2000, the State Department has handled more than 600,000 applications from immigrants, refugees, and asylum seekers. As a result of the war in Syria, over 11,000 Syrians have applied for U.S. refugee status since 2006. The status of these applications varies from month to month and statistics do not accurately depict who remains in the United States and who does not.

The etiology of this worldwide epidemic is clear. It is war that is at the foundation of all human suffering as millions are forced to relocate geographically. This person-made disaster points to the overall lack of respect and empathy for human life perpetrated by brutal governments, religious zealots, and other indigenous tribal warring groups. The known causes are also exemplified by civil and religious armed conflicts, continuous bombing of villages and towns, violence perpetrated by drug warlords, forced sexual prostitution and slavery, human trafficking, imprisonment by the government for possessing the "wrong" sociopolitical or religious beliefs, racism, discrimination, forced isolation/internal displacement, detention camps, deprived access to adequate mental and physical health care, and withholding of the basic food, water, shelter, and clothing for warmth. Overall, it is an incomprehensible task for any one government, organization, or agency to provide assistance for all those in critical need.

## SOCIOCULTURAL FAMILIAL IMPACT OF WAR

Acts of genocide, ethnic cleansing, political persecution, and other atrocities have wounded the soul of indigenous populations. The mental health field is only beginning to understand the impact that war has on cultures and civilian families. Children are especially vulnerable and profoundly affected by war because of long-term exposure to political and cultural violence. In the United States, it is estimated that approximately 43% of all refugees are children (American Psychological Association, 2010). Many families are often forcibly separated or relocated, creating a family crisis accompanied by the loss of family rituals and identity. There is the significant loss of parents, family, friends, homes, schools, and other familiar daily routines. Since the 1990s, there have been well over two million children who have been killed, six million disabled, and 20 million left homeless as the result of war (Stichick & Bruderlein, 2001). The United Nations (2016) reports that between January 2011 and June 2015, about 1,400 boys and girls have been abducted in Iraq by al Qaeda and ISIS. Additionally, over 3,000 children have died as the result of improvised explosive device (IED) explosions.

There are severe mental, physical, social, emotional, psychological, and spiritual consequences to these cultures, which has created a historical trauma that is passed down to many future generations. This humanitarian crisis requires a long-term plan to bridge the gap between Western mental health treatment strategies and adapting culturally relevant approaches for indigenous groups exposed to war (Hanson & Vogel, 2012; Miller & Rasmussen, 2009). The complex trauma acquired by armed conflict, poverty, malnutrition, and displacement into overcrowded and impoverished refugee camps has created mental and physical trauma resulting in permanent disabilities. The destruction of social networks and those who are survivors of forced child military service, sexual assault, and the loss of social and material support, as well as widows and orphans, has created a complex trauma that cannot be addressed purely from Western models of mental health treatment. Rather, exposure to war on civilians requires integrative culturally sensitive approaches to heal the symptoms of posttraumatic stress and the daily stressors of survival on war-affected indigenous populations.

A humanitarian crisis of epic proportions exists on a global basis for immigrants, refugees, internally displaced persons, and asylum seekers from war-torn countries. The complex global security both at home and abroad has far-reaching implications for the sociocultural and psychosocial health, safety, and welfare of all the planet's populations. The complex trauma experienced by immigrants, refugees, and asylum seekers appears to be a silent epidemic for most Americans. The critical challenges for these indigenous/ethnic groups rarely come into the consciousness of "things to worry about" for most Americans, unless of course one or more of these groups live in your community. It certainly becomes an issue for Americans who identify or belong to the ethnic heritage of these groups. The reality is that there is no amount of money or donations that can heal the suffering of foreign nationals, which can be viewed on the nightly news and other 24-hour electronic media news outlets.

Additionally, fear and ignorance are easily spread by some U.S. politicians who misuse language (i.e., illegal aliens, Muslim terrorists), which ultimately stigmatizes ethnic minority groups. Truly, language has the potential to harm or heal. Stigmatizing language communicated about different minority groups has the potential to perpetrate overt acts of prejudice, discrimination, and intentional/unintentional racism. Misuse of language by well-intentioned U.S. lawmakers who have created legal terms such as *Hispanic* also has the potential to stigmatize minorities because it does not consider cultural identity (i.e., Latina[o], Columbian, Mexican American) and within-group differences. The various terms we use to describe other cultures tend to seep into the unconsciousness of many Americans. Consequently, we normalize the stigmatizing language used to describe different minorities and can easily become intolerant of others, which hinders our ability for compassion and empathy.

As mental health professionals, we must deflect the negative attitudes and overt prejudices that are sustained in the larger society. The groups most affected have sustained enough harsh treatment for one lifetime. Thus, we have an ethical obligation to build

cultural awareness, knowledge, and skills to work with others who are culturally different. Unfortunately, the majority of practitioners do not have training to work with the
complex trauma experienced by immigrants from war-torn countries (Stebnicki, 2015).
Despite training in multicultural counseling, most practitioners do not have the language skills and cultural knowledge to work with these indigenous populations. This
should not prevent mental health professionals from responding to the humanitarian
need in an empathic way of being. Accordingly, special training is required to work competently and ethically with immigrants from places in the far reaches of the globe, which
is discussed later in this chapter.

## GOVERNMENT-DRIVEN DISASTER RESPONSE AND STRATEGIC INITIATIVES

There is a human cost to living in an unpredictable world that has experienced person-
made disasters perpetrated on defenseless and disempowered civilians who are exposed
to war. There are no peaceful political resolutions in many scenarios. As a consequence,
there are always civilian casualties as a result of war. Historically, there has always been
a humanitarian response in times of large-scale disasters. So, having some faith there
will always be humanitarian efforts, as well as compassion for others, requires a determined, hopeful, positive, and optimistic view of the world.

Humanitarian efforts are seen in many corners of the Earth where agencies and organizations have mobilized to cobble together basic services for food, clean water, shelter,
clothing, and medical health care. It may be the nature of humans that every nonprofit
agency, faith-based organization, or government entity has its own conceptual idea of
assisting with food, clean water, shelter, clothing, health care, and financial support.
However, it is critical that some organizations can take charge of planning, coordinating,
organizing, and leading a unified coalition of care providers and volunteers to be effective in large-scale disaster response, such as the masses of immigrants, refugees, and
asylum seekers fleeing their homelands and geographically relocating all over the world.

The Strategic Foresight Initiative (SFI) action plan developed by the Federal Emergency Management Agency (FEMA, 2012) is one example of an agency that has stepped
up to the challenge of addressing the needs of immigrants, refugees, and asylum seekers
in the United States and has projected and anticipated potential crisis outcomes up to
the year 2030. Although FEMA's mission is not humanitarian in nature, the SFI action
plan provides a comprehensive crisis response plan for handling the influx of indigenous/
ethnic populations. This transformative crisis response and disaster plan is intended to
advance strategic planning at the local, county, state, and federal government levels to be
prepared for potential associated risks of epidemics, pandemic health, illness and disease
concerns, biological risks, and other crises that might erupt as a result of populations
from war-torn countries arriving to the United States.

The guideposts presented in FEMA's SFI report explore and highlight other critical
areas of epidemic concerns such as the (a) increasing complexity and decreasing predictability of living in a secure homeland environment; (b) evolving mental, medical,

and physical health care needs of all Americans and at-risk populations; and (c) future resource constraints of fiscal, technological, and highly trained personnel to work at the epicenter of disaster. An abbreviated list of SFI scenarios includes understanding the preparation, prevention, protection, and disaster response in dealing with the health care of older aging adult populations, persons with chronic illnesses and disabilities, technology, terrorism in the homeland, pandemics, drought, and multiple other critical incidents that deal with the strain of economic resources, the deteriorating infrastructure, and other major threats that are person-made and biological in nature.

The United States is the world's strongest nation enjoying the advantages of civil rights for all cultural minority groups (e.g., persons of racial/ethnic diversity; persons with disabilities; persons that identify as lesbian, gay, bisexual, and transgender [LGBT]), state–federal programs for disability benefits (e.g., workers compensation, supplemental security income [SSI], Social Security disability insurance [SSDI]), technology, energy, and alliances and partnerships with other countries to decrease security threats on multiple levels. Despite these strengths, there are countries, governments, and other dark entities that would like to undo the benefits and progress afforded to Americans.

For example, the 2015 report of the military's contribution to national security (Joint Chiefs of Staff et al., 2016) identifies threats to our national security. These include, but are not limited to: (a) Russia—which has repeatedly demonstrated a lack of respect for the sovereignty of its neighboring countries and other actions that violate multiple human rights agreements; (b) Iran—which also has interest in pursuing nuclear and missile delivery technologies and state-sponsored terrorism, and has undermined stability in Middle Eastern countries such as Israel, Lebanon, Iraq, Syria, and Yemen; (c) North Korea—which also is in very active pursuit of nuclear weapons, ballistic missile testing, and cyber-attacks and has repeatedly and contentiously confronted and bullied Korea and Japan with harm; and (d) China—which has added much anxiety and tension to the Asia-Pacific region not only militarily, but by claiming its territories include nearly the entire South China Sea.

The key point is that the government and antigovernment groups that make up these suppressive cultures have unpredictable behaviors that threaten the health, safety, and welfare of Americans and all other reasonable countries' indigenous populations around the world. Regardless of your political, moral, and philosophical beliefs regarding the engagement in war, the presence and actions of the U.S. military, its allies, and its partners are critical to deter aggression and defeat extremist groups in key global hot spots.

History has shown that the real victims of war are defenseless and disempowered civilians. As a result of enduring national interests, national security, and a plethora of international critical incidents and issues, one gets the impression that the United States has multiple and complex concerns that are a potential threat to the health, security, and overall well-being of the homeland.

Presently, we have incurred multiple limitations that exceed our resources in responding to complex multiple critical events occurring simultaneously (e.g., terrorism, conflict/war, cyber security, natural disasters, biological threats). From some sociopolitical perspectives, issues related to immigrants, refugees, and asylum seekers have become low priority for government agencies and present a challenge of epic proportions. Thus, it is critical that we set an example of service and respond to the humanitarian needs of others, creating opportunities for healing the mind, body, and spirit of critical populations.

## GUIDELINES FOR MENTAL HEALTH SCREENINGS FOR NEWLY ARRIVED REFUGEES AND ASYLUM SEEKERS

The Centers for Disease Control and Prevention (CDC, 2016) and the Division of Global Migration and Quarantine published guidelines in June 2015 for evaluating the mental and physical health needs of newly arrived refugees and asylum seekers. The long journey of refugees and asylum seekers is a testament to their psychological, emotional, and physical resiliency. However, many die along this perilous journey. Exposure to profound stressors and traumatic events predisposes refugees and asylum seekers to a life of chronic and persistent mental and physical health conditions, causing permanent disability. More specifically, the chronic and persistent risk factors that predispose refugees and asylum seekers to a lifetime of disabilities include depression, posttraumatic stress symptoms, anxiety and panic attacks, substance use disorders, somatization, and traumatic brain injuries.

The etiology and underlying cause of refugees' and asylum seekers' mental and physical conditions are well documented in the literature (CDC, 2016; Craig, MacJajua, & Warfa, 2009; Fazel, Wheeler, & Danesh, 2005; Hanson & Vogel, 2012; Higson-Smith, 2013; Miller & Rasmussen, 2009; Pells & Treisman, 2012). It is unimaginable for most Americans to understand the horrific life that some have endured. This includes, but is not limited to, exposure to war and combat at an early age, state-sponsored violence and oppression, torture, internment camps, human trafficking, displacement from one's home and country, loss of family members and prolonged separation, the stress of adapting to a new culture, and living in poverty and unemployment. Indeed, the process of resettlement and psychosocial adjustment to living in a new country does in fact require medical and mental health interventions.

### Triage of Refugees and Asylum Seekers

Under the authority of the INA and the Public Health Service Act, the Secretary of Health and Human Services and the CDC's Division of Global Migration and Quarantine outline regulations for medical and mental health screenings of refugees seeking admission to the United States. Other government agencies involved in the medical and mental health screenings are the Department of State (DOS) and the USCIS. The process and regulations are quite complex. Thus, the reader should consult the References section for a more comprehensive review.

One of the first steps in this process is developing health clinics in the homeland and overseas for the purpose of triaging refugees and asylum seekers. Clinicians perform a variety of medical and mental health evaluations using medically trained American-born interpreters and bicultural interpreters. Based on the severity of symptoms presented by the refugee patient and his or her ability to function in daily life, the medical evaluations are triaged into three separate groups. Group I includes those refugees with chronic, serious, and acute health conditions that require immediate follow-up. Group II includes refugees with less acute mental health or psychiatric symptoms that only require routine follow-up care. Group III involves refugees without any identified mental or physical symptoms that require routine or immediate care.

## Refugees' Mental and Physical Assessment

Guidelines and procedures for the mental and physical assessment are comprehensive and mandatory for all refugees and asylum seekers coming to the United States. The goal is to prevent, detect, and intervene in mental or physical health conditions that require urgent or immediate attention and to generally assess those refugees that require referral and follow-up care with other providers. The following are mandatory evaluations completed by medical and mental health professionals:

- ▶ Review of any available premigration medical and mental health records from the refugees' country of origin
- ▶ Current medical history, physical exam, use of prescription medications, allergies, and particularly screening for such neurological conditions as traumatic brain injury
- ▶ Exposure to any occupational hazards as many indigenous minority groups have worked in agriculture, mining, and factory occupations that have a high-risk exposure to toxins
- ▶ The level of exposure to combat and other traumatic events, particularly screening for symptoms of posttraumatic stress
- ▶ Screening for other mental health conditions such as depression, anxiety, and substance use disorders. Screenings for drug and alcohol use also include any use of traditional herbal indigenous substances such as khat
- ▶ Specialized child screenings that include childhood immunizations, vaccinations, allergies, any malnutrition, maltreatment, scars, physical deformities, the child's patterns of normal development, level of education, and any somatic complaints
- ▶ Social–familial–cultural history, educational, occupational, or literacy levels

If significant positive findings emerge from any of these assessments, it is quite typical that follow-up clinical observations and assessments are warranted. All critical information is provided to resettlement agencies so that individual needs can be met. It is particularly important that upon initial assessment vulnerable populations are identified because of some unique needs requiring follow-up care. Some vulnerable populations include the following individuals: (a) pregnant women and infants, (b) severely disabled individuals and those who have chronic illnesses, (c) those who exhibit chronic and persistent psychiatric symptoms, (d) those who are developmentally disabled and those who possess other neurocognitive conditions, and (e) those who are aged, elderly, or frail.

## CULTIVATING A WORKING ALLIANCE WITH REFUGEES: CONSIDERATIONS FOR MENTAL HEALTH PROFESSIONALS

It is of paramount importance that mental health professionals use culturally sensitive approaches when interacting with refugees, many of whom are significantly culturally different from the professional's background. Rapport building is at the foundation of cultivating a strong working alliance. The use of culturally appropriate empathy and other therapeutic techniques is discussed in more detail in other chapters of the book. However, mental health professionals should anticipate some level of difficulty during rapport building, which is a natural artifact of working with immigrants, refugees, and asylum seekers. Some examples of these difficulties exist because:

► Many cultural groups distrust Americans because they were taught to fear them by their country of origin.

► The U.S. military may have invaded their country, which destabilized their government and destroyed their homeland.

► Americans are many times viewed as violent people as portrayed in movies and other electronic media.

► Some indigenous groups may view mental health professionals as an extension of their previous punitive government.

► Some indigenous groups may not understand the American lifestyle behaviors as portrayed in the electronic and social media.

► Most indigenous groups do not have a mental health provider system such as the United States and many do not endorse mental health counseling because they were taught not to disclose personal problems and issues to strangers.

Facilitating culturally sensitive approaches with refugees and asylum seekers also requires some knowledge, awareness, and skills in the following areas:

► Knowledge of the geographic location and salient aspects of the refugee's culture (i.e., religious and spiritual beliefs, occupations, daily lifestyle habits, form of government, system of health care and education)

► Competencies in the use of cultural empathy (i.e., use of eye contact, nonverbal language, spatial distance, time orientation)

► Administration and use of all assessments (standardized and nonstandardized) and an understanding that most assessments were not culturally normed on the population being served

► The mental health professional's overreliance on Western mental health counseling theories and techniques

► The mental health counselor's overuse of diagnosing and treating mental health disorders as they relate to *Diagnostic and Statistical Manual of Mental Disorders* (5th ed.; *DSM-5*; American Psychiatric Association, 2013) criteria

## First Steps in Cultivating a Working Alliance

Many refugees and asylum seekers want to escape their countries of origin because of mental and physical torture, mass violence and genocide, witnessing the killings of family members and friends, sexual abuse, kidnapping of children and women to be used in forced sexual prostitution, looting of personal possessions by the government/military, starvation, and deprivation of food, shelter, and clothing. The acts of brutality perpetrated on these indigenous groups have created distrust among almost everyone except the friends and family whom they journeyed with to find safe haven. Accordingly, mental health professionals can cultivate a working alliance possessing awareness, knowledge, and skills in the following areas:

▶ Use language interpreters when necessary for communicating and always attend to the person you are speaking to, not the interpreter. It is preferable to use an interpreter from the indigenous group you are serving.

▶ Find a tribal leader, elder, or some other member of the refugee group who has knowledge of the specific culture and the needs of his or her own people.

▶ Collaborate, support, and coordinate services working through one or two persons who are indigenous to the culture, which can help build trust among others in the group.

▶ Understand that "silence" does not imply resistance. Rather, many refugees have a natural reluctance toward Americans or engage in Western models of therapeutic services from someone outside their culture.

▶ Understand how to interpret the emotions and cognitions of refugees, which is critical to engaging in therapeutic alliances. For instance, many refugees may exhibit feelings of rage and anger. This should not be anthologized. Rather, anger and rage are many times experienced as inconceivable betrayal by the government they once trusted. There are many other emotions that require other interpretations.

▶ Use natural spaces or the natural environment to build a rapport and working alliance with someone. An office space or building can potentially intimidate many indigenous populations and may retraumatize these individuals as a representation of the brutal government from which they fled.

## Second Steps in Cultivating a Working Alliance

There are no words to describe the horrific trauma that many refugees have experienced. A seasoned humanitarian mental health professional understands the refugee's risk factors and long-term mental health problems, and knows how to reduce further traumatic exposure by creating a *circle of trust*. This trust can potentially be developed by the strategies offered in the First Steps in Cultivating a Working Alliance section and can be strengthened by the following therapeutic culturally endorsed interventions:

▶ Mental health professionals should view refugees as "survivors" rather than "victims." There are extraordinary stories of survival that can help build resiliency among others in the refugee groups. Shared storytelling among group members that are matched appropriately (men to men; women to women) is critical. Individual therapeutic interactions for many indigenous groups are not a natural way of healing. Thus, the group is only as strong and resilient as those that comprise the group. Refugee groups can draw to one another because they have earned the circle of trust.

▶ The numbness and shock of being a survivor of the horrific extraordinary stressful and traumatic events experienced by the refugee may linger much longer than anticipated. Everyone heals at his or her own rate and pace; however, the level of intensity and posttraumatic stress symptoms may endure for months after an arrival to a safe haven country.

## CONCLUDING REMARKS

The etiology of the worldwide epidemic of immigrants, refugees, and asylum seekers is clear. It is war that is at the foundation of all human suffering as millions are forced to relocate geographically. This epidemic of person-made disaster points to the overall lack of respect and empathy for human life perpetrated by brutal governments, religious zealots, and other indigenous tribal warring groups. The known causes are also exemplified by civil and religious armed conflicts, continuous bombing of villages and towns, violence perpetrated by drug warlords, forced sexual prostitution and slavery, imprisonment by the government for possessing the "wrong" sociopolitical or religious beliefs, racism, discrimination, forced isolation/internal displacement and detention camps, deprived access to adequate mental and physical health care, and the withholding of basic food, water, shelter, and clothing for warmth. Overall, disaster mental health responders who commit to work with specific indigenous populations of global cultures require a much different approach to provide culturally sensitive interventions and strategies. This chapter offers some guidelines to mental health professionals to begin working globally with the new culture of immigrants, refugees, and asylum seekers.

## REFERENCES

American Psychological Association. (2010). Resiliency and recovery after war: Refugee children and families in the United States. Retrieved from http://www.apa.org/pubs/info/reports/refugees-full -report.pdf

American Psychiatric Association. (2013). *Diagnostic and statistical manual of mental disorders* (5th ed.). Arlington, VA: American Psychiatric Publishing.

Centers for Disease Control and Prevention. (2016). Guidelines for mental health screening during the domestic medical examination for newly arrived refugees. Retrieved from http://www.cdc.gov/ immigrantrefugeehealth/pdf/mental-health-screening-guidelines.pdf

Craig, T., MacJajua, P., & Warfa, N. (2009). Mental health care needs of refugees. *Psychiatry, 8*(9), 351–354.

Fazel, M., Wheeler, J., & Danesh, J. (2005). Prevalence of serious mental disorder in 7,000 refugees resettled in Western countries: A systematic review. *The Lancet, 365*, 1309–1314.

Federal Emergency Management Agency. (2012). Crisis response and disaster resilience 2030: Forging strategic action in an age of uncertainty. Progress report highlighting the 2010 to 2011 insights of the Strategic Foresight Initiative. Retrieved from http://www.fema.gov/media-library-data/20130726-1816-25045-5167/sfi_report_13.jan.2012_final.docx.pdf

Genocide Intervention Network. (2016). Annual report 2008. Retrieved from http://endgenocide.org/wp-content/uploads/sites/4/2013/02/GI-NET-Annual-Report-Final.pdf

Hanson, E., & Vogel, G. (2012). The impact of war on civilians. In L. L. Levers (Ed.), *Trauma counseling: Theories and interventions* (pp. 412–433). New York, NY: Springer Publishing.

Higson-Smith, C. (2013). Counseling torture survivors in contexts of ongoing threat: Narratives from sub-Saharan Africa. *Journal of Peace Psychology, 19*(2), 164–179.

Homeland Security. (2016). Definition of terms. Retrieved from http://www.dhs.gov/definition-terms#permanent_resident_alien

Joint Chiefs of Staff, Unified Combatant Commands, & Office of the Secretary of Defense. (2016). *The national military strategy of the United States of America 2015: The United States military's contribution to national security.* Retrieved from http://www.jcs.mil/Portals/36/Documents/Publications/2015_National_Military_Strategy.pdf

Mercy Corps. (2016). Top stories. Retrieved from https://www.mercycorps.org

Miller, K. E., & Rasmussen, A. (2009). War exposure, daily stressors, and mental health in conflict and post-conflict settings: Bridging the divide between trauma-focused and psychosocial frameworks. *Social Science & Medicine, 70*, 7–16.

Pells, K., & Treisman, K. (2012). Genocide, ethnic conflict, and political violence. In L. L. Levers (Ed.), *Trauma counseling: Theories and interventions* (pp. 389–411). New York, NY: Springer Publishing.

Physicians for Social Responsibility. (2016). Body count: March 2015 report. Retrieved from http://www.ippnw.de/commonFiles/pdfs/Frieden/Body_Count_first_international_edition_2015_final.pdf

Stebnicki, M. A. (2015, October). *The psychosocial cost of war on non-military civilian populations: A global perspective.* Presentation made at the Annual Conference of the Licensed Professional Counseling Association of North Carolina, Raleigh, NC.

Stichick, T., & Bruderlein, C. (2001). Children facing insecurity: New strategies for survival in the global era. Harvard program on humanitarian policy and conflict research. Retrieved from http://reliefweb.int/sites/reliefweb.int/files/resources/F067BD96BAD2F990C12571D900437781-Harvard-May2001.pdf

United Nations. (2016). New UN report warns of "abhorrent violations" against children in war-torn Iraq. Retrieved from https://childrenandarmedconflict.un.org/new-un-report-warns-of-abhorrent-violations-against-children-in-war-torn-iraq

United Nations High Commissioner for Refugees. (2016). World refugee day: Global forced displacement tops 50 million for the first time in post-WWII era. Retrieved from http://www.unhcr.org/53a155bc6.html

U.S. Citizens and Immigration Services. (2016a). Immigration and Nationality Act. Retrieved from https://www.uscis.gov/laws/immigration-and-nationality-act

U.S. Citizens and Immigration Services. (2016b). Policy manual. Retrieved from https://www.uscis.gov/policymanual/HTML/PolicyManual.html#introduction

U.S. Citizens and Immigration Services. (2016c). Refugees and the refugee process. Retrieved from https://www.uscis.gov/humanitarian/refugees-asylum/refugees

U.S. State Department (2016). Diplomacy in action. Retrieved from http://www.state.gov

War Chronicle. (2016). Estimated war dead World War II. Retrieved from http://warchronicle.com/numbers/WWII/deaths.htm

Wiist, W. H., Barker, K., Arya, N., Rhode, J., Donohoe, M., White, S., . . . Hagopain, A. (2014). The role of public health in the prevention of war: Rationale and competencies. *American Journal of Public Health, 106*(4), 34–37. http://dx.doi.org/10.2105/AJPH.2013.301.778

# CHAPTER 15

# Military and Disaster Mental Health Counseling*

Mental health counselors are challenged with providing disaster and trauma counseling services to a variety of populations, some of whom may be culturally different. Active duty military and many veterans who have been exposed to combat have a much different experience and response to such trauma and disaster, significantly more so than civilians. It is of paramount importance for counselors to understand the unique cultural differences between military and civilian mental health. This chapter elucidates the unique cultural characteristics in regard to diagnosing and treating posttraumatic stress symptoms (PTSSs) and other mental health conditions that result in cumulative and repeated exposure to overseas deployments while being at the epicenter of combat, violence, and a host of other traumas.

A great deal of counselor education and research has been developed that focuses on preparing professional counselors in understanding the unique cultural attributes of a diversity of cultural groups (e.g., Arredondo, Gallardo-Cooper, Delgado-Romero, & Zapata, 2014; Balcazar, Suarez-Balcazar, Taylor-Ritzler, & Keys, 2010; Corey, Corey, Corey, & Callanan, 2015; Ivey, Bradford Ivey, & Zalaquett, 2010; Lee, 2013; Murphy & Dillon, 2011; Pedersen, 2000; Ratts & Pedersen, 2014). The military is clearly recognized in the counseling and psychology literature as a culture unto itself because of its language, rituals, organizational structure, values, mission, and the within-group difference in the various branches of the military (e.g., Army, Air Force, Navy, Marines, Coast Guard, National Guard, Reservists). In fact, many of the newer multicultural counseling textbooks now include a chapter on military counseling. The importance cannot be overstated in knowing how to establish a rapport and build an optimal working alliance with those who identify themselves as active duty, veterans, disabled veterans, or a family member.

*Adapted from Chapter 77, Stebnicki (2016), in *The Professional Counselor's Desk Reference* (2nd ed.), © Springer Publishing Company.

Assessment, diagnosis, and treatment issues are both similar and different when counseling military versus community or civilian populations. Some of these notable differences relate to the (a) psychosocial response to combat and trauma versus civilian types of traumatic experiences; (b) types of injuries and disabilities acquired on the battlefield (e.g., blast wounds, traumatic brain injury [TBI]); (c) occupational status between enlisted and officer ranks; (d) resiliency, coping skills, and posttraumatic growth required to maintain alertness and mission-ready status; (e) mission and specialty operations performed within each branch of service; (f) psychosocial adjustment issues related to acquired traumatic mental and physical conditions; (g) the military response to PTSSs versus the civilian response; (h) understanding the deployment cycle; and (i) reintegration and transition from active duty to civilian life, particularly with acquired mental and physical health conditions (Stebnicki, 2016).

## MENTAL HEALTH AND DISASTER TRAINING WITH MILITARY POPULATIONS

In a national survey of military counseling content and curriculum in Council on Rehabilitation Education (CORE, 2014) and Council for Accreditation of Counseling and Related Educational Programs (CACREP, 2014) accredited master's programs (Stebnicki, Clemmons-James, & Leierer, 2016), none of the program directors/coordinators surveyed indicated that they have a specialty-track, concentration, or degree program that relates to military counseling. Only one program indicated it offered a 12-semester-hour certificate program in military and trauma counseling. Less than 5% of respondents indicated that they had a military course as an elective. Most counselor education programs reported that military counseling-related issues were infused in other course work throughout the 60-semester-hour curriculum (i.e., professional issues, mental health assessment and treatment, orientation to the profession). Overall, military mental health counseling issues have been sparsely undertaken in terms of curriculum development or student engagement activities. Thus, it may be difficult for preprofessional mental health counselors to develop their skills as they relate to treating trauma and disaster within military populations. Receiving continuing education opportunities in military trauma counseling may in fact be difficult for licensed mental health professionals; training may not be readily available, making it difficult to have a cultural understanding of active duty, veterans, veterans with disabilities, and their family members (Helwig & Schmidt, 2011).

## MILITARY CULTURE

Each of the military's different branches has its own operational language, rituals, values, mission, organization, and sociopolitical structure. It meets the definition of a culture unto itself (Stebnicki, 2016). The U.S. Department of Defense (DoD, 2016a) has its own military dictionary: officer ranks and insignias (DoD, 2016d); enlisted ranks and insignias (DoD, 2016b); its own laws and code of conduct (DoD, 2016c); and many other life areas that define the mission and operations within the different branches of the service (e.g., Army, Air Force, Navy, Marines, Coast Guard, National Guard, Reservists).

Adler and Castro (2013) suggest that no other occupations exist where the demands of killing, avoiding being killed, caring for the wounded, and witnessing death and injury are all required parts of training, except for the job of military service. There are frequent geographic relocations; separation from family, friends, and loved ones; and 24/7 availability where one is always on call. It is within this culture where service members' lives, health, and safety depend on one another to be optimally mentally and physical fit for duty. This close-knit group of active duty personnel and veterans creates a type of extended family that is not typically seen in most work environments.

One fundamental difference between the military and civilian response to trauma is again delineated by Adler and Castro's (2013) Occupational Mental Health Model for the military. They suggest that service members are not passive "victims" of being at the epicenter of extraordinary stressful and traumatic events. Rather, military personnel train for the physical and psychological demands of combat on a frequent basis, whereas civilians do not. Thus, the reaction to trauma for military personnel is to aggress, not stress. In civilian life, most individuals react as "victims" because they are not prepared mentally and physically to be confronted with such unpredictable traumatic events. Thus, in civilian trauma, the individual typically experiences an acute onset of the full range of PTSSs, such as intrusive, intense, and prolonged traumatic memories; persistent avoidance of the trauma triggers; hypervigilance; detachment; isolation; and withdrawal.

When military personnel witness catastrophic injury or death on the battlefield, it is "mission forward" because the life and safety of their brothers and sisters are dependent on how well they perform physically and mentally. It is not possible to begin the grieving process while one is fighting for survival. Thus, military personnel may not experience the full range of PTSSs or feel the symptoms of loss and grief while in a state of high alert. Consequently, PTSSs may be delayed and the full mental health effects may not be experienced until postdeployment. For some veterans, these PTSSs are transient; they go through periods of exacerbation and remission. However, many are chronic and persistent throughout one's lifetime with varying degrees of intensity.

Even though military personnel experience extraordinary stressful and traumatic events at a significantly greater frequency than civilians, the mental health needs are the same. However, the psychosocial adjustment to trauma is somewhat different between military personnel and civilians. For example, many civilians have immediate access to mental health services early on in the aftermath and recovery of traumatic events. Additionally, civilians typically do not experience the stigma attached to seeking mental health treatment as is found in military culture (Stebnicki, 2015).

In contrast, military personnel rarely seek mental health counseling, especially during deployment. In the hypermasculine culture of the military, active duty personnel are trained to "suck it up." If active duty personnel, regardless of rank, seek mental health counseling and are diagnosed with a mental health condition such as posttraumatic stress disorder (PTSD) or substance use disorder (SUD), the service member is at risk for losing his or her rank, career promotions, security clearances, and overall can be isolated by unit members because unit command will lose trust in his or her ability to perform in dangerous environments. In a worst case scenario, the service member may be medically discharged or receive a dishonorable or less-than-honorable discharge.

The important point here for mental health counselors is that military personnel per-form a very mentally and physically challenging occupation or career that demands the use of multiple coping and resiliency skills, some of which may be healthy (i.e., talking to someone) or unhealthy (i.e., drinking heavily). Most military personnel do not live within a culture that endorses mental health screening, assessment, and treatment on a regular and ongoing basis. As a consequence, these individuals may be at risk for a variety of undiagnosed conditions that could manifest in the months and years to come. Thus, there may be lost opportunities for psychotherapeutic approaches in which medi-cation alone cannot heal the wounds of war.

## THE DEPLOYMENT CYCLE

As a natural artifact of serving in the military, there are significant life events that emerge within the cycle of deployment (Basham, 2013; Pincus, House, Christenson, & Adler, 2014). Mobilizations can occur in the continental United States (referred to as CONUS) or overseas, typically referred to as "deployment." Some military personnel are mobi-lized or deployed for humanitarian missions while others are in support of combat troops. Some deployments are in combat zones (referred to by Navy personnel as "com-bat space") where troops are down range, or operate strategically in a command and control or forward operating base (FOB). Other deployments may be on a base overseas (rear base such as a Naval or Army hospital). The deployment cycle as discussed in the literature basically is a theoretical stage model of psychosocial adaptation and adjust-ment that predicts the anticipated physical, psychological, emotional, psychosocial, and family reactions to being deployed, redeployed, and reintegrated to either military or civilian life. Mental health counselors who are familiar with the different phases or stages of the deployment cycle can choose specific mental health strategies and approaches such as critical incident stress debriefings or short-term solution-focused therapy to decrease the symptoms of trauma, substance abuse, depression, and other significant mental health conditions that decrease mental and physical functioning.

Despite varying interpretations in the literature of the phases within the deployment cycle, most models are described in three phases: recovery, resiliency, and reintegra-tion. Theoretically, transitioning successfully through each of the phases requires mul-tiple support systems and coping and resiliency skills that are both internal and external to the individual. It is beyond the scope of this chapter to comprehensively discuss the deployment cycle. The resources in this chapter provide an excellent and comprehensive resource for helping professional counselors understand the difficult challenges that military personnel must navigate during various stages of their deployment cycle (see Defense Centers of Excellence [DCoE], 2016; Military One Source, 2014; Pincus et al., 2014). This is particularly an issue for service members who transition from active duty to civilian life, which requires career and vocational counseling (Farley, 2010, 2013).

Mental health professionals who do not understand the unique aspects and chal-lenges of service members within the deployment cycle may not understand military culture. Consequently, some counselors may inaccurately assess, diagnose, and treat individuals based on the traditional training they received from their counselor education programs. Knowing the unique aspects of the deployment cycle assists mental health counselors in gaining therapeutic leverage and developing appropriate goals with active duty military, veterans, and/or family members. The following is a brief description of unique characteristics within the deployment cycle:

▶ *Predeployment:* The service member receives a "warning order" for deployment where he or she leaves his or her state-side base. Deployments can vary from 3 to 15 months, depending on the mission. Unique characteristics with this stage include (a) the possible anticipation or denial of loss of life or separation from family; (b) training up for combat involving intense exercises; (c) getting all affairs in order; (d) mental and/or physical distancing from family, spouse/partner, and loved ones; and (e) decreased communication and intimacy with spouse/partners and emotional insulation from family members.

▶ *Deployment:* This stage can last a month. Military spouses/partners report feelings of abandonment with a major life shift in all household and family responsibilities. Unique characteristics with this stage include (a) mixed emotions of anxiety, depression, and relief; (b) feelings of disorientation and being overwhelmed; (c) emotional sense of loneliness, sadness, numbness, detachment, and isolation; (d) sleep disturbances; and (e) feeling secure in a new environment.

▶ *Sustainment:* This stage can last between 2 and 5 months. It is marked by a period of establishing new resources for support with a heavy reliance on the family readiness officer (FRO). The FRO is typically a civilian spouse of the deployed who serves in a professional capacity as the primary coordinator of activities, events, and communications from command on the progress of the mission. As challenges arise, spouses/partners and family members realize that they have developed some coping resources. Life is somewhat back to balance again, but only in a new and different way.

▶ *Postdeployment:* This stage is marked by the intense anticipation of a "homecoming" and the spouse's/partner's thoughts of whether he or she is the same mentally, physically, and psychologically as before deployment. Exact return dates from deployment can vary from weeks to months, making things very intense and frustrating for family members. Some military units go through 1 to 2 weeks of debriefing before going back to their home station/base or family members. This time is spent in psychological stress/debriefings, physical examinations, and other activities to prepare the individual to reintegrate into the mix of military–civilian life. Some postdeployment programs include spouse/partners in therapeutic and informational activities.

▶ *Reintegration:* Time frames for this stage are variable, depending on the family coping skills and resiliency traits. It is common that many military personnel desire their own space and can only handle short periods of family time/family togetherness and may not feel any intimacy between their spouse/partner. Many bases require follow-up support services for the service member such as follow-up mental and medical health appointments, command briefings, family readjustment activities, and other programs and services to assist with reintegration.

The following comprehensive resources provide an excellent guide to professional counselors who are dealing with military clients who have issues related to deployment, recovery, resiliency, and reintegration.

## COMBAT EXPOSURE

Some of the more familiar "war stories" as told by active duty or combat veterans include phrases such as "my head was always on a swivel"; "I only got 2 hours of sleep"; "I saw some of my unit buddies blown up and burned alive"; and countless other stories that depict the mental, emotional, psychological, and physical horrors of war. In an occupation where injury and casualty notifications are given to troops and family members on a frequent basis, good battlefield medicine makes the difference between life and death. For some, survivor guilt and witnessing death and injury become the motivation for hunting down combatants.

Clearly, exposure to combat increases the risk for chronic and persistent mental and physical health problems throughout one's life. Operation Enduring Freedom (OEF; Afghanistan 2001), Operation Iraqi Freedom (OIF; Iraq 2003), and Operation New Dawn (OND; Afghanistan 2001) have seen about two million troops deployed overseas with up to 100,000 injuries and over 6,825 fatalities at the time of this writing (Department of Defense [DoD], 2014). The signature injury of the current conflict is TBI that affects 13% to 25% of military personnel. These injuries typically occur from mortar, rocket, artillery, small arms, roadside bombs, improvised explosive devices (IEDs), sniper attack, and blast wounds. High rates of mental health conditions are also associated with TBI such as posttraumatic stress (PTS; 15%–60%), depression (23%), anxiety (43%), and SUDs (10%–34%).

## MILITARY PTSD

Another condition related to combat exposure is PTSD. Many service members do not like this diagnostic category because of the stigma attached to having a "disorder." Moreover, having a medical record of PTSD can hinder one's career, such as receiving promotions, losing security clearances, and not being able to carry a weapon; these are integral to the military occupation. The terms *PTS* or *PTSSs* are preferable when addressing mental health problems in this area. The term *PTS* normalizes the combat exposure experience for many service members who can relate with being in a state of hypervigilance, having intrusive thoughts and memories of unit members being blown up, and having the intense prolonged mind–body effects that are associated with being in the epicenter of combat. PTS is much less clinically oriented, which helps build rapport with clients and suggests that the counselor is treating the individual, not the diagnostic category.

The diagnostic category of PTSD as observed in the new *Diagnostic and Statistical Manual of Mental Disorders* (5th ed.; *DSM-5*; American Psychiatric Association, 2013) is no longer subsumed under anxiety disorders. Rather, PTSD is listed within its own separate category (see *DSM-5* 309.81). Military PTSD researchers suggest that some of their criteria and diagnostic features may not fit well or be relevant with the reactions of the service members affected (Adler & Castro, 2013; Kilpatrick et al., 2013; Roitman, Gilad, Ankri, & Shalev, 2013). For instance, the *DSM-5* does not consider multiple traumas experienced on a regular and ongoing basis while being exposed to multiple combat missions. Further, the persistent avoidance of the traumatic triggers, intrusive thoughts, dissociative reactions, or flashbacks may have a delayed response in military life. The mind–body or sympathetic–parasympathetic response for most military personnel exposed to combat is that of survival and "mission forward." Service members cannot afford a "flight" response. Rather, the life, safety, and health of their brothers and sisters depend on the "fight" or "aggress-not-stress" response. Overall, there is a direct correlation between chronic and persistent PTSSs and the level of combat exposure. Accounting for individual resiliency factors, those who have had low or no exposure to combat have a much lower chance of being diagnosed with PTSD.

To further understand how military life differs from civilian life, Algoe and Fredrickson (2011) suggest that being in the military prompts changes in the service member's social structure that reflect a change from independence in civilian life to interdependence within a strict sociocultural hierarchy of rank. The men and women who train to become mission ready, deploy and are transported long geographic distances together, live and eat in close quarters, and share the requirements of mental and physical toughness, must be intentionally focused in varying degrees of mental and physical readiness. Overall, the demands of being trained to kill combatants, avoiding being killed, caring for the wounded, and witnessing death and injury have a psychological cost. Military service is not just an occupation; rather, it is a culture integrated into the individual's mind, body, spirit, and mission readiness that cannot easily be "turned off" after departure and reintegration into civilian life.

The diagnostic category of PTSD itself has been redefined in some of the military literature and is often referred to as *complex PTSD*. This is because of the coexisting physical and mental health-related conditions associated with trauma experienced in combat. This includes, but is not limited to, SUDs, depression, anxiety, TBI, sleep disorders, and other chronic medical health conditions. It can be anticipated that most military personnel who have acquired any of the aforementioned mental health conditions, particularly PTSS, likely do not seek treatment. This is because of the (a) stigma attached to seeing a mental health professional while on active duty; (b) perception that those military personnel who seek treatment may be viewed as weak, not possessing leadership qualities, or could lack focus and concentration during high-stress critical incidents such as combat; (c) hypermasculine traits represented in military life with the expectations to conform (i.e., "suck it up", "mission forward", "mission first"); and (d) the impact that seeking treatment has on rank, career promotions, and maintaining security clearances.

## DEPRESSION IN THE MILITARY

Depression has reached epidemic proportions in the United States. It is the most reported medical and mental health condition seen in primary care physicians' offices. Approximately 30% of patients seen by family or internal medicine physicians in civilian populations are diagnosed with depression. The majority of patients (70%–80%) present with physical symptoms only. Thus, the primary treatment involves medication only. Few patients receive comprehensive care such as receiving psychotherapy and medication. Obviously, physicians are not practicing psychotherapists. However, even those trained in the role of prescriber (i.e., psychiatrists, nurse practitioners) do not typically engage in long-term psychotherapy with their patients. In the general civilian population, 15% to 20% of individuals are treated for depression, with an 80% recovery rate. Approximately 22% of individuals diagnosed with depression have a relapse of symptoms within the first year of treatment.

Dr. Andrew Weil, an integrative medicine physician and director of one of the nation's first medical schools of integrative medicine (University of Arizona), talks extensively about the epidemic of depression in *Spontaneous Happiness* (Weil, 2011). He has been a researcher and practitioner in mind–body medicine for over 40 years. According to many researchers, depression will be the second most disabling condition in the United States by 2020. There are multiple factors that account for depression but at least half of all patients with depression are undiagnosed and untreated. Dr. Weil suggests that in his research and physician practice, the majority of patients with depression can be treated without any pharmaceutical products. A small percentage of patients actually benefit from short-term use of antidepressant medications. The majority can heal with behavioral lifestyle changes that are learned in counseling and psychotherapy, or with proper exercise and nutrition, herbal remedies, and other integrative approaches.

Regardless of military or civilian populations, the incidence and prevalence of major depressive disorders increase exponentially based on exposure to trauma, chronic illness, and disability. Depression is a natural artifact of exposure to extraordinary stressful and traumatic events such as exposure to combat. It is comorbid with other diagnosed mental health conditions such as PTSD, generalized anxiety disorders (GADs), and SUDs, and exists in the downward cycle of bipolar disorders. Depression is particularly present during medical conditions such as chronic pain, TBI, neurocognitive disorders, spinal cord injury, traumatic amputation, stroke, cancer, rheumatoid arthritis, Parkinson's disease, and many other conditions. Many of the chronic medical illnesses are acquired long after exposure from moderate to high levels of combat. The residual functional deficits are seen in many VA clinics and other health care practices in veteran populations 10 to 20 years after discharge from military service.

## SUBSTANCE USE DISORDERS

The DoD substance use personnel policy (DoD, 2016e) requires all branches of service to conduct random urinalysis drug testing to detect and deter drug use among active duty service members. If a service member does test positive, the commander should refer him or her for further drug and alcohol assessment. After an SUD assessment is completed by a qualified professional, a determination is made according to the DoD's problematic substance abuse policy. The response from the service personnel's command can range anywhere from mandatory treatment to dishonorable discharge.

The research on co-occurring mental health conditions such as PTSD and SUDs indicates that there is a strong association between trauma exposure and SUDs. However, mental health counselors should not make assumptions regarding this link. Recently, researchers in trauma and addiction suggest that having such a co-occurring mental health condition can precede each other, follow each other, contribute to the development or course of PTSD, or arise independently of one another (Burke & Curruth, 2012). Thus, exposure to trauma per se and the development of PTSD do not necessarily increase the risk of developing drug and alcohol addiction. Substance use patterns must be viewed as a biopsychosocial issue where there are many contributing factors.

The National Center for PTSD (NCPTSD, 2016) provides a clinician's guide to deal with substance abuse issues during deployment. The reader may want to consult the References section as a recommended resource for an in-depth comprehensive approach to deal with SUDs for active duty military and veterans.

## SUICIDE IN THE MILITARY

Suicide in the military and among veterans has reached epidemic proportions. The Department of Defense Suicide Prevention Office (DoD, 2015) reports a significant increase in the incidence and prevalence of suicide ideation, threats, attempts, and completions across all branches of the military. In fact, suicide completions in the military during 2012 surpassed that of casualties on the battlefield in 2011. Suicide risk in the military depends on multiple factors stated as follows:

▶ Younger active duty males who have had combat exposure have at least a three times higher risk than active duty females to have a suicide attempt or completion. Note: In civilian populations, older White males (veterans) are at four times higher risk than females to have a suicide attempt or completion.

▶ Suicide behavioral health assessments include assessing risk factors such as age, medical/physical conditions, exposure to combat, and other comorbid psychiatric conditions. Military members that have comorbid conditions such as depression or bipolar disorder are at the highest risk, followed by those with SUDs, PTSD, and TBI.

▶ Among OEF/OIF veterans, those who have screened positive for PTSD are over four times more likely to have frequent episodes of suicidal ideation than those without PTSD.

▶ Veterans who have both PTSD and TBI are at three times higher risk (than those with TBI alone) to have suicide attempts.

## Suicide Assessment

Traditional suicide mental health assessments, as seen in civilian community mental health clinics, must be adjusted for active duty personnel or military veterans. This is primarily because of the: (a) hypermasculine culture of the military, which does not endorse, support, or reinforce disclosure of feelings, emotions, and cognitions related to depression, posttraumatic stress symptoms, and other mental health conditions; (b) stigma associated with mental health counseling while active duty because of the fear of losing promotions, security clearances, and confidence as a stable leader; (c) mission-forward, aggress-not-stress culture that requires constant attention to the life and safety issues related to the combat environment; and (d) secrecy, shame, and confusion of disclosure of multiple and complex trauma exposure. Consequently, the mental health practitioner or medical health care provider may underestimate the lethality of both active duty military and veterans due to lack of disclosure.

The Department of Veterans Affairs (2016) provides multiple resources for mental health practitioners who work with military veterans. One particular source readers may want to consult is the Safety Plan Quick Guide for Clinicians, which delineates warning signs of suicide and assesses intent and some of the other symptoms associated with suicide lethality.

Table 15.1 compares and contrasts the traditional community mental health assessment with a military service member and veteran suicide assessment. Overall, it is important to distinguish the differences between community-based and military-based mental health assessments. This includes the interpretation and consideration of structured and unstructured, formal and informal mental health assessments.

Overall, suicide assessment requires a competent professional who can evaluate specific cultural factors related to military and veteran populations. All suicide ideation and threats should be taken seriously. However, some community mental health providers may overreact because of the stigma attached with being in the military (e.g., the perception that all military personnel are angry, prone to violence, and are a risk to others around them).

## MILITARY INTAKE INTERVIEW

The intake interview is critical to understanding the current status and needs of service members, whether they are active duty or veteran clients. The personal interview is one of the more powerful means by which to assess the individual's mental health functioning. Diagnostic tools and standardized assessments may provide good data to professional counselors. However, competent and ethical mental health counseling approaches to build rapport and connect with clients face to face may be the best approach to assessment and diagnosis. The content revealed within each of the questions in the following list should yield many relevant details about the individual service member's background. This should ultimately assist in developing the client's treatment plan and identify resources and unused opportunities.

## TABLE 15.1 Traditional Community Mental Health Versus Military Mental Health Suicide Assessment

| Traditional Community Mental Health Assessment | Military/Veteran Mental Health Assessment |
|---|---|
| 1. Does the individual communicate an intent to harm self or others? | MIL/Vet may be emotionally detached or choose not to disclose personal feelings, emotions, and cognitions because of stigma, fear of losing career promotions and trust by other unit members, or may need to be in a constant state of mission ready, mission forward. |
| 2. Has the individual devised a detailed plan? (Are any weapons accessible—is there a history of anger, aggression, violence?) | MIL/Vet may not disclose a plan but has been trained to aggress not stress, has displayed use of weapons, may feel internal anger, and has certainly been exposed to violence. |
| 3. Does the individual have a history of any suicide ideation, threats, and/or attempts? | MIL/Vet may have no record of mental health treatment because of stigma involved with counseling. |
| 4. Are there any specific life stressors that the individual experienced recently (e.g., loss of a loved one, chronic illness/disability, legal issues, incarceration)? | MIL/Vet combat exposure places the person in a high-risk category of witnessing and experiencing loss, death, and life-threatening injury. Issues with complex PTSD complicate exposure to life stressors within the deployment cycle. |
| 5. Does the individual have any current mental health risk factors (e.g., depression, bipolar, PTSD, SUDs, TBI)? | MIL/Vet who has combat exposure likely has undiagnosed/untreated mental and physical health risk factors. |
| 6. What type and level of support does the individual have (family, friends, other)? | MIL/Vet, due to overseas deployment or geographic relocation (CONUS), may lack family support. Their unit may offer some support, but if mental health risk factors go unrecognized by command, this increases the suicide risk. In particular, those guards or reservists who do not live on base/in garrison lack the natural supports because after deployment they typically go back to their hometowns and rarely do others know what they have been exposed to. |

CONUS, continental United States; PTSD, posttraumatic stress disorder; SUD, substance use disorder; TBI, traumatic brain injury.

A word of caution should be noted during the intake interview. The professional counselor should not expect or even anticipate full disclosure of all details. This is because service personnel cannot disclose many categories of information related to national security interests. Some categories include, but are not limited to, geographic location of their mobilization, deployment, or mission; the nature and extent of their work and what they did on their mission; and the types of tools, knowledge, machinery, weaponry, computer programs, or other materials they dealt with while on the job.

Additionally, it is of paramount importance to understand that women in the military have a much different experience than men. Female service members are more likely to experience military sexual trauma (MST), physical assault, and intimate partner violence (IPV) at much higher rates than men in the military (Iverson, Mercado, Carpenter, & Street, 2013). The intake interview for female service members should integrate questions related to the exposure of any previous interpersonal violence, particularly incidents of childhood or adult sexual abuse, sexual harassment, or assault by males during training or while deployed. Sexual trauma questionnaires in the military oftentimes include questions such as: "While in the military have you/did you receive uninvited and unwanted sexual attention such as touching or cornering, pressure for sexual favors, or verbal remarks?" and "Did someone ever use force or the threat of force to have sexual contact with you?" If the person responds in the affirmative to any of these questions, then the professional counselor must also consider these traumatic events in treatment planning.

The following list of questions should assist professional counselors in understanding the active duty member or veteran's background as it relates to his or her particular culture. Each of these questions may merit follow-up probes.

- What is your MOS (military occupational service for Marines, Army, Air Force)?
- What is your RATE (Navy pay grade) or Rating (Navy occupational service)?
- Where did you do your basic training?
- What advanced training do you have?
- Any experiences that you remember that caused negative or disturbing memories?
- Have you talked to anyone about these experiences?
- Are you (were you) married during your time in the service (or during your deployment)?
- Do you (have you ever) used the VA for services?
- When you were deployed overseas were you in a combat zone? FOB?
- Have you ever been surrounded by the enemy? Blown up? Under fire?
- Have you witnessed the death or serious injury of anyone in your unit?

## MEDICAL AND PSYCHOSOCIAL ASPECTS

As a result of medical advances, improved body armor, and battlefield life-saving medicine, there are more active duty military and veterans who have survived traumatic injuries than ever before (Jackson, Thoman, Suris, & North, 2012). Besides being at a much higher risk for mental health issues (i.e., PTSS, SUDs, depression) during deployment and combat operations, researchers suggest that many servicemen and servicewomen have significantly more visits to their medical health care providers (Lehavot, Der-Martirosian, Simpson, Shipherd, & Washington, 2013; Wachen et al., 2013). Additionally, professional counselors should anticipate a high incidence of MST among female active duty and veteran clients, which places this group in an even higher risk category of mental and physical health problems. Overall, both men and women who have served in the military are at risk for acquiring chronic and persistent health-related conditions throughout their lifetime.

## Health Concerns of Military Veterans

The following is a list of frequently reported symptoms of military personnel and veterans that are recognized among health care providers (Lehavot et al., 2013; Wachen et al., 2013). They are divided into specific body systems. It should be noted that women who screen positive for PTSD have more frequent visits to their medical providers and report poorer physical health than their male counterparts.

- ▶ *Cardiovascular:* chest pain
- ▶ *Dermatological:* skin disorders (rashes, eczema, psoriasis, unexpected hair loss, scalp problems)
- ▶ *Gastrointestinal:* frequent diarrhea, recurrent abdominal pain, recurrent nausea
- ▶ *Genitourinary:* sexual difficulties or discomfort, loss of bowel and bladder control
- ▶ *Musculoskeletal:* loss of strength, joint and muscle pain, joint stiffness
- ▶ *Neurological:* recurrent migraines, numbness, difficulty speaking, tinnitus, eye and vision problems
- ▶ *Pulmonary:* wheezing, coughing, shortness of breath, frequent coughing

## Blast Wounds and TBI

TBI experienced by explosions is divided into three areas: primary (changes in atmospheric pressure caused by a blast wave), secondary (blast injuries occurring as a result of objects accelerated by energy of the explosion striking the victim), and tertiary (injury as a result of the victim's body being thrown by the blast; Warden, 2006; Wightman & Gladish, 2001). All blast injuries involve high-explosive detonations where the person is exposed to some level of inhalations of dust, smoke, carbon monoxide, chemicals, burns from hot gasses or fires, and in some cases having a penetrating wound or being thrown against a hard surface. Regardless of having an open or closed head brain injury, the nature of such experiences results in complex TBI. The mild classification of TBI (referred to sometimes as postconcussive syndrome) accounts for about 85% of all TBIs. Consequently, the service member may experience the following symptoms: an altered state of consciousness for up to 30 minutes; reduced concentration, focus, short-term memory, and ability to learn new tasks; persistent headaches, vertigo, tinnitus, and sleep disturbance; and depression, irritability, and anger.

As the medical and health care community is equipped to work with the medical–physical injuries of servicemen and servicewomen, professional counselors must step up and become mission ready to work with those who have mental and psychosocial health needs. Overall, understanding psychosocial adjustment issues related to chronic illness and disability (Marini & Stebnicki, 2012), as well as working with clients who have psychiatric, substance abuse, and mental health issues (Levers, 2012), are essential in healing traumatic experiences.

## THE WOUNDED WARRIOR AND MORAL INJURY

Military personnel return from deployment with severe wounds that are invisible. Many refer to this as *moral injury*. Dr. Edward Tick (2014) has written extensively on moral injury. He is author of many books including the *Warrior's Return: Restoring the Soul After War*. Dr. Tick offers multiple resources to veterans and family members in the transformational journey to restoring the soul after the soul-wounding experienced by those who have been at the epicenter of combat and war. Dr. Tick has worked with veterans regarding the treatment of military PTSD for over 40 years. He is a cofounding member, along with his wife, of the nonprofit organization "Soldier's Heart."

In fact, an entire category of invisible wounds exist besides moral injury. This includes, but is not limited to, TBI, MST, GAD, SUDs, and PTSD. Moral injuries cause a range of symptoms and behaviors that also include insomnia, nightmares, anger, rage, flashbacks, hypervigilance, and difficulty with concentration and focus. Consequently, the residual functional capacity of moral injury involves a crippling combination of scars that prevent veteran men and women from engaging in social and intimate relationships, occupations and careers, educational opportunities, recreational activities, and living life optimally.

Indeed, moral injuries are invisible wounds that have no identifiable clinical medical–physical findings. The war fighter's psychological–emotional battle wounds are not visible by others outside of the military culture. Rather, the etiology appears to lie in the existential and spiritual realm, which requires a transformation after finding meaning and purpose in the reintegration of the wounded soul. As a consequence, many veterans are not recognized for their heroism because stories are rarely if ever shared with others outside the circle of trust (e.g., selected family members, former unit buddies, VFW mentors). Many veterans have internalized their PTSSs. Yet, they are experienced as shame, denial, and loss of meaning and purpose in civilian life overall. The long-term effects of these types of traumatic experiences result in chronic illnesses, depression, SUDs, anxiety disorders, suicide ideation, and suicide completions.

Some veterans do not use the term *moral injury*. However, they might remark that "my trauma didn't happen from combat . . . it happened when I was confronted by killing enemy combatants and realizing they were another human being." Some would say that the mission itself had no meaning and may remark, for example, that "we fought hard in the Korengal Valley for a year and now we just left it." Some state that "I left this country a warrior thinking I was protecting American lives, but when I returned home from Iraq I realized that I became merely a mercenary for corporations."

Exposure to war causes more than physical injuries. In some ways, the traumatic experiences of veterans have been reflected as a betrayal of what is right and wrong; good and evil; what is supposed to be spiritual and sacred. Some veterans do not want to recognize the frequency and intensity of these traumatic experiences as they relate to such feelings and cognitions. This is because moral injury is somewhat of an ambiguous loss, a loss without meaning and purpose, a soul wounding.

Dr. Tick suggests that issues related to moral injury have become exacerbated around 2009 when the DoD decided that PTSD alone did not meet the criteria for receiving a Purple Heart. This award was designated for primarily physical wounds caused by "outside forces or agents." In many ways, the absence of a combat service medal (other than the general medals associated with being deployed in-country of operations such as Iraqi/Afghanistan) sends the message to the military veteran that the mission has very little meaning and does not validate his or her combat experiences. Overall, the DoD position suggests that one's wounds must be visible, there must be blood spilled and physical injuries sustained to be a true "wounded warrior." Many veterans have interpreted the Purple Heart policy as a betrayal by a nation that holds them responsible for their own internal invisible suffering.

In Native American tradition, wounds were not hidden while the warrior returned home. The wounds of many Indian tribes were painted, decorated, and displayed on their horses and on themselves. Some veterans today who have come back from war as amputees proudly display their prosthetic devices. In summary, moral injuries are described as a type of "soul wound" where the epicenter is that of "the tortured soul" that is violating the morals, principles, ideology, and truth of human existence—or what being human is all about. The individual cannot be healed by medicine or surgery. Rather, the psychosocial and psychospiritual aspects of healing a moral injury begin from recognizing the ambiguous nature of this invisible, yet very lethal wound that is not sustained by physical injury. Then the person needs to go through a ritual, initiation, or healing process that leads to rebirth of the soul. Native healers call this a "soul retrieval." Many advocate that the veterans' experiences must be made public, validated, and not remain invisible. To live in a shroud of secrecy and shame only deepens the pain and suffering of the tortured soul.

## CONCLUDING REMARKS

One fundamental difference between the military and civilian response to trauma is that military service members are not passive "victims" of being at the epicenter of extraordinary stressful and traumatic events. Rather, military personnel train for the physical and psychological demands of combat on a frequent basis, whereas civilians do not. Thus, the reaction to trauma for military personnel is to aggress, not stress. In civilian life, most individuals react as "victims" because they are not prepared mentally and physically to be confronted with such unpredictable traumatic events. Thus, in civilian trauma, the individual typically experiences an acute onset of the full range of PTSSs such as intrusive, intense, and prolonged traumatic memories; persistent avoidance of the trauma triggers; hypervigilance; detachment; isolation; and withdrawal. In military life, however, the physiological and psychological reactions tend to be muted and delay the full range of symptoms related to complex PTSD. Overall, military personnel have had a higher exposure to trauma, particularly cumulative trauma. If mental health counselors want to work at optimal levels with active duty service members, veterans, and family members, it is critical that they have awareness, knowledge, and skills to work with this unique culture.

## REFERENCES

Adler, A. B., & Castro, C. A. (2013). An occupational mental health model for the military. *Military Behavioral Health, 1,* 41–51.

Algoe, S. B., & Fredrickson, B. L (2011). Emotional fitness and the movement of affective science from lab to field. *American Psychologist, 66*(1), 35–42.

American Psychiatric Association. (2013). *Diagnostic and statistical manual of mental disorders* (5th ed.). Arlington, VA: American Psychiatric Publishing.

Arredondo, P., Gallardo-Cooper, M., Delgado-Romero, E. A., & Zapata, A. L. (2014). *Culturally responsive counseling with Latinas/os.* Alexandria, VA: American Counseling Association.

Balcazar, F. E., Suarez-Balcazar, Y., Taylor-Ritzler, T., & Keys, C. B. (2010). *Race, culture, and disability: Rehabilitation science and practice.* Sudbury, MA: Jones & Bartlett.

Basham, K. K. (2013). Facilitators and barriers in effective clinical practice with postdeployment military couples and families. *Military Behavioral Health, 1*(22), 22–30.

Burke, P. A., & Curruth, B. (2012). Addictions and psychological trauma: Implications for counseling strategies. In L. L. Levers (Ed.), *Trauma counseling: Theories and interventions* (pp. 214–230). New York, NY: Springer Publishing.

Corey, G., Corey, M. S., Corey, C., & Callanan, P. (2015). *Issues and ethics in the helping profession* (9th ed.). Stamford, CT: Cengage.

Council for Accreditation of Counseling and Related Educational Programs. (2014). Accredited programs. Retrieved from http://www.cacrep.org/directory/?state=&dl=&pt_id=&keywords=&sub mitthis= Author

Council on Rehabilitation Education. (2014). Accredited programs. Retrieved from http://www.core -rehab.org/AccreditedPrograms Author

Defense Centers of Excellence. (2016). Deployment health clinical center: Recovery, resiliency, and reintegration. Retrieved from http://dcoe.mil

Department of Defense. (2014). U.S. casualty status: Updated death and injury rates of U.S. military personnel during the conflicts in Iraq and Afghanistan. Retrieved from https://www.cbo.gov/sites/ default/files/113th-congress-2013-2014/workingpaper/49837-Casualties_WorkingPaper-2014-08_1 .pdf

Department of Defense. (2016a). Dictionary of military and associated terms. Retrieved from http:// www.dtic.mil/doctrine/dod_dictionary

Department of Defense. (2016b). Enlisted rank insignias. Retrieved from http://www.defense.gov/ about/insignias/enlisted.aspx

Department of Defense. (2016c). Code of conduct: Guide to keeping the faith. Retrieved from http:// archive.defense.gov/news/newsarticle.aspx?id=42786

Department of Defense. (2016d). Officer rank insignias. Retrieved from http://www.defense.gov/about/insignias/officers.aspx

Department of Defense. (2016e). Problematic substance use by DoD personnel. Retrieved from http://www.dtic.mil/whs/directives/corres/pdf/101004p.pdf

Department of Veterans Affairs. (2016). Safety plan quick guide for clinicians. Retrieved from http://www.mentalhealth.va.gov/docs/va_safetyplan_quickguide.pdf

Farley, J. I. (2010). *Military-to-civilian career transition guide: The essential job search handbook for service members* (2nd ed.). Indianapolis, IN: JIST Works/JIST Publishing.

Farley, J. I. (2013). *Quick military transition guide: Seven steps to landing a civilian job.* St. Paul, MN: JIST Works/JIST Publishing.

Franklin, K. (2015). Department of Defense quarterly suicide report, calendar year 2015, 3rd quarter. Retrieved from http://www.dspo.mil/Portals/113/Documents/DoD-Quarterly-Suicide-Report-CY2015-Q3.pdf

Helwig, A. A., & Schmidt, L. L. L. (2011). Content analysis of 32 years of American Counseling Association convention programs. *Journal of Counseling & Development, 89,* 148–154.

Iverson, K. M., Mercado, R., Carpenter, S. L., & Street, A. E. (2013). Intimate partner violence among women veterans: Previous interpersonal violence as a risk factor. *Journal of Traumatic Stress, 25,* 767–771.

Ivey, A. E., Bradford Ivey, M., & Zalaquett, C. R. (2010). *Intentional interviewing and counselling: Facilitating client development in a multicultural society* (7th ed.). Belmont, CA: Brooks/Cole.

Jackson, J., Thoman, L., Suris, A. M., & North, C. (2012). Working with trauma-related mental health problems among combat veterans of the Afghanistan and Iraq conflicts. In I. Marini & M. A. Stebnicki (Eds.), *The psychological and social impact of illness and disability* (6th ed., pp. 307–330). New York, NY: Springer Publishing.

Kilpatrick, D. G., Resnick, H. S., Milanak, M. E., Miller, M. W., Keyes, K. M., & Friedman, M. J. (2013). National estimates of exposure to traumatic events and PTSD prevalence using *DSM-IV* and *DSM-5* criteria. *Journal of Traumatic Stress, 26,* 537–547.

Lee, C. (2013). *Multicultural issues in counseling: New approaches to diversity* (4th ed.). Alexandria, VA: American Counseling Association.

Lehavot, K., Der-Martirosian, C., Simpson, T. L., Shipherd, J. C., & Washington, D. L. (2013). The role of military social support in understanding the relationship between PTSD, physical health, and healthcare utilization in women veterans. *Journal of Traumatic Stress, 26,* 773–775.

Levers, L. L. (2012). *Trauma counseling: Theories and interventions.* New York, NY: Springer Publishing.

Marini, I., & Stebnicki, M. A. (2012). *The psychological and social impact of illness and disability* (6th ed.). New York, NY: Springer Publishing.

Military One Source. (2014). *Military deployment guide.* Retrieved from http://download.militaryonesource.mil/12038/Project%20Documents/MilitaryHOMEFRONT/Troops%20and%20Families/Deployment%20Connections/Pre-Deployment%20Guide.pdf

Murphy, B. C., & Dillon, C. (2011). *Interviewing in action in a multicultural world* (4th ed.). Belmont, CA: Brooks/Cole, Cengage.

National Center for PTSD. (2016). Substance abuse in the deployment environment. Retrieved from http://www.humana-military.com/library/pdf/substance-abuse-in-deployment.pdf

Pedersen, P. (2000). *A handbook for developing multicultural awareness* (3rd ed.). Alexandria, VA: American Counseling Association.

Pincus, S. H., House, R., Christenson, J., & Adler, L. E. (2014). The emotional cycle of deployment: Military family perspective. Retrieved from http://www.military.com/spouse/military-deployment/dealing-with-deployment/emotional-cycle-of-deployment-military-family.html

Ratts, M. J., & Pedersen, P. B. (2014). *Counseling for multiculturalism and social justice: Integration, theory, and application* (4th ed.). Alexandria, VA: American Counseling Association.

Roitman, P., Gilad, M., Ankri, Y. L. E., & Shalev, A. Y. (2013). Head injury and loss of consciousness raise the likelihood of developing and maintaining PTSD symptoms. *Journal of Traumatic Stress, 26,* 727–734.

Stebnicki, M. A. (2015, March). *Military and trauma counseling: Treating the mind, body, and spirit of active duty military and veterans.* Presentation made at the Annual Conference of the American Counseling Association, Orlando, FL.

Stebnicki, M. A. (2016). Military counseling. In I. Marini & M. A. Stebnicki (Eds.), *The professional counselor's desk reference* (2nd ed., pp. 499–506). New York, NY: Springer Publishing.

Stebnicki, M. A., Clemmons-James, D., & Leierer, S. (2016). A survey of military counseling content among CORE and CACREP-accredited programs. *Rehabilitation Research, Policy, and Education.* [manuscript accepted]

Tick, E. (2014). *Warrior's return: Restoring the soul after war.* Boulder, CO: Sounds True.

Wachen, J. S., Shipherd, J. C., Suvak, M., Vogt, D., King, L. A., & King, D. W. (2013). Posttraumatic stress symptomatology as a mediator of the relationship between warzone exposure and physical health symptoms in men and women. *Journal of Traumatic Stress, 26,* 319–328.

Warden, D. (2006). Military TBI during the Iraq and Afghanistan wars. *Journal of Head Trauma Rehabilitation, 21*(5), 398–402.

Weil, A. (2011). *Spontaneous happiness.* New York, NY: Little, Brown.

Wightman, J. M., & Gladish, S. L. (2001). Explosions and blast injuries. *Annals of Emergency Medicine, 37*(6), 664–678.

# CHAPTER 16

# The Trauma of Terrorism and Disaster Mental Health Counseling

The September 11, 2001, terrorist attacks on New York City and the Pentagon may have illuminated the face of terrorism in America. We have not felt free, safe, and secure since. We can no longer go back in time to the agrarian, rural, and small-town way of life existed in 1800s and 1900s America. Terrorism now has become the new reality television show for the 21st century. The danger with this new reality is that our stress and anxiety levels have risen. Presently, we are in unchartered territory and, somehow, with all our technology and clandestine intelligence-gathering agencies and personnel, we cannot predict what will occur in our future. The only real predictive intelligence we have is something really big could happen if we are not vigilant.

Homeland security and counterterrorism experts were right again. It happened on June 12, 2016, when an American-born citizen who pledged his allegiance to the Islamic State in Iraq and Syria (ISIS) killed 49 people and seriously injured 53 others at the Pulse nightclub in Orlando, Florida, the deadliest attack on Americans since 9/11. The club appeared to be targeted by the lone gunman because it was often frequented by the lesbian, gay, bisexual, and transgender (LGBT) community, a population already vulnerable to stereotypes, discrimination, bullying, fear, and hatred.

Metaphorically, we are all victims and survivors of terrorism in America. Consequently, there are, in fact, clinically significant mental health symptoms associated with how we live our daily routines. In some symbolic way, we all share the same ancestry in the world community of trying to stay safe and secure and live a peaceful existence. One common thread is the evil that has lain in the soil, beneath our feet, which has surfaced and reared its horrid character and has rendered us feeling extremely vulnerable.

The word *terror* is from the Latin word *terrere*, which basically means *to frighten*. Brutal dictators, kings, and warlords have known for centuries the psychological aspects of how to intimidate its peoples through threats of violence, torture, and death. The Romans, Crusaders, Nazis, and ISIS, as well as participants in the thousands of wars fought over centuries, are just a few examples that spark terror into the hearts and minds of all who have walked the Earth. The goal of terrorism is to create mass catastrophic human tragedies that generate panic, fear, anxiety, and a sense of helplessness. Terrorism and terrorist networks have a social, financial, occupational, and travel significance. In essence, terrorism, or the perceived threat of terrorism, is built on radical views of power and control to the most extreme degree imaginable.

## MENTAL HEALTH IMPACT OF TERRORISM

The beginning of the 21st century in the United States has seen an unprecedented shift in the decline of Americans' mental health and the related symptoms of extraordinary stress, worry, and anxiety. This may be because of threats and perceived threats of person-made mass violence such as terrorism (e.g., use of biological, viral, nuclear, radiation, and improvised explosive devices, as well as small arms; Stebnicki, 2001, 2007). Studies that have investigated the decline in mental health functioning (e.g., levels of happiness, satisfaction, wellness) and rise in psychopathology (e.g., depression, anxiety, substance abuse) suggest the data are divided into the prevalence and incidence of symptoms among (a) the general population that exhibited mental health symptoms, and (b) those that are estimated by formal clinical diagnostic evaluations, most of which are collected from hospitals, clinics, and other mental health treatment practices and programs (Whalley & Brewin, 2007). There is indeed a psychological threat, whether real or perceived, when terrorists elect to target and single out other humans who do not pledge to the same political, religious, and cult-like ideology.

The consequence of terrorism on the psychological and mental health of individuals was seen in the September 11, 2001, attacks that left emotional, physical, spiritual, and environmental scars upon the mind, body, and spirit of many Americans. We are still paying the price for this catastrophic event by engaging enemy combatants around the globe in one of the longest conflicts: Operation Iraqi Freedom (OIF), Operation Enduring Freedom (OEF), and Operation New Dawn (OND). Collectively, these wars have resulted in over 6,825 American service member deaths, with 50,000 to 100,000 permanent mental and physical disabilities (Stebnicki, 2016). The mental and physical costs are not only seen among active duty personnel and veterans, but also among families. Since the September 11 terrorist attack and deployment of 2.5 million military that answered the call to fight terrorists, divorce rates among military personnel and veterans increased 50%, as have contributing factors that lead up to divorce, such as domestic violence, alcoholism, depression, posttraumatic stress, and other clinically significant mental health issues related to children and adolescents (Ysasi, Silva, & Becton, 2016). The indirect mental health impact of fighting terrorism on civilian populations is difficult to measure. However, one can be certain that there is a spillover effect in the mental and physical health of civilians in the United States and the culture as a whole.

The violence associated with terrorism in particular may give rise to higher levels of psychopathology, more so than natural disasters (Alexander & Klein, 2005; Suris & North, 2012). This is particularly relevant for those living in large populated areas such as New York City, which was ground zero for the September 11 terrorist attacks (Schlenger et al., 2002; Schuster, Stein, & Jaycox, 2001). The Schlenger et al. (2002) study in particular used a sample size of 2,273 participants living in New York City and its metropolitan area, as well as Washington, DC. This study showed significantly higher levels of posttraumatic stress symptoms and other clinically significant psychological distress 1 to 2 months after the terrorist attacks, in comparison to other large metropolitan areas around the country.

These clinically significant symptoms were not only centered at ground zero. Rather, in the first month following the September 11 terrorist attacks, there was a rise in clinically significant mental health symptoms from populations far away from New York City (Knudsen, Roman, Johnson, & Ducharme, 2005). Research data appear to be insufficient to demonstrate a significant comparison between the different types of disasters (i.e., person-made, natural, technological), particularly terrorism. Underlying this problem is the inadequate sample size and the use of uniform methods to demonstrate these relationships empirically (Suris & North, 2012). Overall, current data suggest that 30% to 40% of those individuals directly involved in acts of terrorism will require formal mental health treatment and 20% will require treatment 2 years later (Knudsen et al., 2005).

Extraordinary stressful and traumatic events, both person-made and natural disasters, have accelerated worldwide over the past 16 years, which may contribute to the decline in mental health functioning in world cultures. A cataclysmic event that took place on December 26, 2004, was a tsunami and earthquake, registering 9.0 off the west coast of northern Sumatra, that claimed the lives of 500,000 and disabled one million other people. To date, thousands have not been found in countries that were affected, such as Sri Lanka, India, Indonesia, Malaysia, and Thailand. In regard to terrorist attacks, there have been significant increases in both threats and attacks in countries such as France, India, Iraq, Israel, Russia, Spain, Sri Lanka, and the United Kingdom (Whalley & Brewin, 2007).

Fear, anxiety, and distress are natural responses to hostile acts of terrorism (Stebnicki, 2005, 2006, 2016b). As mental health professionals, we are in a constant state of disaster preparedness. Maintaining operational status in critical incident response, particularly for person-made mass catastrophic events, requires ongoing disaster preparedness, response, and recovery. Mental health professionals do not have an option to "stand down" when there are multiple threats in the environment. While the military, law enforcement, and medical personnel all prepare for the medical/physical rescue, mental health professionals must prepare for the mental health rescue.

Acts of war and terrorism threaten the independence, autonomy, and overall lifestyle of all cultural groups. Such acts stimulate feelings of fear and helplessness. Terrorism provokes thoughts and feelings of fear, worry, and panic because of the visual images of destruction and harm to self and loved ones. The nightly news and other electronic media assist in stimulating and reinforcing these images that are mapped into our physical, mental, emotional, and spiritual body. Many of the mental health symptoms turn into images that evoke feelings of helplessness and acts of rage and anger. Acts of terrorism indeed are cowardly and violent acts that are random, unprovoked, and intentionally directed at defenseless citizens. Many who were closest to ground zero during the terrorist attacks of September 11 experienced a multitude of losses, including the loss of: (a) having control over life, (b) faith in one's God or higher power, (c) a sense of fairness or justice in the world, (d) security and emotional well-being, (e) physical and mental health, and (f) careers, education, and overall lifestyle. Consequently, when these people try to cope cognitively with these irrational traumatic events, this sets off a chain of psychological responses that goes beyond ordinary comprehension. Many are left with feelings of vulnerability, fearfulness, and helplessness, and become overwhelmed by grief.

Because our emotional and psychological foundation has been shaken, we may react with extreme anger against all Muslims, Arab Americans, or others who look like extremists or Middle Easterners. This type of fear can be transmitted through families and cultures. Some may want to take vigilante justice into their own hands, seeking retribution in an irrational manner. Others will take on the role of a bully perpetrator and engage in acts of oppression, discrimination, and overt hatred toward all those they perceive to be a threat.

As mental health professionals, it is vital to be aware of the unhealthy coping responses some individuals may exhibit, particularly as they relate to acts of terrorism. It is quite healthy and normal to be angry at perpetrators of violence, although turning into the perpetrator and organizing violence against particular cultural groups is not normal and healthy. This type of retaliation and revenge only serves to increase mental health symptoms.

The quest to defeat evil such as terrorism is strong. Americans are resilient and have much greater resources and an advantage over other countries related to disaster preparedness, response, and recovery. The U.S. government under the Department of Homeland Security, private security contractors, and the U.S. Armed Forces have a well-developed, coordinated, and collaborative effort both at home and overseas to respond to acts of terrorism. Despite current political debates and whichever side of politics one ascribes, the advantages of having the largest military and homeland security budget and resources significantly outweigh the situation in poorer nations, those that are defenseless and vulnerable geographically.

## TERRORISM: A NEW TYPE OF DISASTER MENTAL HEALTH RESPONSE

The desolation left in the aftermath of natural, person-made, and technological disasters has created a sort of historical trauma among world cultures, particularly Westerners who have not had to fight enemy combatants on our home soil since the Revolutionary War. Americans now have daily reminders of the threats of war and terrorism. Terrorism and the constant perceived threats of terrorism have created a new type of trauma among world cultures. The new bullies of the world now have well-trained militias and terrorist networks, well-funded war chests, an ideology that believes death to self and others is the only solution to their cause, and a propaganda strategy that recruits mentally competent and able-bodied Americans to their mission of "kill all those who are not believers."

The persistent fears, chronic anxiety, and uncertainty about our future confrontations with terrorists and enemy combatants is a normal response to an abnormal cultural group that cares nothing at all about the sanctity of life itself.

Many medical and mental health practitioners are now observing an increased frequency in both persistent and transient physical and psychological symptoms that are associated with anxiety and acute stress-related disorders. Although the symptoms of stress and anxiety may not fit the level of intensity and chronicity noted as the prototypical classification in a manual of mental health disorders (i.e., *Diagnostic and Statistical Manual of Mental Disorders* [5th ed; *DSM-5*; American Psychiatric Association, 2013]) or psychological assessment, these symptoms appear to have the same pathways that may lead to more chronic and persistent symptoms of stress and anxiety-related disorders. From a self-care perspective, it is critical to deal with these early on because the cumulative and long-term nature of stress and anxiety can lead to higher levels of impaired functioning, depression, anxiety, and substance abuse disorders, just to name a few.

We appear to be in the midst of a paradigm shift in the mental health and health care professions when it comes to dealing with American lives under the threat of terrorism and war. Understanding the epidemiology of the new anxiety and stress-related conditions as it relates to mental health issues requires a shift in thinking using a biopsychosocial approach to prevention and treatment. Accordingly, planning and preparing for disaster mental health scenarios regarding acts of terrorism involve not only the medical needs of the individual, but also the psychological and psychosocial needs. The sections that follow are offered as psychoeducational materials that may be used for a range of individuals and groups (e.g., mental health clients, employees in an organization, adults and adolescents in the community) with the intention of therapeutic engagement. More specifically, the intent is to (a) educate students, faculty, and staff in school systems, employees in private businesses and organizational settings, government workers, and those in faith-based settings about the normal responses to abnormal events such as the persistent threats of terrorism and war; (b) minimize exposure to the anxiety and traumatic stressors associated with the perception of living in an unsafe world; and (c) provide resources and advice for coping and communicating with students, coworkers, family members, and an extended community of care volunteers.

## What Are Healthy and Unhealthy Feelings as They Relate to Terrorism?

There are a host of psychological and behavioral responses to the threats of terrorism and war. It is okay to feel these emotions because this just means that we are human. Psychologists and mental health professionals suggest that some of our basic human needs in life are to feel some sense of safety, security, and love. Currently, our sense of safety and security may be challenged, as well as our moral sense of what we believe to be right or wrong, good and evil in the world. Consequently, some students, coworkers, and family members may have alterations in their moods and emotions that include, but are not limited to:

► Anger toward the government
► Hatred toward Middle Eastern cultural groups

- Spiritual confusion and disbelief about long-held religious/spiritual values
- Increased levels of anxiety and fear toward our future
- Persistent or transient feelings of irritability and hyperactivity
- A numbing sensation or detachment from current events in America
- Disruption in our sleep patterns
- Increased use of alcohol, caffeine, tobacco, or food intake

For most individuals who have successfully coped with stressful life events in the past, many of these feelings resolve over time. However, for those individuals who have poor coping skills and who have not effectively dealt with a past life crisis, these psychological and behavioral changes may require help from a close family member, a spiritual or religious advisor/clergy member, a support group, or a mental health professional. Finally, it is important to remember that: (a) we should not place a value on our emotions as "good emotions or bad emotions," because we are all human and negative emotions can tell us if we need to be taking care of ourselves better, and (b) the most dysfunctional emotion that we can have is not feeling any emotion at all.

## Threats of Terrorism and War Are Everywhere: What Can I Do to Decrease My Stress and Anxiety?

There is no doubt that the horror of September 11 has created significant stress and anxiety in the lives of many Americans focusing on terrorism and war, especially when public figures and government officials tell us that "freedom and fear are at war" and that "the goal of terrorism is to kill and destroy Americans and the American way of life." Consequently, many Americans possess feelings that they have never experienced before. There is the perception by some that we could be traumatized physically, mentally, emotionally, psychologically, and/or spiritually. These threats and fears are exacerbated by our daily exposure to acts of terrorism in the world. We are overwhelmed by the electronic and print media, repeated discussions with family members and friends, conversations at school and work, and other socially reinforced reminders that increase our level of fear, anxiety, and uncertainty about our future. We should not allow the current scenarios or images of threats of terrorism and war to undermine our abilities to function and pursue goals in our daily lives. It would be foolish to ignore real evidence of terrorism in our environment, just as it would be foolish to ignore things that trigger our stress and anxiety about this topic. Thus, the following recommendations can be used as guidelines for reducing levels of anxiety and stress:

- Go about your daily routine as normally as possible and do not become overexposed to the news media's spin on terrorism and war.
- Limit your discussions with others about terrorism and war; do not let this dominate routine social activities, meetings with coworkers, and family mealtimes.

▶ Redirect your thoughts about terrorism and war to focus on the tasks that require your attention in the here and now; concentrate on daily routine tasks at work, school, and home.

▶ Do the things in life that you do well in order to feel a sense of internal accomplishment and control, being aware of things in your life that you can and cannot control.

▶ Strengthen your resiliency to stress and anxiety by exercising; getting enough rest; performing stress reduction activities; monitoring your food, caffeine, and tobacco intake; participating in creative pursuits; and using spiritual and/or religious practices to build your coping abilities.

## Why Do I Have Fears of Terrorism? Are They Rational?

Psychologists and mental health professionals have studied the emotion of fear for quite a long time. They tell us that we ordinarily fear things that we: (a) are taught to fear, because fear is a learned behavior; (b) cannot control in life, such as being a passenger in an airplane; (c) perceive to be an immediate danger to ourselves; and (d) have had recent negative experiences with in our lives. It is normal to have fears of uncertainty about future events that may disrupt our daily routines. Changing one's perspective to match the proportion of the actual threat can help keep the fear of "what is going to happen next" from growing out of proportion to the actual risk. There is no doubt that the aim of terrorism is to induce psychological fear and anxiety in individuals and to disrupt the American way of life.

Despite threats to American citizens that may be real, it is critical that we respond to these events in a rational manner. Looking at these issues from a statistical or actuarial perspective, we find that the National Safety Council (NSC; 2016) data state that the number one cause of death in the United States is unintentional drug overdose from illicit drugs, pharmaceutical products, and poisoning. The odds of dying from (a) heart disease and cancer is one in seven; (b) motor vehicle crash is 1 in 113, (c) discharge of a firearm is 1 in 7,944 (except for Chicago and other large cities); (d) cataclysmic storm is 1 in 63,679, or (e) struck by lightning is 1 in 174,426.

According to the Centers for Disease Control and Prevention (CDC, 2016), October 2001 was the first inhalational anthrax case in the United States aside from one episode in 1976. From October to November 2001, only 22 cases of bioterrorism-related anthrax poisoning were reported and investigated, with five of these cases being fatal. It is unknown how many others could have been exposed to anthrax, but did not acquire any of the related symptoms. Compare the anthrax virus to the HIV/AIDS virus, where 4,000 persons are diagnosed each month and worldwide and over 50 million have died.

One of our most critical public health concerns (CDC, 2016) is cardiovascular disease, the number one fatal disease that affects over six million Americans and results in approximately 1.5 million heart attacks annually. An additional concern of critical importance is the number of intentional deaths due to firearms, where the CDC reports that during 2001 to 2013, the number of Americans who died totaled an alarming 406,495.

The number of U.S. citizens killed as a result of terrorist acts overseas totaled 350 during this same reporting period as reported by the state department. The National Consortium for the Study of Terrorism and Responses to Terrorism (2015) indicates that between 2004 and 2013, 80 Americans (non-military) died as a result of terrorist attacks. This did not account for the terrorist attacks of September 11. The majority of these attacks took place in Iraq and Afghanistan. Of those 80 Americans, only 36 died on U.S. soil.

Reviewing these disease statistics alone should prompt us to ask ourselves, *Do we fear the appropriate things in life?* From a rational perspective and from a public health and epidemiological concern, a smallpox or anthrax attack may not be as detrimental to Americans as HIV/AIDS, smoking, cancer, cardiovascular diseases, road accidents, or episodes of violence and crime in our cities.

## How Do I Talk to Children and Adolescents About Fears of Terrorism and War?

Regardless of the child's age, the threats of war and terrorism can provoke much anxiety and stress. The impact on children and adolescents especially becomes intensified when they sense high levels of anxiety and stress among the adults they are around, such as teachers, parents, and other family members. All kids require some interventions that include calming, protection, holding, and hugging, as well as an outlet that can provide an open, honest expression of the child's fears and anxiety. It is important to remember that children's/adolescents' psychological reactions differ depending on their age. Adults should only discuss issues of terrorism and war at the child's/adolescent's level of understanding and comfort. Children/adolescents most affected by fears of terrorism and war are likely to be those who have family members in the armed forces. The dynamics within this special group require more intensive therapeutic support to help family members cope with the issues associated with marital distress, separation, divorce, and the possible loss of a parent.

Adolescents who are especially affected by the events of war and terrorism on a persistent and long-term basis may exhibit one or more of the following reactions:

▶ Recurring thoughts and emotions relating to incidents of terrorism

▶ Difficulty concentrating and maintaining focus with important daily routines

▶ Persistent feelings that are sometimes very intense or unpredictable

▶ Difficulty in expressing their emotions about the attacks on America

▶ Becoming afraid of their regular everyday routine, not wanting to leave the house, or perhaps isolating themselves

▶ Decreasing or ceasing their typical or daily routines (e.g., exercise, diet, job, hobbies)

▶ Feelings of "survivor guilt" (e.g., why did I survive while others perished? I should not be enjoying my vacation at the beach)

▶ Feelings of a sense of loss or chronic sadness

- ► Interpersonal relationships that often become strained; perhaps more frequent arguments with family members and coworkers

- ► Changes in personality, attitudes, or behavior such as crying, anger, frustration, externalized hostility, denial of the event, or constant negativity Physical symptoms that may include dizziness, diarrhea, constipation, headaches, loss of appetite, restlessness, fatigue, inability to sleep, or a preexisting health-related condition that may be exacerbated

- ► Beginning to use or increasing the use or abuse of tobacco, caffeine, alcohol, and other addictive substances

If these symptoms persist for more than 1 month, these may be emotional and psychological indicators that the adolescent should seek help from a psychologist, counselor, or mental health professional.

Like the school-yard bully, terrorists use intentional psychological assaults to intimidate, dominate, disrupt, and threaten violence to our American way of life. The ongoing psychological threats of terrorism among American children are unprecedented. Studies regarding resiliency, hardiness, and coping have focused primarily on posttraumatic stress adjustment after critical incidents such as the September 11, 2001, terrorist attacks on New York City and Washington, DC; school shootings; and various other crimes, hurricanes, floods, and earthquakes. However, studies on coping with the continuous psychological threat of terrorism in our homeland have not been an issue for Americans.

The current literature on promoting resiliency among children exposed to ongoing threats of terrorism has primarily involved studies done with the children of Northern Ireland, Israel, and Bosnia. This research suggests that kids exposed to the condition of posttraumatic stress and those who have direct exposure to a traumatic event through physical harm, loss of home, and/or seeing a family member die will have a much poorer posttrauma adjustment.

The following guidelines can be used to discuss the threats of terrorism and war with children/adolescents.

- ► Assume that children/adolescents have heard a lot about terrorism from television, radio, their friends, and teachers at school. Consequently, kids will likely have some misinformation about world events, which could create confusion and misunderstanding and trigger needless fears and anxiety. It is important to be available and approachable to let your child know that it is okay to talk about unpleasant events in the world. Ultimately, you may need to provide your child with more factual information at his or her level of understanding of world events.

- ► Most adults feel a certain level of stress and anxiety about the threats of terrorism and war, and kids typically sense these fears in adults. It is important that you share your feelings in a rational manner without magnifying or overgeneralizing your own emotions. This helps normalize your child's feelings and emotions when he or she knows that you also have some of the same fears and concerns. Once you and your child's/adolescent's emotions have been acknowledged and responded to in an empathic manner, deal with these emotions in a solution-focused manner. Your goals should be to work together on a plan where the whole family can feel some sense of personal safety and emotional security.

▶ Identify for your child/adolescent what other people are doing to protect Americans, such as the local police officers who help protect the town; National Guard officers who help protect people in the state; doctors who help prevent illnesses; firefighters who help protect the town's houses and schools; and emergency personnel and other volunteers who are trained and prepared to answer emergency calls wherever we are.

▶ Remind your child/adolescent that in response to the September 11 trauma, the United States has had much support from others around the world. There are people in many other countries who also do not want to see Americans hurt through war and terrorism. Some of these countries also want to protect Americans.

## What Should I Be Doing to Prepare Myself for the Possibility of a Terrorist Attack?

Coping with the persistent and recurrent fears of terrorism has been a challenge for many cultures throughout the centuries. The Roman Empire sought to dominate the world through political, military, religious, social, biological, and other actions and influences. Viking and Pirate raiders have plundered the coasts and navigable rivers of both North America and the British and Celtic coastline. Acts of terrorism have been perpetrated by the sociopolitical ideology of revolutionary guerillas in Central and South American countries. Fortunately, Americans have not had to live their lives by the fear and control of institutional and systemic terror.

The majority of Americans cannot begin to understand the minds of Islamic extremists and the violence they advocate against Westerners. However, let there be no doubt that many cultures in the world are envious of America's independence, autonomy, open-market and capitalistic economy, advances in health and medical technology, and how we nourish justice, democracy, and human rights. Since those cultures that wish to harm us cannot send armies and troops to U.S. soil, they do so covertly by attempting to attack our government and financial symbols, threatening our transportation systems, and perpetrating other violent acts. Terrorism is all about disrupting the American lifestyle and spirit. One of the most important lessons that we can learn from centuries of violence in the world is how to live as survivors rather than as victims.

Preparing oneself for dealing with the ongoing stress and anxiety of terrorism and war begins with understanding your own psychological resiliency and personal hardiness. The research on the psychosocial aspects of living with a chronic life-threatening illness can perhaps provide some important analogies concerning prevention, coping, and survival, with the psychological threat of war and terrorism. Understanding the psychosocial aspects of living life in this new age of terrorism requires a significant shift in thinking and an awareness of living life between different government threat levels. Here are a few ways to cope:

▶ Form a rational understanding of things you can and cannot control in the world. For example, you can control your exposure to the news of terrorism by deciding what you read in the newspaper, watch on television, or listen to on the radio. You can also control how much and at which level of threat you choose to prepare for your physical safety.

▶ Spend time with family and friends. It is okay to discuss your stress and anxiety about terrorism with others, but do not allow this to be the focus of your togetherness with friends and family. Family and friends can help remind you of what is important in your life and help you feel love and security.

▶ Terrorism and war is not a single event that has a beginning, middle, and end. The emotional aftermath of September 11, 2001, lives on in the minds of many Americans. The stress and anxiety you may be feeling in this aftermath may be persistent and ongoing. Individuals who are resilient do not allow themselves to drift toward a destructive indifference about their place in the world. Healthy survivors acquire a capacity for gaining experience with handling their stress and anxiety so their life does not become unhealthy or dysfunctional. Thus, take care of your body and mind and cultivate your spirit in a variety of ways to nourish your soul for daily functional living.

▶ Empower yourself by organizing a plan of physical safety and the prevention of anxiety and stress. Find out what you can do in your school, work, and home environment to keep you and your family safe.

▶ The most important resource we have is each other. This is not the time to isolate and withdraw from life. In today's world, our heightened anxiety and stress about terrorism are a normal response to abnormal events. Take responsibility by continuing with your daily activities.

## CONCLUDING REMARKS

There are many world cultures envious of America's independence, autonomy, and open-market and capitalistic economy, as well as the United States' advances in health and medical technology and the way it nourishes justice, democracy, and human rights. Since those cultures that wish to harm us cannot do so militarily by sending armies and troops, they attempt to attack our government and financial symbols and transportation systems by perpetrating acts of violence. Terrorism is all about disrupting the American lifestyle and spirit. One of the most important lessons that we can learn from centuries of violence in the world is how to live as survivors rather than as victims. Preparing oneself for dealing with the ongoing stress and anxiety of terrorism and war begins with understanding your own psychological resiliency and personal hardiness. These chronic and persistent thoughts and feelings undermine our overall mental, physical, psychological, emotional, and spiritual well-being. Overall, mental health professionals are well trained and qualified to work with the unique attributes of the person-made disasters of terrorism.

## REFERENCES

Alexander, D. A., & Klein, S. (2005). The psychological aspects of terrorism: From denial to hyperbole. *Journal of the Royal Society of Medicine, 98*(12), 557–562.

American Psychiatric Association. (2013). *Diagnostic and statistical manual of mental disorders* (5th ed.). Arlington, VA: American Psychiatric Publishing.

Centers for Disease Control and Prevention. (2016). Emerging infectious diseases. Retrieved from http://wwwnc.cdc.gov/eid/article/8/10/02-0389_article

Knudsen, H. K., Roman, P. M., Johnson, J. A., & Ducharme, L. J. (2005). A changed America? The effects of September 11 on depressive symptoms and alcohol consumption. *Journal of Health and Social Behavior, 46*, 260–273.

National Consortium for the Study of Terrorism and Responses to Terrorism. (2015). *American deaths in terrorist attacks*. Retrieved from https://www.start.umd.edu/pubs/START_AmericanTerrorismDeaths_FactSheet_Oct2015.pdf

National Safety Council. (2016). Injury facts 2016 is your source for safety data. Retrieved from http://www.nsc.org/learn/safety-knowledge/Pages/injury-facts.aspx

Schlenger, W. E., Caddell, J. M., Ebert, L., Jordan, B. K., Rourke, K. M., Wilson, D., . . . Kulka, R. A. (2002). Psychological reactions to terrorist attacks: Findings from the national study of Americans' reactions to September 11th. *Journal of the American Medical Association, 288*(5), 581–588.

Schuster, M. A., Stein, B. D., & Jaycox, L. H. (2001). A national study of stress reactions after September 11th terrorist attacks. *New England Journal of Medicine, 345*, 1507–1512.

Stebnicki, M. A. (2001). The psychosocial impact on survivors of extraordinary stressful and traumatic events: Principles and practices in critical incident response for rehabilitation counselors. *Directions in Rehabilitation Counseling, 12*(6), 57–71.

Stebnicki, M. A. (2005, September). *Disaster mental health interventions: A crisis response plan for North Carolina*. Presentation made at the Annual Licensed Professional Counseling Association of North Carolina (LPCANC) Conference, Greensboro, North Carolina.

Stebnicki, M. A. (2006, January). *The disaster mental health plan for North Carolina*. Presentation made at the Licensed Professional Counseling Association of North Carolina (LPCANC) mini-conference, Greenville, North Carolina.

Stebnicki, M. A. (2007). *What is adolescent mental health: Helping disconnected and at-risk youth to become whole*. Lewiston, NY: Edwin Mellen Press.

Stebnicki, M. A. (2016a). Military counseling. In I. Marini & M. A. Stebnicki (Eds.), *The professional counselor's desk reference* (2nd ed., pp. 499–506). New York, NY: Springer Publishing.

Stebnicki, M. A. (2016b). Disaster mental health response and stress debriefing. In I. Marini & M. A. Stebnicki (Eds.), *The professional counselor's desk reference* (2nd ed., pp. 439–447). New York, NY: Springer Publishing.

Suris, A. M., & North, C. S. (2012). Mental health preparedness for terrorist incidents. In I. Marini & M. A. Stebnicki (Eds.), *The psychological and social impact of illness and disability* (6th ed., pp. 461–478). New York, NY: Springer Publishing.

Whalley, M. G., & Brewin, C. R. (2007). Mental health following terrorist attacks. *The British Journal of Psychiatry, 190*(2), 94–96.

Ysasi, N. A., Silva, I., & Becton, A. D. (2016). Counselling families of active duty military and returning veterans. In I. Marini & M. A. Stebnicki (Eds.), *The professional counselor's desk reference* (2nd ed., pp. 409–413). New York, NY: Springer Publishing.

# CHAPTER 17

# The Psychosocial Impact of Environmental and Natural Disasters*

*Mark A. Stebnicki and Irmo Marini*

Any discussion of "Earth's destructive power" must include factors related to the influence that humans have on the environment. There are three simple words that best describe the psychosocial response to natural and environmental disaster: *prediction, preparation,* and *prevention.* As a consequence of environmental and natural disasters, there are far-reaching physical, mental, cognitive, social, emotional, and spiritual implications that are challenging our overall well-being. This chapter discusses the psychosocial influences of environmental and natural disasters on individuals and communities. Psychosocial issues will be offered to mental health counselors intervening in specific natural disaster scenarios.

Truly, we are in the midst of a paradigm shift in the helping professions as environmental and natural disasters have accelerated globally in the past 20 years. While medical professionals, police, and other first responders all prepare for the medical–physical rescue in a host of disaster scenarios, professional counselors are called upon to provide the mental health rescue. Our feelings of safety and security have compromised our mind, body, and spirit. The perimeter surrounding our natural environment has been breached by poor and sometimes toxic water, air, and agricultural and food products. Diseases brought on by the Zika, Ebola, and HIV/AIDS viruses have changed medical science's uncertainty regarding the diagnosis and treatment of these pandemic viruses.

There are also multiple unknown and unnamed viruses awaiting analysis in the laboratory. Many health officials warn of a global pandemic causing mass causalities as the result of viruses with ambiguous etiologies and narrow choices for treatment. The H7N9

*Adapted in part from Chapter 92, Stebnicki & Marini (2016), in *The Professional Counselor's Desk Reference* (2nd ed.), © Springer Publishing Company.

and H5N1 avian flu virus is one example of a pandemic virus that was first identified in Southern China, March 2013 (Finkelstein et al., 2007). These pandemic influenza viruses have adapted themselves to humans. It has drawn the attention of global health organizations for research and urgent medical care. The severe acute respiratory syndrome (SARS), mad cow disease, and Ebola virus are all examples of viruses that have created high stress, anxiety, and fear among the world's populations. They are disruptive to global commerce, cause major economic loss, and have jeopardized diplomatic relations around the world (Karesh & Cook, 2005).

Many in the United States and across the globe may not feel prepared for the next pandemic that will be linked to environmental or natural disasters. The Centers for Disease Control and Prevention, Department of Homeland Security, Environmental Protection Agency, and the multiple other state and federal government agencies that monitor our human and natural resources are on call 24/7/365 with critical incident response teams standing ready to protect us in times of biological, environmental, and natural disasters. However, the security of nations and their citizens are not guaranteed. Humankind has some responsibilities not to perpetrate environmental and natural disasters. This must be monitored and evaluated on a day-to-day or moment-to-moment basis so as to not compromise our mental and physical well-being.

## PERSON–ENVIRONMENT INTERACTION EFFECTS

Trauma and disaster are two opposing realities with how we want to live our lives in peace and comfort. Throughout the history of humankind, we have had multiple opportunities to choose peace over violence or choose quality of the Earth's natural resources over amassing wealth. There has been a shift in consciousness reported in the medical, social, psychological, and humanistic sciences. It appears closely aligned to the horrific terrorist attacks of Tuesday, September 11, 2001. Many Americans have felt vulnerable since. Another example is the Boston Marathon bombings of April 15, 2013, which triggered multiple traumatic physical, mental, and psychological conditions such as the traumatic memories of September 11 . The Boston Marathon bombings triggered traumatic memories for some living in and around the New York City–DC metropolitan area. Indeed, these tragedies speak to the resiliency of the human spirit. However, the journey to healing trauma is not found in a textbook or 45-minute therapy session. It requires transforming meaning and understanding into the everyday practice with the identity of "I am a survivor."

More recently, the terrorist attacks in Paris on January 7, 2015, and terrorist attacks globally have affected the safety and security of many Europeans and Americans as well. In the United States, gun-related deaths occur on a daily basis, with 10,495 firearm-related deaths reported in 2014 (Centers for Disease Control and Prevention [CDC], 2014). Chicago, Illinois, is one example that stands out with gun-related violence. In one of the most deadly weekends in Chicago, Memorial Day 2016, four people died and 53 were wounded. Between January 1 and June 1, 2016, gun violence in Chicago increased by 50% with at least 1,492 shot and 250 persons killed (*Chicago Tribune*, 2016). By comparison, the deaths in Afghanistan between 2001 and June 2016 totaled 3,517 battlefield casualities among U.S. military personnel and all coalition forces.

Catastrophic events, whether natural or person-made, just never seem to cease. They create a historical trauma among the culture. Even though disasters of terrorism and gun violence are unnatural and person-made, it has changed our internal and external environment. They are closely aligned with our mental, physical, and spiritual health.

Environmentally in natural or person-made disasters, the air and water quality changes with burning steel, plastics, tires, oil, and other materials. Disposal of toxic materials becomes an environmental challenge. Eagle (2003) tells a story from the Chumash Native North American tribe that begins with a worm being eaten by a bird. The bird is eaten by a cat that is then killed and eaten by a very mean dog. The dog is then killed by a grizzly bear. The grizzly bear is killed by a hunter who then climbs a mountain to proclaim his superiority over all the Earth. The hunter dies atop the mountain, and as his body decomposes a worm crawls out of his body. The point is that ancient indigenous wisdom has many lessons to teach us about the life cycle, humankind's strengths and limitations, and how we become out of balance within our environment.

The person–environment threat is real when it comes to environmental or natural disasters. For example, the use of nuclear weapons historically has proved they can inflict casualties in significant numbers with a cost to both the person and environment. There has never been a time in our history when at least nine countries (i.e., United States, Russia, United Kingdom, France, China, India, Pakistan, Israel, and North Korea) are in possession of known and tested nuclear weapon systems, as reported by the International Campaign to Abolish Nuclear Weapons (ICAN, 2015).

In addition to the global power and control of nuclear threats, there are many war-torn countries that practice ethnic genocide and perpetrate acts of political violence. The request for assistance draws in other countries to provide not just security operations, but also to assist with the medical, physical, emotional, and spiritual rescue. There are enormous strains on the food, water, waste treatment, and housing needs for populations of bordering countries that can offer humanitarian assistance. Consequently, there is a "domino effect" as populations of refugees, immigrants, and asylum seekers shift geographically, creating an imbalance of the Earth's natural and human resources. Prior to such disruptions, many indigenous groups had a natural balance for hundreds and even thousands of years.

When evil forces are present, power, control, and balance shift to those who choose to climb to the top of the mountain and proclaim superiority over all humankind. Brutal dictatorships, rebel military groups, and politicians threaten the foundations of civil and human rights. Many in the United States have become complacent, desensitized, and disassociate themselves from changing world events. However, the next environmental and natural disaster sits at our doorstep. Americans can monitor disasters in their living rooms while watching TV media coverage that spans 24 hours a day. The average person may not feel a sense of internal control over his or her environment. Rather, there is a sense of external control with the perception that there are multiple life areas that cannot be changed (i.e., sociopolitical, physical–environmental, economic). Consequently, learned helplessness and disempowerment become a way of life for many. American psychologist and Harvard Professor Walter Cannon (1871–1945) devoted his life's work to his theories and assertions of the fight-or-flight and learned helplessness responses.

The interested reader should refer to Cannon's exhaustive work in this area. The point is that these syndromes are relevant today as we are confronted and challenged with a combination of environmental, natural, and person-made disasters.

It is difficult for the average American to challenge or confront the "bully," a label some would assign to terrorist groups, sociopolitical domination, Wall St. billionaires bankrupting savings accounts and retirement funds, social injustice and civil rights violators and perpetrators, or hardline fanatical or conservative religious groups. All of these individuals, organizations, and systems have extraordinary control over other human beings, which can create a strain on natural resources disrupting the environment. The psychological cost to this is enormous.

Environmental and natural disasters are envirobiopsychosocial by nature. Many times there are contributing factors involving substantial interaction effects between the person and the environment with which he or she lives. Thus, it is of paramount importance for mental health professionals to recognize that disaster survivors do in fact have some degree of control and responsibility over their internal and external environment for healing traumatic experiences.

## PREDICTION, PREPARATION, AND PREVENTION

Humankind has the power to destroy itself at so many levels globally. We do in fact have some degree of control over our environment. However, it requires a high level of social and humanitarian consciousness for (a) *predicting* the consequences of our actions, (b) *preparing* for worst case scenarios after the process of self-destruction has already begun, and (c) possessing the awareness, knowledge, and skills for *preventing* and perhaps reversing the reckless regard for human life.

Environmental and natural disasters that are typically reflected in the literature relate to hurricanes/tsunamis, earthquakes, floods, and chemical and nuclear power plant disasters. However, acts of terrorism, ethnic genocide, and political acts of violence have created environmental disasters for the victims and survivors. The use of chemical weapons, threats of a nuclear arsenal, bombing of dams causing forced flooding, deep drilling in earthquake-prone zones, and criminal acts of arson creating massive wildfires are just a few examples of person-perpetrated acts of violence posing as naturally occurring events. Consequently, the need for survival is immense for those at the epicenter when considering depleted water supplies, lack of sanitary waste water treatment, an infrastructure to handle toxins that create life-threatening diseases, and agricultural and food supplies decimated by warring factions and by natural means. One may never be able to predict a hostile takeover of his or her geographic region of the world or be empowered to deny a permit to a toxic chemical plant that predictably will compromise water, air, and food/agricultural environments. However, preparing for such events requires being educated and attuned to all the warning signs.

The metaphor of "disease prevention" through lifestyle and behavioral health changes illustrates how disaster preparation and prevention can be theoretically applied to the natural environment. Historically, there has been a medical focus in disaster preparation. This has ranged from biomedical interventions, emergency medical treatments, and screenings that focus on injury, infection, and exposure to related illnesses (Yun, Lurie, & Hyde, 2010). However, the mental health cost to environmental and natural disasters requires attention, particularly to symptoms and conditions related to mood, anxiety, and substance use disorders. Insurance companies and health care providers spend hundreds of millions of dollars each year on smoking cessation programs, educating others on good nutrition and promotion of regular aerobic/exercise activities using health-promotion strategies, as well as social–emotional peer support groups and other wellness connections. Hence, integrating these same principles could benefit the complex combination of problems sparked by environmental and natural disaster preparation and prevention. Cultivating a caring community, connecting with natural support systems, and partnering with nonprofit organizations and local businesses assist in forming preparation and prevention networks.

We appear to be in a constant cycle of *prediction, preparation, and prevention* for the next environmental and natural disaster. In the aftermath of environmental and natural disasters, a type of historical trauma has been created among Westerners. These experiences of various natural and human-made disasters appear to be shared cross-culturally on a global basis. For instance, in the United States, Hurricane Katrina, which came over land August 29, 2005, left emotional, physical, spiritual, and environmental scars upon our minds, bodies, and souls. Year-round there is a great frequency and intensity of forest fires, tornadoes, and now super-tornadoes that have been acknowledged by climate scientists as the new normal. As a consequence, there is a consciousness shift within the helping professions that must address the psychosocial impact of individuals, communities, organizations, systems, and particularly those most vulnerable during trauma and disaster events.

As a consequence of the ongoing environmental and natural disasters, we are simply emotionally, socially, physically, spiritually, and occupationally exhausted from hearing, seeing, feeling, and sensing the same persistent and transient physical, mental, and psychological symptoms as our clients, many of whom have been at or near the epicenter of such critical incidents. This is especially relevant for those professionals who serve military personnel and veterans, many of whom have been deployed in hostile regions globally or have been mobilized for humanitarian missions. As mental health professionals dealing with trauma and disaster, we are at risk of empathy fatigue and becoming a profession of *wounded healers* (Stebnicki, 2016).

## PSYCHOSOCIAL HEALING

Regardless of how far we are from the epicenter of global disaster and other catastrophic events, many individuals are affected at some level of consciousness, particularly as it relates to how far out of balance their internal and external worlds have become. Consequently, it requires some level of psychosocial healing to get back to balance as disaster unfolds. The defining moment of psychosocial healing in environmental and natural disasters may relate to our perception or assessment of the particular threat and understanding of our coping and resiliency resources (Stebnicki, 2001).

Clearly, extraordinary stressful and traumatic events have negative consequences on our physical and mental health. Stress researchers report that one of the hallmarks of the stress response, particularly in traumatic stress, is the complex physiological changes that occur in our mind–body from a systemic level, which places us at risk for chronic illnesses and disability, as our immune system becomes less capable to ward off disease (Lazarus, 1999; Sapolsky, 1998; Tomko, 2012; Wachen et al., 2013; Weil, 1995). The impact of sudden traumatic disability, for instance, has profound implications mentally, physically, socially, emotionally, and vocationally, and can hinder one's level of independence in all life areas (Livneh & Antonak, 2005; Marini, 2012). In many ways, chronic illness and disability trigger a grief and loss response, which may be associated with the loss of physical, mental, emotional, cognitive, and independent functioning. Consequently, the individual's ability to adjust and adapt relates much to his or her coping and resiliency resources.

## Common Mental Health Symptoms

Extraordinary stressful and traumatic events compromise our medical and physical health, but what about our mental health? Stress researchers have made it abundantly clear that there are mental health consequences to trauma and disaster (Stebnicki & Marini, 2016). Accordingly, disaster mental health counselors can expect a variety of thoughts, behaviors, and emotions related to survivors' experience of environmental and natural disasters. For instance, Tang, Liu, Liu, Xue, and Zhang (2014) conducted a meta-analysis of risk factors in adults and children following natural disasters. They reported a prevalence rate of depression following natural disasters ranging from 5.8% to 54% among adults, and 7.5% to 44% among children. Major depressive episodes can occur weeks or months postdisaster and persist for years if untreated. Risk factors include being single, being female, poor education, prior trauma, injury, losing employment or property, bereavement during the disaster, and house damage. Epidemiological studies of posttraumatic stress symptoms and the disorder itself (PTSD) indicate a prevalence between 5% and 60% postnatural disasters (Bell & Robinson, 2013).

Madianos and Evi (2010) report on 40 years of earthquake data in Greece, noting massive acute stress reactions, posttraumatic stress disorder, depression, and anxiety are common for individuals who have been exposed to serious material losses. Shinfuku (2002) similarly discusses the social and economic support systems that are abruptly disrupted as major contributing factors to experienced trauma by survivors. Williams and Spruill (2005) describe the sudden situational abnormality for survivors as they face loss of their jobs, loss of their homes, devastated neighborhoods, loss of material and sentimental possessions, and most particularly the loss of life. Survivors are faced with the uncertainty of rebuilding, long-term unemployment, whether to stay or leave the area for fear of another natural disaster, the sudden loss of lifestyle, and whether/if they will connect with neighbors and family members again. Boss (1999) describes such uncertainty as "frozen grief" because the grieving process is stalled when families cannot find all members and the loss has no resolution or closure. Boss describes the concept of *ambiguous loss* to describe an unclear loss without closure.

Boss (1999) discusses two types of ambiguous loss: (a) where the individual is psychologically present but physically absent, and (b) where the individual is physically present but psychologically absent or emotionally unavailable. Figley (2006) identifies four phases of natural disaster coping: (a) anticipation and preparation; (b) disaster impact; (c) immediate postdisaster impact; and (d) long-term postdisaster impact. The first phase is described as a work of worry as individuals prepare for impact. The second phase is the impact itself and the uncertain fear regarding anticipated loss of life and material possessions. The third phase immediately following the disaster involves coping with the overwhelming enormity of devastation. Figley indicates survivors are desperate to return to some sense of normalcy, and notes parents should try to establish some sense of predisaster routine ritual. Finally, the long-term impact of natural disasters varies depending on the amount of devastation, whether lives are lost, and whether any unresolved or frozen grief exists.

## ENVIRONMENTAL AND NATURAL DISASTERS: EARTHQUAKES, FLOODS, HURRICANES, AND TORNADOES

Environmental and natural disasters are common experiences of many U.S. citizens and people around the world. From 2010 to June 2016 in the United States alone, the Federal Emergency Management Agency (FEMA, 2016) reported 753 natural disasters. While there are various environmental and psychosocial stressors that deeply affect the mental and physical well-being of Americans such as all types of pollution, ecosystem degradation, resource depletion, and diminished fresh water supplies, *climate change* is the major disruptive environmental force challenging the emergency management system in the United States (FEMA, 2016). There are multiple government agencies responsible for reducing the environmental impact of natural, biological, and other environmental cataclysmic events that create economic hardship on the basic infrastructure in the United States. However, the mental and physical health care cost to humankind has enormous pain and suffering.

The section that follows addresses commonly occurring environmental and natural disasters and offers disaster mental health counselors important issues for consideration based on the typology of each disaster. Four major events are discussed (listed in alphabetical order): earthquakes, floods, hurricanes, and tornadoes. Understanding that there are a multiplicity of other environmental and natural disasters that occur upon this Earth such as atmospheric disturbances (i.e., drought, heat waves, wildfires, ice storms) and dynamic geological events (i.e., volcanoes, tsunamis), there are many commonalities associated with all of these critical events. Thus, practical considerations and psychosocial issues are discussed following the four primary typologies of disasters.

### Earthquakes

The Earth's brittle crust supports all continents of the world. It goes through phases and processes described by some as the Earth floating, ramming into, sideswiping, or pulling apart from the semi-molten mantle that was formed more than 250 million years ago. Natural forces deep within the Earth's crust exert a tremendous amount of pressure on the Earth's plates and rocky seams. After months and years of pressure, the strain builds up on the Earth's slabs and then lurches forward in what is known as an "earthquake" (Gibson, 2007).

The frequency of earthquakes has accelerated astronomically in some geographic areas of the United States and overseas. During May to June 2016, 248 earthquakes have been reported worldwide. These earthquakes have ranged from 2.5 to 7.2 on the Richter scale. In the United States alone, from 2000 to 2012, there have been a total of 3,365 earthquakes with a total of 15,049 worldwide (United States Geological Survey [USGS], 2012). The largest concentration of earthquakes in the United States is currently in the state of Oklahoma where CBS News (2016) reported 230 earthquakes in 2014 with a magnitude of 3.0 or greater. Alarmingly, in 2015, over 900 earthquakes were documented. Prior to 2008, Oklahoma recorded an average of one earthquake per year. The Oklahoma story exemplifies how humankind can perpetrate environmental and natural disasters. Geologists in the state have linked the increased frequency of earthquakes with the state's oil and gas industry. The earthquake fault line had essentially laid dormant for over 300 million years until Oklahoma's oil and gas industry began extracting natural gas from underground wells and pumping waste water from oil and gas production back into the ground (CBS News, 2014).

Earthquakes have the potential to be a primary cause of flooding. Our understanding of earthquake disasters was again ignited by the cataclysmic event that took place on December 26, 2004, in which a tsunami generated by an earthquake registering 9.0 off the west coast of northern Sumatra claimed the lives of over 230,000 people (International Federation of Red Cross and Red Crescent Societies, 2009). This catastrophic event affected a total of 14 countries such as Sri Lanka, India, Indonesia, Malaysia, Thailand, and nine others. The whole world watched as this environmental and natural disaster unfolded on television and through some survivors' cell phone video camera recordings as human lives were swept away by the ocean's fury. Few television viewers could possibly understand the psychological and traumatic impact on the cultures of peoples.

## Floods

From the vantage point of space and the outer stratosphere, the Earth looks bright blue as about three quarters of the planet is composed of water. Every body of water is capable of breaking its boundaries and breaching its banks, causing catastrophic flooding under the right conditions. All humans, plants, and animals need water for survival. It is part of our ecosystem. However, too much of a good thing, especially distributed in the wrong places, can crush homes, ruin the agricultural environment, decimate buildings and other structures, and drown humans and animals. Gibson (2007) suggests that whether we are confronted by a hurricane, tsunami, monsoon, or shifting ocean currents, all waterways eventually overflow. Cataclysmic floods have been recorded throughout history, from Noah's 40 days and 40 nights of rain that flooded all the Earth to the August 1998 and July 1999 Bangladesh floods killing over 1,500 people. There was also the great Mississippi River flood of 1927, and the "500-year flood" of 31 Texas counties in May and June 2016. In 1931, the great flood of China's Yangtze River killed more people than any other natural disaster up until that time, considering it has flooded 1,500 times over its 3,500-year history (Gibson, 2007). The death toll, recorded in various documents, was upward of 4 million souls lost to the 1931 flood.

Both ancient and modern humankind have made multiple attempts at engineering dikes, levees, dams, ponds, lakes, and canals to avert, trap, and channel water away from human beings and the places that they chose to live. Multiple attempts have been made along coastal regions and other geographic areas prone to flooding. Thus, it may be humanity's spiritual need to live close to water, real estate developers' need to build ocean-front properties, or the illusion that we can control Earth's natural resources that recycles the devastating effects of the person-made environmental disasters. From a psychological vantage point, we may attribute this to a healthy sense of internal locus of control. From a reality and historical perspective, humankind has been down this river before and has lost the battle to hold back the mighty Mississippi or the surge of ocean waters with human feats of engineering. The natural elements of water and wind eventually prevail. The environmental advantage is given to the natural structures, physical properties, and quantum mechanics that rule by natural laws and principles. (e.g., gravity, wind, air temperature).

The primary point as it relates to disaster mental health response is to understand that the impacts of *climate change* are expected to increase in severity and frequency, creating extreme droughts, floods, rise in sea levels, and precipitating patterns that affect all who live on the planet (FEMA, 2016). The most visible impacts are seen in deaths due to flooding and life-threatening diseases and viruses caused by polluted and toxic water sources. Climate change affects the core emergency management systems and the mental and physical health care response to individuals and communities during times of floods. Indeed, prediction, prevention, and preparation are all within our capable spirit. However, it requires examination of complementary and alternative methods to mitigate flood disaster relief. Population displacement, migration to other geographic regions placing strains on local and regional resources, and public health risks are among the core mission in this illusion that we can "hold back the water" or at least intelligently live within the natural environment, cope, adjust, and be resilient to this particular environmental and natural disaster.

## Hurricanes

Most hurricanes in North America form off the west coast of Africa. Although they vary depending on the water temperature, time of year, and other meteorological and natural factors, all hurricanes start as tropical disturbances or thunderstorms, then progress to subtropical features, leading to full-blown named tropical systems that have wind speeds between 39 and 73 miles per hour. Thankfully, most systems die off before coming into the warm gulf waters of the mid- and southeast Atlantic region of the United States. Hurricane season runs from June 1 to November 30. In 2010, the end date was extended one month to accommodate some of the recently formed tropical and hurricane systems affecting the United States throughout the month of November.

The Saffir–Simpson scale, developed in 1969 by civil engineers Herbert Saffir and Bob Simpson, was adopted by the National Hurricane Center (2016) to measure characteristics and provide an estimate of the potential property and flooding damage resulting from hurricanes. The categories are primarily based on the following wind speeds: Category 1 (winds 74–95 mph), Category 2 (winds 96–110 mph), Category 3 (winds 111–130 mph), Category 4 (winds 131–155 mph), and Category 5 (winds greater than 155+ mph). Even though tornadoes generally have higher wind speeds, hurricane systems typically reach 500 miles across and maintain sustained winds for hours and days that beat coastal zones, natural vegetation, beach areas, and building structures, and create devastation among humans and animals. The real damage with hurricanes is with flooding that most always results in the loss of both human life and livestock.

In favorable conditions, hurricanes feed off of warm ocean temperatures of 80°F and more. That is why hurricane season begins on June 1. Once a hurricane comes over a land mass or mountain range, such as in the Caribbean island chains (i.e., Aruba, Bonaire, Curacao, Barbados, Dominican Republic), it begins to lose energy, but not until it unleashes its fury to coastal and inland areas. As a travel tip, you may want to reschedule your island, beach, or cruise ship vacation plans either in high-risk months (August and September) or until the end of hurricane season. Container cargo ships do not have such a luxury because of shipping contracts.

Some of the most deadly hurricanes in U.S. history occurred prior to the science of the Saffir–Simpson scale or naming these deadly storms. They include the 1900 Galveston, Texas, hurricane where roughly 8,000 souls were lost by a Category 4 hurricane; the 1928 southeast Florida/Lake Okeechobee hurricane where approximately 2,500 people were killed, and Hurricane Katrina in 2005 where 1,200 deaths occurred due to a Category 3 hurricane (Weather Channel, 2016).

The first author personally experienced Hurricane Floyd on September 14, 1999, less than 2 months after moving to the coastal region of North Carolina. Hurricane Floyd, a Category 4 hurricane, was the state's largest disaster in financial terms, considering it left behind billions of dollars in damages. It also ranked 15th overall in the United States on the list of most deadly hurricanes. Hurricane Dennis, a Category 2 hurricane, arrived to the coastal Carolinas 2 weeks prior. Dennis was larger than usual for mid-Atlantic hurricanes. It was both erratic and intense with its rainfall; although it never reached land, it hugged the coast for several days. The storm was an unwelcomed guest that would not leave. The coastal erosion, high surf conditions, swollen rivers and streams, and heavy wind and rains made conditions just ripe for Hurricane Floyd.

There were immense opportunities for the wisdom I acquired after being at the epicenter of these naturally occurring events while living on the coast. One lesson I learned in the aftermath of Hurricane Floyd was the physics of wind speed and what 30 inches of rain could do to the environment. I gained a new respect for wind speeds of 80 miles per hour sustained for hours, wind gusts over 100 miles per hour, and the damage that 17 feet of water above flood stage could do environmentally. I was blessed; I only required a new roof on my house. Hurricane Floyd provided me with the opportunity to be both the survivor and the disaster mental health responder to a variety of individuals, businesses, and government agencies.

Everyone who lives near the southeast coast of the United States and even New Jersey has a hurricane story to tell. The point of this personal testimonial is to highlight the valuable experiences of disaster response and the complicating conditions that tremendously strained the human resources, emergency management systems, infrastructure, and local communities that were decimated as a result of deadly hurricanes. These catastrophic events also caused flooding, damage to the agricultural environment, and over 100,000 deaths of livestock: turkey, chickens, and hogs. The population displacement, the migration of displaced people to other geographic regions, thereby placing strains on local and regional resources, and public health risks are familiar signs of the weakness and frailty present within the various systems that are responsible for disaster relief. Dynamic partnerships are critical to the future of emergency management systems. It begins with individuals and communities that have weathered the storms of past disasters and can predict, prepare, and plan for reoccurring environmental and natural disasters. The key is ongoing evaluation and a commitment not to be complacent with disaster preparedness.

## Tornadoes

Tornadoes have the fastest and strongest winds of any storms. Scientists still do not know exactly what triggers tornadoes, twisters, or funnel clouds. Tornadoes have measurable wind speeds up to 315 miles per hour and are generally short-lived, lasting an average of 30 minutes or less (Gibson, 2007). The National Weather Service uses the Fujita scale to classify wind speeds of tornadoes, predicting the strength and damage that can potentially occur. Tornadoes range on a scale from 0 to 5 and are categorized as follows: F-0 (40–72 mph), F-1 (73–112 mph), F-2 (113–157 mph), F-3 (158–206 mph), F-4 (207–260 mph), and F-5 (261 + mph). The majority of tornadoes occur in the Great Plains region of the United States in Texas, Oklahoma, Nebraska, Kansas, Iowa, Illinois, Missouri, and Arkansas. Tornadoes will often spawn during hurricane events, particularly when they come over land. One of the worst tornadoes in history occurred across the globe in Bangladesh. It was April 26, 1989, that an F-5 tornado killed 1,300 people; it also left 12,000 seriously injured and 80,000 homeless.

In the United States, one of the worst tornadoes recorded occurred March 18, 1925. Known as the "Tri-State Tornado," it cut a path 219 miles long stretching from Missouri to Illinois to Indiana, killing 747 people and causing $1.65 billion in damage. Murphysboro, Illinois, was particularly hit hard this fateful day as the storm killed 17 children, bringing the town's death toll to 234 people. This tornado destroyed about three quarters of the town. The first author lived in Carbondale, Illinois, for over 16 years, about 15 minutes from Murphysboro. Every tornado season seemed to challenge the 1925 tornadic event. The author had multiple opportunities to work with hurricane survivors, particularly in Arkansas where literally whole towns were destroyed as if by air-dropped or ground-launched cluster bombs. Stories about these tragedies were handed down family to family, which kept the date March 18 fresh in the community's consciousness during tornado season.

## PRACTICAL ISSUES AND PSYCHOSOCIAL CONSIDERATIONS

Time seems to be marked by the season in flood, hurricane, and tornado-prone regions of the United States. As a result of climate change, environmental and natural disaster preparedness has no season. Naturally occurring events are like unwanted neighbors or family members who show up to your house and just do not leave. Hurricanes are one example of naturally occurring events that stay longer than anticipated. As noted earlier, hurricane season has been extended to the end of November because of the warming gulf waters of the Atlantic. Tornadoes may occur during March, which is the astronomical season of winter. Flooding does not appear to have a season because it occurs through year-round rain and snowfall. Accordingly, environmental and natural disasters require year-round prediction, preparation, and prevention planning to maintain the safety and security of human life.

Television and other electronic media educate the public for prevention and preparation, school children practice drills for safety, and many families have developed a backup plan in cases of emergencies. It has become a way of life along the Mississippi Delta, the low country of the Carolinas, and on the wind-swept Great Plains and in the hot and humid air mass of the Deep South. The cultures in these areas are resilient because communities and disaster management systems have determined how to survive over the years.

The following issues are offered for consideration when predicting, planning, and preparing for environmental and natural disasters such as earthquakes, floods, hurricanes, and tornadoes. Disaster mental health (DMH) counselors must plan and prepare for the practical and psychosocial issues related to environmental and natural disasters.

▶ *Disruption of transportation and communication systems:* DMH counselors may not be able to intervene immediately because of rescue worker efforts. For those DMH counselors embedded at "ground zero," there may be opportunities to facilitate emotional support with survivors. However, accessibility to the disaster site may not be possible for days and weeks after the critical event. Alternative transportation may have to be established (e.g., helicopter, four-wheel drive, walking long distances to the disaster site).

▶ *Disruption of community and economic system:* DMH counselors can anticipate that family members, friends, and other community supports may be cut off due to transportation and communication infrastructure. Tent cities and homeless shelters provide the advantage of survivors being in all one space, engaging in natural supports and therapeutic interactions by DMH counselors with disaster survivors.

▶ *Disruption of daily routines:* Depending on the severity of the environmental or natural disaster, DMH counselors can anticipate there will be both short- and long-term implications for persons returning to their work environment, school, faith-based organization, social outings, and other routine activities. This especially becomes an issue if there are disabling mental and physical conditions preventing return-to-work efforts. The business or organization itself may have been damaged during the environmental or natural disaster, which affects employment and causes financial disruption for many in the community affected by the disaster.

▶ *Decreased participation and attendance in social and faith-based activities:* DMH counselors should anticipate a reduction in the number of social, community, and faith-based activities that the person may attend regularly. Aside from accessibility and disruptions in communication systems, the lingering psychological and emotional effects of environmental and natural disasters may preclude individuals from returning to their normal routines.

▶ *Cultural and civil unrest:* DMH counselors should prepare for the community itself that may be in turmoil. The major disruption in daily routine and connections creates concerns regarding the community's overall mental and physical well-being. Given the tremendous stress and pressure the community feels to get back to balance there is the potential for anger and violence, which may require law enforcement and state National Guard intervention.

▶ *Intermittent disruption in power and other utility services:* Many persons, particularly in the United States, live life with the expectation that there will always be electricity, gas, water, telephone, cable TV, Internet, and other utilities available. For most, a disruption in the power and other utility services leads to no use of heating and cooling and the inability to communicate with others. Loss of refrigeration means loss of food supplies. Intermittent or total disruption of communications systems leads to isolation, particularly for those in rural areas. The disruption in power and utility services creates feelings of psychological and emotional unease. Especially for those who have an overdependence on the use of the Internet and cable television, life without these technologies can lead to withdrawal of a biopsychosocial nature.

▶ *Destruction of architecture and physical properties:* The destruction of the physical environment is disorienting to most and can create high levels of stress and anxiety. Schools, churches, cultural centers, sports complexes, and other physical attributes of architectural significance create a sense of disorientation and major disruption in the daily routine of communities. Temporary structures that can be set up such as schools, churches, and other cultural centers of significance can assist in reducing and disrupting the person's and community's normal daily routines.

▶ *Historical trauma and trauma triggers:* Particular seasons of the year in many geographic regions are marked by naturally occurring events reminiscent of past disasters. Storm season (e.g., hurricanes, tornadoes) may trigger stress, anxiety, and emotional and psychological difficulties. This is especially relevant if the population or communities sustained catastrophic losses and grief associated with the death of loved ones or personal injuries, illnesses, or disabilities. The remnants of physical destruction incurred by disasters can hinder an individual's or community's quality of life within their familiar environment. A sense of safety and security may compromise one's mental and physical well-being. Much like the treatment for seasonal affective disorders, mental health counselors can assist historical trauma survivors to prepare for such conditions and events.

▶ *Exhaustion of mental and physical health care systems:* It is indeed a real possibility within hours or days of a disaster that there is a strain on the medical and mental health care system of providers. Overcrowded emergency departments, doctors and nurses who cannot access clinics and hospitals because of inaccessible roadways, and disruption in communications, power, and utilities all create a catastrophic scenario. In the event that temporary medical structures and health care systems are in place, there may not be enough resources for appropriate medical technologies, surgical interventions, and pharmaceutical products that could save lives. Thus, higher casualties can be anticipated. The U.S. military has an advantage over civilian populations. In the past several decades, there have been improvements in battlefield medicine, better body armor to prevent serious injuries, infantry personnel trained in first aid, and rapid response teams that can predict, prepare, plan, and intervene in times of serious injuries.

## GLOBAL WISDOM FOR THE NEW AGE

The enormous loss of human life, psychological grief, physical pain, and spiritual suffering experienced by the survivors of natural disasters are replayed on the nightly news, by quick-release Hollywood-style movies, in the print media, and over the Internet. Our global community has become increasingly accessible through the use of satellite radio and television, video cellular phones, and all technology the Internet has to offer. In real time, we can watch global, regional, and local tragedies unfold in the comforts of our living room. The disaster scenarios that take place on the global media stage add another dimension of reality that negatively fuels our experience of empathy fatigue.

Overall, the epidemiological significance of global disaster means that we must be in a constant state of "mission readiness" for service to assist others that may be affected locally, regionally, or nationally. In a divine sense, the human mind, body, and spirit were not designed to sustain this level of stress and sympathetic nervous arousal. Thus, as mental health professionals, it is difficult to turn off the human heart of compassion and empathy.

Smith and Jankoski (2012) point out that disaster response is not a 9 to 5 occupation. There is nothing routine about responding to disasters that are natural, human-made, or terroristic in nature. Thus, partnering with like-minded individuals, organizations, institutions, and systems can provide opportunities to work as key allies in disaster prevention and response. We must be open to the idea of working with other professionals such as school systems, government social services, hospitals and medical centers, mental health clinics, faith-based programs, volunteer operations, and a host of other organizations and institutions that provide disaster mental health response. Surely, as professional helpers, we can become our own best support system.

We are at a time in our history where the collective wisdom of some of the planet's tribal elders, wisdom keepers, new-age social scientists, spiritual–religious teachers, and progressive political and cultural leaders are available to provide rich opportunities for opening our eyes to healing solutions in global disasters. Integrating such belief systems in the 21st century requires an understanding and openness to various cultural worldviews on health, healing, and living life optimally. Thus, it is our intention to offer some foundational principles by which to guide mental health professionals who serve those individuals and groups that have been at or near the epicenter of extraordinary stressful and traumatic events.

- ▶ Psychosocial response, adaptation, and adjustment to disaster create a dynamic, individualized, and subjective experience. Thus, individuals heal at their own pace within their own cultural belief system of health and healing. Building a person- and culturally centered therapeutic environment can go a long way in establishing trust and rapport with the individual, family members, and the communities where they live, which are essential elements for optimal healing.

- ▶ Psychosocial models of adaptation and adjustment to disaster are theoretical platforms by which professional helpers can conceptualize working with individuals and groups along various phases of healing. Thus, healing of the mind, body, and spirit is a very individualized process that glides on a continuum. There are no definitive beginning and ending points, only theoretical stages of psychosocial adjustment.

- ▶ The use of culturally focused compassion and empathy can build rapport and sustain therapeutic interactions. Traditional psychotherapy techniques and group interventions may not be culturally appropriate for those disaster survivors. The nature and types of the extraordinary stressful and traumatic events and the time frame in which they have occurred, as well as other individual factors, help determine how you approach, listen, and respond empathically to the individual or group.

- ▶ In the aftermath of environmental and natural disasters, it is important for parents to demonstrate being patient and calm with their children. Modeling this behavior can provide a calming effect with children as well. It is also important for adults to try to establish some routines similar to or the same as what occurred predisaster; for example, reading a book or telling a story before bedtime, helping prepare food, brushing teeth, and so on. If the devastation precludes some of these activities, encourage children to take up a new activity or continue with their current one if feasible. Engaging in helping others is not only rewarding, but helps distract one from one's own problems.

- ▶ Attempt to reestablish some old or new social events and activities. This may be difficult during extreme devastating events; however, seeking out others is more comforting than isolation.

- ▶ Try and cultivate natural supports with individuals and groups in disaster events. This includes family, friends, extended family, neighbors, community, social, spiritual, and religious support, as well as many other unused opportunities.

▶ Disaster mental health professionals should seek assistance for personal self-care of the mind, body, and spirit. Sustain a daily or weekly practice with your social and professional support to share your experience of empathy or compassion fatigue.

▶ Cultivate resiliency and coping skills with the intention of personal and professional growth. Try out new creative opportunities that promote natural health and healing of the mind, body, and spirit. Try new and unfamiliar activities such as yoga, tai chi, going on a weekend spiritual retreat, reading a good book, or joining a social or therapeutic support group; these can increase your quality of life.

## CONCLUDING REMARKS

For many, planet Earth does not appear to be a safe place to live because of the multitude of critical events that have the potential to create mass casualties. Indeed, there are lingering effects that have a psychosocial impact for years following environmental and natural disasters. The increased frequency and severity of climate change and resulting natural disasters, in addition to terrorism and political violence, threaten humankind globally. We are in a constant state of existential fear and arousal that many in the United States repress or disassociate. We see such events unfold before our eyes on a daily basis by electronic and print media. How easily we become desensitized to such events and subconsciously develop a copy strategy of learned helplessness.

Mental health conditions of posttraumatic stress, fear, depression, and anxiety from witnessing such events at the epicenter or vicariously are becoming more commonplace for many individuals. Mental health counselors may best serve clients involved in environmental and natural disasters by being culturally attuned. Reestablishing a sense of routine and normalcy for safety, security, and proper resources (e.g., food, water, shelter, health care and safety) is temporary relief in an acute crisis. Long-term adjustment requires dealing with ambiguous loss, frozen grief, and real or imaginary fears of future crisis events. Thus, prediction, preparation, and prevention require envirobiopsychosocial approaches to healing trauma.

## REFERENCES

Bell, C. H., & Robinson, E. H. (2013). Shared trauma in counseling: Information and implications for counselors. *Journal of Mental Health Counseling, 35*(4), 310–323. http://dx.doi.org/10.17744/mehc.35.4.7v33258020948502

Boss, P. (1999). *Ambiguous loss: Learning to live with unresolved grief.* Cambridge, MA: Harvard University Press.

CBS News. (2014, June 27). What's behind Oklahoma's surge in earthquakes? Retrieved from http://www.cbsnews.com/news/increase-in-oklahoma-earthquakes-raises-concerns-over-fracking-and-wastewater-injections

CBS News. (2016, January 4). What is causing Oklahoma's record earthquakes? Retrieved from http://www.cbsnews.com/news/is-fracking-causing-oklahomas-earthquakes

Centers for Disease Control and Prevention. (2014). Assault or homicide. Retrieved from http://www.cdc.gov/nchs/fastats/homicide.htm

*Chicago Tribune.* (2016, June). Memorial Day weekend shootings add to a violent May in Chicago. Retrieved from http://www.chicagotribune.com/news/local/breaking/ct-chicago-shootings-violence-memorial-day-weekend-met-0531-20160530-story.html

Eagle, R. (2003). *Native American spirituality: A walk in the woods.* Zanesfield, OH: Rainbow Light.

Federal Emergency Management Agency. (2016). Disaster declaration by year. Retrieved from https://www.fema.gov/disasters/grid/year

Figley, C. R. (2006). *Helping the traumatized in post-Katrina Louisiana.* Workshop presented at the Louisiana Association for Marriage and Family Therapy Conference. Baton Rouge, LA.

Finkelstein, D. B., Mukatira, S., Mehta, P. K., Obenauer, J. C., Su, X., Webster, R. G., & Naeve, C. W. (2007). Persistent host markers in pandemic H5N1 influenza virus. *Journal of Virology, 81*(19), 10292–10299. http://dx.doi.org/10.1128/JVI.00921-07

Gibson, C. (2007). *Extreme natural disasters.* Iverington, NY: Collins/Hydra Publishing.

International Campaign to Abolish Nuclear Weapons. (2015). Nuclear arsenals. Retrieved from http://www.icanw.org/the-facts/nuclear-arsenals

International Federation of Red Cross and Red Crescent Societies. (2009). Tsunami five-year progress report (2004–2009). Retrieved from http://www.ifrc.org/Global/Publications/disasters/tsunami/IFRC-Tsunami-5Yrs-Report-Final-Web.pdf

Karesh, W. B., & Cook, R. A. (2005). The human-animal link. Council on Foreign Relations. Retrieved from https://www.nceas.ucsb.edu/~sjryan/PPP/readings/Karesh%20and%20Cook,%202005.pdf

Lazarus, R. S. (1999). *Stress and emotion: A new synthesis.* New York, NY: Springer Publishing.

Livneh, H., & Antonak, R. F. (2012). Psychological adaptation to chronic illness and disability: A primer for counselors. *Journal of Counseling & Development, 83,* 12–20. http://dx.doi.org/10.1002/j.1556-6678.2005.tb00575.x

Madianos, M. G., & Evi, K. (2010). Trauma and natural disaster: The case of earthquakes in Greece. *Journal of Loss and Trauma, 15,* 138–150. http://dx.doi.org/10.1080/15325020903373185

Marini, I. (2012). Cross-cultural counseling issues of males who sustain a disability. In I. Marini & M. A. Stebnicki (Eds.), *The psychological and social impact of disability* (6th ed., pp. 151–165). New York, NY: Springer Publishing.

National Hurricane Center. (2016). Saffir-Simpson Hurricane Wind Scale. Retrieved from http://www.nhc.noaa.gov/aboutsshws.php

Sapolsky, R. M. (1998). *Why zebras don't get ulcers: An update guide to stress, stress-related diseases, and coping.* New York, NY: W. H. Freeman.

Shinfuku, N. (2002). Disaster mental health: Lessons learned from the Hanshin Awaji earthquake. *World Psychiatry, 1,* 158–159.

Smith, J. A., & Jankoski, J. (2012). Disaster behavioral health: Counselors responding to terrorism. In L. L. Levers (Ed.), *Trauma counseling: Theories and interventions* (pp. 454–470). New York, NY: Springer Publishing.

Stebnicki, M. A. (2001). The psychosocial impact on survivors of extraordinary stressful and traumatic events: Principles and practices in critical incident response for rehabilitation counselors. *New Directions in Rehabilitation, 12*(6), 57–72.

Stebnicki, M. A. (2016). From empathy fatigue to empathy resiliency. In I. Marini & M. A. Stebnicki (Eds.), *The professional counselor's desk reference* (2nd ed., pp. 533–545). New York, NY: Springer Publishing.

Stebnicki, M. A., & Marini, I. (2016). The psychosocial impact of global disasters. In I. Marini & M. A. Stebnicki (Eds.), *The professional counselor's desk reference* (2nd ed., pp. 611–615). New York, NY: Springer Publishing.

Tang, B., Liu, X., Liu, Y., Xue, C., & Zhang, L. (2014). A meta-analysis of risk factors for depression in adults and children after natural disasters. *BMC Public Health, 14*, 623–640. http://dx.doi.org/10.1186/1471-2458-14-623

Tomko, J. R. (2012). Neurobiological effects of trauma and psychopharmacology. In L. L. Levers (Ed.), *Trauma counseling: Theories and interventions* (pp. 59–76). New York, NY: Springer Publishing.

United States Geological Survey. (2012). Earthquake facts and statistics. Retrieved from http://earthquake.usgs.gov/earthquakes/eqarchives/year/eqstats.php

Wachen, J. S., Shipherd, J. C., Suvak, M., Vogt, D., King, L. A., & King, D. W. (2013). Posttraumatic stress symptomatology as a mediator of the relationship between warzone exposure and physical health symptoms in men and women. *Journal of Traumatic Stress, 26*, 319–328. http://dx.doi.org/10.1002/jts.21818

Weather Channel. (2016). The most devastating hurricanes in U.S. history. Retrieved from https://weather.com/tv/shows/hurricane-week/news/most-devastating-hurricanes-20130713#/1

Weil, A. (1995). *Spontaneous healing: How to discover and enhance your body's natural ability to maintain and heal itself.* New York, NY: Fawcett Columbine/Ballantine.

Williams, J. M., & Spruill, D. A. (2005). Surviving and thriving after trauma and loss. *Journal of Creativity in Mental Health, 1*(4), 57–70.

Yun, C., Nicole, L., & Hyde, P. S. (2010). Moving mental health into disaster preparedness spotlight. *New England Journal of Medicine, 363*, 1193–1195. http://dx.doi.org/10.1056/NEJMp1008304

# CHAPTER 18

# Trauma and Resiliency in Disaster Mental Health Counseling

The intent of this chapter is to discuss how mental health counselors can cultivate resiliency approaches with individuals, families, and communities that have been at the epicenter of disaster and trauma. I offer both well-researched resiliency approaches, approaches that have cultural-specific meaning, as well as those utilized across a variety of disciplines that may be endorsed by personal testimonial. It is anticipated that seasoned mental health professionals will go beyond the traditional diagnosis and treatment of posttraumatic stress and co-occurring disorders. The overall intent is to offer multiple healing approaches to treat the mind, body, and spirit for integration in everyday life.

Truly, there are multiple challenges during times of mass disaster where populations closest to the epicenter have exposure to the harshest conditions, chaotic situations, and intense images, sounds, smells, and other sensations, which all become mapped and trapped in the mind, body, and spirit. It is important and necessary for the stories of trauma to be told. The cultural and therapeutic communities must participate as witnesses to the journey of healing trauma. Healing the mental, physical, and spiritual wounds of trauma requires the participation of family members and the culture to help cultivate coping and resiliency approaches. Building resiliency and psychological hardiness does not just begin with *day one* of a critical event. Rather, cultivating resiliency occurs in disaster preparation and long-term recovery.

## PRINCIPLES OF RESILIENCY

There are excellent models of cultivating resiliency that can be integrated into programs for healing. For example, the research in posttraumatic growth (PTG; Tedeschi & Calhoun, 1996, 2004; Updegraff & Taylor, 2000), resiliency (Kumpfer, 1999; Siebert, 2005; Wright, 1983), hardiness (Bandura, 1997; Kobasa, 1979), and positive psychology (Csikszentmihalyi & Nakamura, 2002) suggests that many people have the ability to emerge from extraordinary stressful and traumatic experiences and be transformed into a new depth of understanding, establish purpose for their life, and develop a peaceful resolve. Marini and Chacon (2012) explored significant factors related to trauma and resiliency as they relate to chronic illness and disability. There are factors of subjective well-being, optimism, self-determination, hope, happiness, flow, spirituality, and the use of adaptation mechanisms that create the characteristics or composite of individuals who possess higher levels of resiliency.

Indeed, new and emerging areas of resiliency research have devoted much attention to the models of assessing resiliency and constructs related to positive psychology, wellness, subjective well-being, and environmental influences such as social support, a sense of belonging, faith in a higher power, and basically living harmoniously. The intent of this chapter, however, is focused primarily on applied approaches to cultivate resiliency. The interested reader should consult the References section for a complete literature review that explores these competing concepts.

Resilience has been defined by the American Psychological Association (APA, 2016) as "the process of adapting well in the face of adversity, trauma, tragedy, threats or significant sources of stress" (p. 1). Even though there is no one accepted definition of resiliency, most researchers suggest that there are foundational principles that play a key role in how resiliency is felt and expressed. A consistent finding in resiliency psychology research suggests that a person's attitudes and beliefs play a key role in the degree of resiliency that is exhibited or expressed. Resilient individuals appear to be internally directed, self-motivated, and thrive in adverse conditions.

So, what can mental health practitioners gain from understanding how to cultivate resiliency skills among individuals, family members, and communities healing from trauma? First, having the awareness that all individuals have the capacity to bounce back from adversity. Mending the mind, body, and spirit has much to do with developing one's resiliency traits, finding meaning and purpose in life, and transforming one's character and heart to fight a new battle for optimal well-being. The following principles of resiliency are derived from anecdotal, self-report measures, personal testimonials, and well-designed empirical studies:

▶ *Attitudes and beliefs:* Individuals who exhibit or express resiliency almost always appear to be positive thinkers, possess an internal locus of control, are inwardly directed and self-motivated, and seem to thrive in adverse conditions as a result of positive attitudes and beliefs.

▶ *Making conscious choices:* Resilient individuals choose healthy thoughts, emotions, and behaviors. They consciously choose to take responsibility for their emotional, cognitive, physical, and spiritual well-being. Resilient individuals manage to balance self-defeating and destructive lifestyle behaviors with more healthy habits.

▶ *Positive thinking:* The power of positive thinking is about cultivating a purpose-driven life, believing in yourself, having faith in your abilities, and having a high level of confidence that you can affect a positive outcome with self and others. As many individuals struggle with intense daily stressors and posttraumatic symptoms, bouncing back from adversity requires living life with a positive attitude and gratitude. Resilient individuals know how to practice positive thinking patterns that are genuine and richly conscious of how to integrate positive practice into their daily routines for a more intentional way of living.

▶ *Taking self-responsibility:* Resilient individuals seek opportunities for making intentional conscious choices in both small and significant life decisions. They "own" the problems that they have created and take on the challenge of responsibility for rehabilitation of self-destructive behaviors and healing their mind, body, and spirit. Taking self-responsibility can be learned and will generalize to other areas of the individual's life.

▶ *Self-motivation:* Resilient individuals find their own unique style of motivating their self across many life areas. Resilient individuals know how to spring forward and pull through adversity because they have had other opportunities for self-motivation. They are persistent with tasks that they take on and have an innate sense for knowing how to achieve their life goals.

▶ *Try out new and different things:* Resilient individuals accept that change is a part of living. There may be certain feelings, emotions, thoughts, cognitions, and behaviors that lead to self-destructive behaviors and hinder mental–emotional well-being. There may be adverse life circumstances (e.g., medical–physical–psychological health) that prevent the individual's career, educational, social, relational, or independent living goals. Thus, resilient individuals take healthy risks, are reality driven and flexible, and do not fear new things that feed their mind, body, and spirit.

## CULTURAL ASPECTS OF RESILIENCY

A resilient and healthy culture can easily be observed by disaster mental health professionals. Communities and cultures that have been at the epicenter of both person-made and natural disasters thrive, not just survive. Healing from disaster combines coping resources with good mental, physical, emotional, and social wellness. Resiliency researchers who have studied mass disasters in communities (Levers, 2012; Norris, Friedman, & Watson, 2002; Stebnicki, 2001; Suris & North, 2012; Walsh, 2007; Walsh & McGoldrick, 2004) report that resilient communities:

▶ Cultivate natural support systems they can draw from within their own families, extended families, and communities as a whole.

▶ Have the leadership and organizational skills to bring together resources through family members, faith-based communities, nonprofit organizations, private businesses, and other social networks to rebuild the mind, body, and spirit of the culture or community.

▶ Know how to facilitate adaptive coping, restore a sense of safety and security, foster hope for the future, nurture those who have been closest to the epicenter of trauma and disaster, and overall promote compassionate connections to restore the mind, body, and spirit of the culture or community.

► Exhibit attitudes of tolerance, openness, and respect for different approaches to the same solutions, and dissolve perceptions of mistrust, victimhood, or discourse within the culture or community.

► Take responsibility for progressively moving forward, developing new infrastructure, revising current organizational plans to find new solutions, accommodate and care for those most in need to help rebuild their future, and communicate common life areas to the culture or community to rehabilitate the meaning and purpose of life within the culture or community.

► Organize memorials and healing rituals, share stories, and cultivate communal emotional, social, cognitive, and spiritual well-being.

From an indigenous cultural perspective, healing trauma begins with an identification and connection with one's cultural rituals and traditions, which reduce cultural stress, anxiety, pain and wounding (McCormick, 2005). The path to resiliency within a cultural context transcends the individual's experience of loss, trauma, and disaster (e.g., "This happened to me . . .") to an understanding of how the critical event impacted the culture as a whole (e.g., "We experienced the loss of . . .").

At the foundation of many cultures are symbols, languages, rituals, and other attributes that bring culturally specific meaning and purpose to individuals. If individuals disassociate themselves from their cultural beliefs, rituals, and worldview, then many times this can become a lonely experience for them, especially if they are trauma or disaster survivors. They begin to lose their identity and have some degree of cultural confusion. This parallels family systems theories that suggest that healthy families can transcend a range of family crises (i.e., chronic life-threatening illness, disability, alcohol and drug addiction, mental illness, physical or sexual abuse). For many who grew up in an unhealthy family system, it may be to their advantage to retain some parts of their family values, beliefs, or rituals and let go of others that were of an unhealthy nature. Overall, having two or more cultural identities (e.g., biracial or multiethnic identity) is quite natural and healthy for some so they can maintain balance, connection, and communication with family, extended family, and cultural members.

Maintaining cultural balance, connection, and communication is an important component of cultural resiliency and is reflected in the Medicine Wheel teaching among native North American Indians (Eagle, 1989, 2003; Tafoya & Kouris, 2003). More modern counseling and psychotherapy versions are reflected in the comprehensive works of Myers, Sweeney, and their colleagues (see Shannonhouse, Myers, & Sweeney, 2016). The Medicine Wheel teachings have a core belief in maintaining a balance of the mental, physical, emotional, and spiritual dimensions within the individual. If the "physical body" becomes ill, then healing can occur within the mental, emotional, and spiritual body. As a specific expression of their religious beliefs, many Native Americans prefer not to have their spiritual body separated or described. Rather, they would prefer to include the mental, physical, emotional, and spiritual body as the unity of their whole self or describe it as a "way of life" or "the way of health." Thus, in native spirituality it is important to live life in constant connection moment by moment, which reflects connection with God, the Creator, or the Great Spirit.

In ancient belief systems, all of creation is filled with *Spirit* that can be found in human beings, animals, plants, minerals, and all of life's substances. When the person or culture loses their *spirits,* this can be a profound depletion and alienation from the Creator and has been termed *soul loss* from ancient teachings (Ingerman, 1991). Today's soul loss is seen in the historical person-made traumas (e.g., ethnic cleansing, slavery, torture, mass shootings) and natural disasters (e.g., tsunamis, flooding, earthquakes) that we have seen in modern centuries. Overall, the individual's dissociation with cultural beliefs, values, and rituals; cultural alienation; disenfranchisement; marginalization; and racial and ethnic suppression is traumatizing and has the potential to harm every aspect of the culture and community.

## RESILIENCY IN THE MILITARY CULTURE

In times of mass destruction and catastrophic events, there is a strong need for survival. Military service members are an example of a cultural group who are for the most part survivors and resilient in the face of trauma (Stebnicki, 2016). This is despite the public stigma and media stereotype of the "wounded warrior" with multiple mental health disorders. The fact that service members are trained to kill enemy combatants, avoid being killed or injured, and be a first responder for those injured in battle (Adler & Castro, 2013) speaks volumes about the resiliency of the human spirit. The U.S. Armed Forces does a great job of preparing men and women for physical and mental toughness. For example, military personnel are trained to run toward gunfire, or to "aggress not stress." In civilian life, however, if you are fired upon, the response is to run for your life, be detached, and isolate primarily. Civilians are not trained for combat operations. Thus, civilian populations that experience extraordinary stressful and traumatic events typically experience the full range of acute and posttraumatic stress symptoms.

Generally during combat operations, service members do not experience the full range of acute stress symptoms. Military personnel are taught to survive and thrive in the face of an adversarial threat. However, there is still a psychological cost to combat exposure and other highly stressful situations. In other words, there is not time to have a disabling condition of fear, panic, or an acute traumatic stress reaction. There is also not time to grieve the loss of your unit buddies if they become severely injured or die while engaging enemy combatants. The life and safety of others in your unit are dependent on your quick and decisive action to neutralize all enemy threats.

The neurobiopsychosocial threats are mapped within the individual, family members, and the military culture itself. This cultural immersion occurs among newly enlisted recruits, ranking officers, and the command structure, and is carried through to separation from the military. Some of the stress and trauma associated with the military culture, for example, include, but are not limited to:

▶ Deployments of 6 months or longer, as well as repeated deployments

▶ Receiving less than 5 hours of sleep in a day

▶ Witnessing death up close of other service members and civilian populations

▶ Physical injury of a serious and life-threatening nature

▶ Losing close friends while in combat

▶ The threat and anticipation of dying or potential threat of the high probability of death

▶ History of untreated mental health conditions (e.g., sexual trauma, substance use disorders, anxiety, depression)

▶ Frequent geographic relocation and family separation

The human response to both military and civilian traumas when confronted with the same or similar threat is generally the same from a physiological perspective. However, it is the cognitive perceptual experience where stress and trauma differ. The body of research throughout *Disaster Mental Health Counseling* reminds us that it is the perception of stress and traumatic stress where we all differ with regard to the individual stress response. In other words, we all differ in terms of the frequency and type of exposure, magnitude and level of intensity, and the overall neurobiopsychosocial response to how we turn on and turn off our stress response. However, the mind, body, and spirit remember the full sensory experience of stress and trauma.

The psychological reaction to trauma as it relates to civilian cultures in war-torn countries is somewhat different where fighting for survival may be a daily occurrence. It is much like the tough streets of Chicago where gang members fight for neighborhoods, illicit drug territories, and try to avoid being killed. Among the major differences between the United States and other countries are the civil rights, freedoms, and responsibilities of the government to protect its citizens from tyranny and civil unrest. The point is that resiliency traits may be linked to the psychological reactions of trauma as experienced by the culture itself. Cultural groups tend to gauge their reaction to loss, grief, death, and the overall experience of trauma by the reaction of their family members, friends, and community. If your cultural identity is to face adversity as "aggress not stress" rather than "run-for-your-life," then perhaps survival for the culture is based on how well they bounce back from harsh conditions, internal locus of control, perception and attitude toward the trauma itself, and other factors leading to a reserve tank full of resiliency.

The incidence and prevalence of posttraumatic stress symptoms in the military population are greater than in the civilian population. One primary reason is that military personnel have a much greater exposure to stress, especially traumatic stress. It is simply the frequency and cumulative aspects of stress, and traumatic stress itself, where the experience of trauma may differ between military and civilian populations. Besides, military personnel are trained to anticipate lethal situations, have the means to protect themselves and others around them, and have a different perception of the highly stressful challenges of combat operations. In fact, many active duty military personnel transitioning to veteran status have a difficult time adjusting to civilian life. Many veterans report that they miss the level of excitement, challenge, meaning, and purpose of an occupation that has the potential of placing them in harm's way. This may be unconceivable to many not associated with the military culture. However, it makes the point that stress and trauma are, in part, one's perception and attitude toward the stressor and suggests that we all turn on and turn off our stress mechanisms differently.

These points are supported by the research that suggests not all "boots-on-the-ground" have the same level of acute and posttraumatic stress symptoms as the result of combat exposure. The research in military-related trauma suggests that 30% to 60% of military personnel will be diagnosed with posttraumatic stress disorder (PTSD) after deployment (Department of Defense [DoD], 2014; Jackson, Thoman, Suris, & North, 2012; Kilpatrick et al., 2013).

So what about the other 40% or so who do not have a diagnosis of PTSD? What is different about this group that we can learn about? Indeed, all branches of the military are concerned with the men and women who volunteer to take an oath to protect the United States and its citizens. The Department of Defense and its government contractors continually seek therapeutic opportunities to build resiliency among its troops. For instance, the Army's Master Resiliency Training and Comprehensive Soldier and Family Fitness Program (CSF2, 2016), Defense Centers of Excellence (DCoE, 2016), Marine Corps Community Services (MCCS, 2016), Real Warriors Program (2016), and many other resiliency programs are directed toward building resiliency skills among the military culture.

There are a host of cognitive, emotional, behavioral, and physiological symptoms and conditions related to the frequency of exposure to stress and traumatic stress. Those who work with active duty personnel and veterans hear the familiar "war stories" such as: "My head was always on a swivel"; "I only got 2 hours of sleep"; "I saw some of my unit buddies blown up and burned alive"; and countless other stories that depict the mental, emotional, psychological, and physical horrors of war.

Resiliency training in the military culture is essential given the exposure to extraordinary stressful and traumatic events that take place with this unique occupation. The military as a whole understands the stress associated with combat operations and training for combat. In the Native American tradition, wounds were not hidden when the warrior returned home. The wounds of many Indian tribes were painted, decorated, and displayed on their horses and on themselves. Some veterans today who have come back from war as amputees will proudly display their prosthetic device. The point is that there are many cultures to learn from with concern for cultivating coping and resiliency skills. The following list includes a combination of well-researched resiliency programs, cultural indigenous approaches, and personal testimonials provided by those who have healed from combat stress and trauma:

▶ Having a realistic view of the combat theater of operations and knowing what to anticipate

▶ Conducting mental and physical training in preparation of stress and traumatic stress

▶ Reviewing previous experience with extraordinary stressful and traumatic events with previous deployment experiences

▶ Having faith in God or a higher power

- ► Having regular and routine spiritual and religious practices
- ► Trusting unit commanders and their leaderships, as well as other peers/service members
- ► Having an optimistic attitude
- ► Talking to someone in the "circle of trust" about fears and anxieties
- ► Having meaning and purpose in the mission

There are also a good number of indigenous approaches facilitated by Native American cultures that tend to serve at a higher rate, proportionately, than other minority groups. These include sweat lodge ceremonies, pipe ceremonies, trauma storytelling, and other rituals and prayers meaningful to tribal members. There are also complementary, alternative, and integrative medicine approaches that have been facilitated by qualified practitioners who have excellent reported testimonials associated with healing trauma. These include, but are not limited to, expressive writing about stress and traumatic experiences, animal-assisted therapy, yoga, mindfulness meditation and stress reduction, and acupuncture.

Overall, resiliency programs among active duty personnel, veterans, and family members are emerging as a growth opportunity for many disaster mental health professionals. Not all military deployments are related to combat operations. There are many in the military culture mobilized within the continental United States (CONUS) during times of natural disasters and civil unrest. There are also those deployed overseas to take part in humanitarian operations. Thus, we have much to learn from the military culture that encounters multiple challenges of stress and trauma as part of its unique occupation.

## EMPATHY AS THE FOUNDATION OF RESILIENCY

The intentional and conscious use of empathy during therapeutic interactions is integral to building client rapport and achieving an optimal working alliance. Developing client trust and rapport is of paramount importance before facilitating any strategies and approaches beyond attending, listening, and empathy as a way of being. Research suggests that some individuals are naturally predisposed to the personality traits (and states) of hardiness, resiliency, and coping skills. Many mental health practitioners ground their work in helping individuals acquire, increase, and maintain hardiness, resiliency, and coping.

It is essential as mental health professionals to help clients cultivate healing approaches and build a deeper level of awareness and insight for optimal healing. The following six elements are offered as a way to achieve an optimal level of therapeutic engagement and assist your client in cultivating resiliency:

1. Experiences, thoughts, and feelings are all interconnected and can affect the medical–physical, emotional, cognitive, and spiritual body. In Western models of mental health care we tend to separate the mind (use of a mental health practitioner), body (use of medical–physical health care providers), and spirit

(religious–spiritual practices led by a priest, pastor, rabbi, indigenous healers) for healing. Many cultural belief systems view the mind–body–spirit as all one healing source. The optimal healing environment for clients involves a coordinated or integrated system of care working with multiple providers achieving the overall well-being of the individual.

2. Thoughts, feelings, and emotions are organically occurring experiences. Embracing this principle lets us know that we are all human beings by nature. Paying attention to how thoughts, feelings, and emotions unfold in our life creates opportunities for awareness, insight, and personal growth as a human being.

3. Experiencing negative and hurtful feelings or painful memories is a natural cue from our mind, body, and spirit that we are not in balance. We should not place any values or judgments on negative emotions; they are all just emotions and we feel these because we are human beings. Specific thoughts or feelings we have do not mean that we have a disorder, that we are defective, or that there is something abnormal about us. This is a normal response to an extraordinary (not normal) stressful and traumatic event. As time goes on, we may never forget about our negative, stressful, or traumatic experiences, but they will not always feel this intense or out of balance. Paying attention to the experiences of our mind–body–spirit provides us with opportunities for optimal growth and well-being.

4. When the time is right for you, verbalizing thoughts, feelings, and experiences to professional helpers and other people you trust improves your overall mental, emotional, physical, and spiritual well-being. Verbalizing thoughts, feelings, and experiences is a way to release unwanted energy. It does not mean you are weak. Sharing at the level you are most comfortable in the present moment is important for healing the mind, body, and spirit.

5. Seeking help from others is quite normal and is a sign of strength and resiliency. As Frankl (1963) noted in *Man's Search for Meaning*: "But there was no need to be ashamed of tears, for tears bore witness that a man had the greatest of courage, the courage to suffer" (p. 44). The first step in any journey is to show up. Everyone needs help with some task throughout life. As humans we rarely live in total independence. We are dependent on others in many life areas (e.g., transportation, housing, food, clothing, work). Holding on, internalizing, and not sharing your thoughts, feelings, and experiences should not be a survival exercise. It is okay to accept help and support from others for a while until you feel more in balance. Even professional helpers need someone to talk with to help them in problem-solving critical life issues with self and others.

6. There are only three things you have to do in life: show up, pay attention, and be open to the outcome. It may take multiple attempts to try and get help but as time goes on, it becomes easier. You first have to show up. Next, pay attention to what your mind–body–spirit has to offer you. Finally, be open to the outcomes of living a healthier life.

# RESILIENCY: BIOPSYCHOSOCIAL AND CULTURAL MODELS

Few studies have emerged that translate resiliency approaches for specific cultural groups. Many in the positive psychology and resiliency movement suggest that there are specific personality traits that may be unique to some persons who have survived traumatic events. Other researchers suggest that one does not have to be born with such resiliency traits. Rather, these attributes can be self-taught and learned. One aspect of building resiliency and positive coping skills is that the individual has the ability to make a conscious choice to do the very best he or she can to survive, cope, and adjust to negative life circumstances no matter how difficult things can be. Much of this is dependent on internal and external environmental resources.

Few studies have been undertaken that examine unique cultural aspects of resiliency. For civilians in war-torn countries, survival means they either have to fight or leave their homeland or become a refugee or asylum seeker. For persons living in gang-infested urban environments, being in a constant state of hyperarousal is a necessity for survival, which is a learned behavior.

Today, a new science is emerging using a biopsychosocial approach to discover resiliency and coping characteristics of those who have survived extraordinary stressful and traumatic events. It is suggested in the research that persons who are more stress hardy and stress resistant have a higher capacity for emotions such as empathy. These individuals possess what Seibert (2005) calls the *resiliency advantage*. Resiliency psychology has identified why some individuals are more stress hardy than others. You may want to begin an exploration of your own fighting spirit by challenging yourself and taking a resiliency self-assessment quiz online (see Al Siebert Resiliency Center, 2016). Using the self-rating scale developed by Siebert and his colleagues, you will be able to ascertain your capacity for resiliency and subjectively measure if you are in the low, moderate, or high range. Despite the subjective nature of this scale, you may check the validity of your score by asking two or more people who know you well to rate you using the same resiliency quiz items.

An abundance of stories concerning inspiration are based on individuals who have overcome adversity on the battlefield, surviving catastrophic injury, floods, hurricanes, earthquakes, and transitioning back from long periods of rehabilitation. For stories of a more up close and personal nature, look at the resiliency traits of your own family members. View YouTube videos of veteran stories, natural disaster survivors, or survivors of mass shootings. Talk to someone in your own community who has encountered adversity such as a combat veteran, traumatic amputee, spinal cord injury or traumatic brain injury victim from a motor vehicle accident, or cancer survivor. There are also those who have transcended such critical incidents as a chronic life-threatening illness or disability; loss of their job and retirement income; the death of a spouse, son, or daughter; or loss of their home in a fire, flood, or hurricane. Did you ever wonder how these individuals survived and were able to cope with adversity better than some others? Herein lies the secret of the prison camp survivors as told by Viktor Frankl.

## Frankl's Search for Meaning

Dr. Viktor Frankl (1963), a psychiatrist who spent World War II in a Nazi concentration camp, was one of the first psychotherapists to discuss extraordinary experiences of people who survived the death camps of Nazi Germany despite hunger, humiliation, fear, deep injustice, and torture. Frankl, an existential theorist who introduced the most significant Western psychological movement of its time through *Man's Search for Meaning*, provided a dramatic narrative of humankind's capacity for coping and resiliency despite the most horrific treatment imaginable. Logotherapy, an original psychotherapeutic approach that Frankl developed, provides a foundation for treating survivors of extraordinary stressful and traumatic events. It may also bring meaning to the professional helper's experience of empathy fatigue.

The key proposition in logotherapy is to find meaning in one's existential pain and suffering. For Frankl, it was all about perception of one's circumstances in life and then changing this attitude toward an unalterable fate (e.g., life-threatening disease, chronic illness, loss of a loved one). As Frankl states: "Suffering ceases to be suffering in some way at the moment it finds a meaning, such as the meaning of sacrifice" (p. 179). He further suggests that one of the basic tenets of logotherapy is not to gain pleasure or avoid pain, but to seek meaning in life. It was through these death camp experiences where he explains that it is critical to find meaning in one's physical, emotional, and spiritual pain and suffering. In Frankl's final analysis, he wrote:

> It becomes clear that the sort of person the prisoner became was the result of an inner decision, and not the result of camp influences alone. Fundamentally, therefore, any man can, even under such circumstances, decide what shall become of him—mentally and spiritually. (p. 105)

Frankl concludes that it is this spiritual freedom and freedom to make choices (i.e., cognitions, thinking, feeling patterns, actions, behaviors) that cannot be taken away even under the most brutal of circumstances. Thus, this is what brings meaning to life—finding meaning and purpose, knowing that we can make a choice in the present moment, and changing our attitude toward a critical life event.

## INTEGRATIVE APPROACHES IN CULTIVATING RESILIENCY

Perhaps there is something to be learned about resiliency from all cultural groups. Having a natural support system predisaster can enhance resiliency. Additionally, an accountability structure within the culture and community is essential to maintain safety and security. The mental, physical, social, emotional, and spiritual well-being is essential to the survival of all cultures and communities. Thus, preexisting coping and resiliency skills must be natural to the person and his or her environment. A circle of trust, genuineness, empathy, and compassion has to be either in place or cultivated by leaders within the culture and community. Overall, resiliency interventions can be facilitated at various levels from groups, organizations, businesses, and a collection of individuals within the culture that has the awareness, knowledge, and skills for healing trauma.

As for disaster and trauma mental health professionals, other chapters in *Disaster Mental Health Counseling* have demonstrated the importance of assessing and facilitating interventions from a culturally sensitive approach. Clearly, exposure to extraordinary stressful and traumatic events has a significant impact on the mind, body, and spirit of the individual, family, and culture. There are challenging psychosocial adjustment issues reflected in loss, grief, illness, injury, and disability caused by trauma and disaster. However, the medical and mental health models of evidence-based treatments may not be consistent with one's individual and cultural values and beliefs. Thus, the intention is not to provide an all-encompassing list of resiliency and trauma resources. Each mental health practitioner who works in disaster and trauma response has been trained in primary counseling theories, strategies, and resources to assist clients within their practice (e.g., cognitive behavioral therapy [CBT], eye movement desensitization and reprocessing [EMDR], mindfulness meditation). Additionally, in many states the Red Cross has trained practitioners in disaster mental health response models. Depending on your occupational setting (e.g., military, law enforcement, schools), there may be specific models of intervention and resources that are utilized.

The following section offers several widely used interventions in the mental health field (listed in alphabetical order under the general category of therapy) that promote resiliency and reduction in posttraumatic stress symptoms. These are listed by category and do not endorse any one particular method or model. These approaches are typically seen in evidence-based models, personal testimonials, and culturally specific approaches that have been implemented to heal trauma survivors.

- ▶ *Acupuncture:* The term itself describes a family of procedures involving the stimulation points or energy vortexes of various body systems. It is an ancient Chinese medicine approach practiced for centuries in China and other Asian cultures. Acupuncture is one of the more scientifically studied integrative medicine approaches, which uses very thin small needles that penetrate multiple energy points with the intention of relieving blocked energy. Research has shown acupuncture to be effective in treating posttraumatic stress symptoms, depression, and particularly musculoskeletal conditions such as chronic pain. Most states require formal training and eligibility for licensure. Some states have restrictions on who can practice as an acupuncturist, such as someone with a medical degree.

- ▶ *Animal-assisted therapy:* Animals have been used for companionship, therapy, and service since ancient times. The K-9 corp of canines has been utilized since World War II. There are multiple uses for these animals: search and rescue, increase independence for persons with disabilities, and provide assistance for those with mental health issues, as well as for veterans.

- ▶ *Behavioral:* These approaches to enhance resiliency are designed to increase coping and self-efficacy. Increased or high levels of coping and self-efficacy predict positive adjustment and resiliency after exposure to a variety of traumatic stressors. Training is geared toward acquiring skills needed to successfully meet a specific challenge. Gradual exposure then reduces the stressful stimuli; more difficult complex tasks can then be acquired and incorporated into the individual's repertoire.

▶ *Biofeedback:* Bioneurofeedback helps persons control heart rate variability, respirations, and muscle tension and other body systems to control their physiology, cognitive, emotional, and mental activities. Many use this system for stress reduction, chronic pain conditions, depression, and posttraumatic stress symptoms. Many states require formal training and eligibility for licensure. Others have restrictions on who can practice in this modality.

▶ *Cognitive behavioral approaches:* These types of interventions are directed at modifying one's appraisal of threat and adversity under different environments and circumstances. Approaches and strategies are utilized to increase attention, maintain cognitive control, and heighten levels of awareness. Mastery of this approach teaches the individual how to selectively direct his or her attention toward more positive and relevant stimuli while filtering out irrelevant negative stimuli.

▶ *Comprehensive programs:* These include a number of comprehensive programs (i.e., CSF2, 2016; Red Cross Disaster Mental Health Response) that focus on enhancing resiliency through stress inoculation, stress reduction, and stress hardiness training. The majority of the comprehensive training programs include placing the individual in a variety of environments including simulated combat and integrates three phases: (a) conceptual and educational, (b) skill acquisition and rehearsal, and (c) live practice. Trainees master one challenge before moving forward to a more complex challenging situation. Overall, much of the research on comprehensive training programs has shown a significant reduction in symptoms related to posttraumatic stress and depression.

▶ *EMDR:* Affirmed by the Department of Defense, Veterans Administration, and APA, as well as other clinical researchers as the first line of treatment for PTSD, there is less reliance on lengthy verbalizations of trauma experiences when using EMDR. Rather, the individual processes the trauma experience cognitively, which provides opportunities to regulate his or her stress and anxiety experiences and to exert more internal control.

▶ *Equine therapy and equine-facilitated psychotherapy (EFP):* These therapeutic approaches use horses as therapy. The approaches differ from recreational and competitive riding. Rather, the focus is to use horses as therapeutic partners to connect with individuals emotionally and physically. Traditional psychotherapy makes use of intensive talk therapy approaches, whereas EFP relies on nonverbal approaches like animal attachment, challenging riders to communicate verbally/nonverbally with their horse and making unique mind–body connections to achieve optimal mental–physical well-being.

▶ *Expressive arts:* A uniform definition of expressive arts is difficult to discern in the literature. However, one distinct difference is that there are arts grounded in one single modality (i.e., dance, pottery, jewelry making), which defines its context, whereas expressive arts draw from multiple art forms, theories, and disciplines using a range of art-based modalities. Many art therapists have formal training, some at 4-year institutions, and some states have credentialing and eligibility processes. The highest credential for this specialty area is the Registered Expressive Arts Therapist (REAT), by which the person may promote himself or herself as an "Expressive Arts Therapist." However, many mental health professionals have had seminars, workshops, and other training where they facilitate art therapy approaches in sessions such as expressive writing, mandala drawing, use of art form using symbolism, and music therapy. The specialty area of music therapy is much like the REAT where there is formal training and credentialing. However, music therapy would fall into the theoretical definition of expressive arts.

▶ *Mindfulness and stress reduction:* These interventions train individuals to focus on their thoughts in the present moment by bringing themselves back repeatedly in the present and noticing what is being experienced in their thoughts, feelings, and emotions. Once this is mastered, the individual chooses what to do with the experience. The essential element in mindfulness is learning how to control where one directs attention, decrease unwanted or negative energy, and modify the appraisal of threat while increasing the capacity to regulate emotions, thoughts, and experiences. Some mindfulness and stress reduction programs incorporate visualization and the many different types of meditation approaches.

▶ *Native American traditions:* Many Native American traditions recognize the relevance of ritual ceremonies within their culture. Rituals such as sweat lodge, Medicine Wheel, pipe ceremonies, circle dances, powwows, and storytelling facilitate therapeutic traditions among First Nations' peoples. They offer guidance, illuminate patterns of non-ordinary states of human consciousness, and deepen the connection with the land, natural Earth elements, rhythms of nature, community, and heightened spiritual experiences. Many Native Americans combine native rituals and traditions with modern counseling and psychotherapy. This has been used for adolescents forced into drug and alcohol treatment centers as well as Native American veterans who have served in the U.S. military.

▶ *Positive cognitive reappraisal:* The therapeutic strategy associated with this technique involves cognitive approaches for reappraising thoughts, feelings, and emotions for enhancing resiliency. This reframe or reappraisal sends signals to the mind–body, which reduces emotional and physiological arousal. This technique has been used in the treatment of depression and anxiety disorders.

▶ *Storytelling:* This ancient art form has been used in many cultures to communicate significant life events such as trauma and disaster. It is a therapeutic form of expression not only for the individual storyteller but also for the participants who can share their own stories. Modern counseling and psychotherapy use the group therapy process to achieve much of the same therapeutic benefits. Storytelling is a very interactive approach that often uses koans, morals, parables, or metaphors to communicate concepts, thoughts, cognitions, feelings, and experiences of disaster and trauma among individuals and groups.

## CONCLUDING REMARKS

Healing journeys begin with culturally relevant approaches that transform the mind, body, and spirit for hardiness, coping, and resiliency. Mental health professionals can assist others across cultures in cultivating resiliency and coping skills that lead to healing emotional/physical pain and offer a path to soul reintegration. Achieving some degree of closure with previous traumatic events does not mean forgetting or disassociating oneself from the pain and suffering that survivors face on a daily basis. Rather, it offers opportunities to integrate traumatic events within a social, emotional, and intrapersonal context.

All therapeutic modalities offer opportunities for healing. Resiliency approaches such as talk therapies, self-help books, intensive inpatient/outpatient programs, retreats, or Native American ceremonies are not goals for treatment. Rather, it is a lifelong process whereby mental health professionals assist clients in acquiring some degree of healthy life success and satisfaction. As professional helpers, we can model good healthy choices by exercising the power of positive thinking, taking responsibility for things that we can control, and motivating ourselves for success.

## REFERENCES

Adler, A. B., & Castro, C. A. (2013). An occupational mental health model for the military. *Military Behavioral Health, 1*, 41–51. http://dx.doi.org/10.1080/21635781.2012.721063

Al Siebert Resiliency Center. (2016). Developing human resiliency around the world to master change, thrive under pressure and bounce back from setbacks. Retrieved from http://resiliencycenter.com

American Psychological Association. (2016). What is resilience? Retrieved from http://www.apa.org/helpcenter/road-resilience.aspx

Bandura, A. (1997). *Self-efficacy: The exercise of control*. New York, NY: W. H. Freeman.

Comprehensive Soldier Fitness 2 (CSF2). (2016). Comprehensive soldier and family fitness training. Retrieved from https://www.army.mil/standto/archive_2013-04-04

Csikszentmihalyi, M., & Nakamura, J. (2002). The concept of flow. In C. R. Snyder & S. J. Lopez (Eds.), *Handbook of positive psychology*. New York, NY: Oxford University Press.

Defense Centers of Excellence. (2016). Deployment health clinical center: Recovery, resiliency, and reintegration. Retrieved from http://dcoe.mil

Eagle, B. M. (1989). The circle of healing. In R. Carlson & J. Brugh (Eds.), *Healers on healing* (pp. 58–62). New York, NY: Tarcher.

Eagle, R. (2003). *Native American spirituality: A walk in the woods*. Zanesfield, OH: Rainbow Light.

Frankl, V. E. (1963). *Man's search for meaning*. New York, NY: Pocket Books.

Ingerman, S. (1991). *Soul retrieval: Mending the fragmented self*. San Francisco, CA: Harper San Francisco.

Jackson, J., Thoman, L., Suris, A. M., & North, C. (2012). Working with trauma-related mental health problems among combat veterans of the Afghanistan and Iraq conflicts. In I. Marini & M. A. Stebnicki (Eds.), *The psychological and social impact of illness and disability* (6th ed., pp. 307–330). New York, NY: Springer Publishing.

Kilpatrick, D. G., Resnick, H. S., Milanak, M. E., Miller, M. W., Keyes, K. M., & Friedman, M. J. (2013). National estimates of exposure to traumatic events and PTSD prevalence using *DSM-IV* and *DSM-5* criteria. *Journal of Traumatic Stress, 26*, 537–547. http://dx.doi.org/10.1002/jts.21848

Kobasa, S. C. (1979). Stressful life events, personality, and health: An inquiry into hardiness. *Journal of Personality and Social Psychology, 37*, 1–11.

Kumpfer, K. (1999). Factors and processes contributing to resiliency: The resiliency framework. In M. D. Glantz & J. L. Johnson (Eds.), *Resilience and development: Positive life adaptations* (pp. 179–224). New York, NY: Kluwer Academic/Plenum Publishers.

Levers, L. L. (2012). *Trauma counseling: Theories and interventions.* New York, NY: Springer Publishing.

Marine Corps Community Services. (2016). Combat operational stress. Retrieved from http://www .mccscp.com/combatstress

Marini, I., & Chacon, M. (2012). Positive psychology, wellness, and post-traumatic growth implications for rehabilitation counselor education. In I. Marini & M. A. Stebnicki (Eds.), *The psychological and social impact of illness and disability* (6th ed., pp. 377–393). New York, NY: Springer Publishing.

McCormick, R. (2005). The healing path: What can counselors learn from Aboriginal people about how to heal? In R. Moodley & W. West (Eds.), *Integrating traditional healing practices into counseling and psychotherapy* (pp. 293–304). Thousand Oaks, CA: Sage Publications.

Norris, F. H., Friedman, M. J., & Watson, P. J. (2002). 60,000 disaster victims speak: Part II. Summary and implications of the disaster mental health research. *Psychiatry, 65*, 240–260. http://dx.doi .org/10.1521/psyc.65.3.240.20169

Real Warriors Program. (2016). Real warriors, real battles, real strength. Retrieved from http://www .realwarriors.net

Shannonhouse, L. R., Myers, J. E., & Sweeney, T. J. (2016). Counseling for wellness. In I. Marini & M. A. Stebnicki (Eds.), *The professional counselor's desk reference* (2nd ed., pp. 618–223). New York, NY: Springer Publishing.

Siebert, A. (2005). *The resiliency advantage: Master change, thrive under pressure, and bounce back from setbacks.* San Francisco, CA: Berrett-Koehler Publishers.

Stebnicki, M. A. (2001). The psychosocial impact on survivors of extraordinary stressful and traumatic events: Principles and practices in critical incident response for rehabilitation counselors. *New Directions in Rehabilitation, 12*(6), 57–72.

Stebnicki, M. A. (2016). Military counseling. In I. Marini & M. A. Stebnicki (Eds.), *The professional counselor's desk reference* (2nd ed., pp. 499–506). New York, NY: Springer Publishing.

Suris, A. M., & North, C. S. (2012). Mental health preparedness for terrorist incidents. In I. Marini & M. A. Stebnicki (Eds.), *The psychological and social impact of illness and disability* (6th ed., pp. 461–478). New York, NY: Springer Publishing.

Tafoya, T., & Kouris, N. (2003). Dancing the circle: Native American concepts of healing. In S. G. Mijares (Ed.), *Modern psychology and ancient wisdom: Psychological healing practices from the world's religious traditions* (pp. 125–146). New York, NY: Haworth Integrative Healing Press.

Tedeschi, R. G., & Calhoun, L. G. (1996). The posttraumatic growth inventory: Measuring the positive legacy of trauma. *Journal of Traumatic Stress, 9*, 455–471. http://dx.doi.org/10.1002/jts.2490090305

Tedeschi, R. G., & Calhoun, L. G. (2004). Posttraumatic growth: Conceptual foundations and empirical evidence. *Psychological Injury, 15*(1), 1–18. http://dx.doi.org/10.1207/s15327965pli1501_01

Updegraff, J. A., & Taylor, S. E. (2000). From vulnerability to growth: Positive and negative effects of stressful life events. In T. H. Harvey & E. Miller (Eds.), *Loss and trauma*. Philadelphia, PA: Brunner-Routledge.

Walsh, F. (2007). Traumatic loss and major disasters: Strengthening family and community resilience. *Family Process, 46*, 207–227.

Walsh, F., & McGoldrick, M. (2004). Loss and the family: A systemic perspective. In F. Walsh & M. McGoldrick (Eds.), *Living beyond loss: Death in the family* (2nd ed., pp. 3–26). New York, NY: W. W. Norton.

Wright, B. A. (1983). *Physical disability: A psychological approach* (2nd ed.). New York, NY: Harper & Row.

# CHAPTER 19

# From Empathy Fatigue to Empathy Resiliency*

In traditional Native American philosophy, it is told that each time you heal someone you give away a piece of yourself. The journey to become a medicine man or woman requires an understanding that the healer at some point in time will become wounded and requires healing (Tafoya & Kouris, 2003). Nouwen (1972) refers to this experience as *the wounded healer* where the helper may detach or withdraw into himself or herself, creating a space for no one else to enter. As in Native American culture as well as others who discuss professional fatigue syndromes, many counseling professionals in the West also encounter a wounded healer type of experience. I refer to this phenomenon as empathy fatigue. It results from a state of psychological, emotional, mental, physical, spiritual, and occupational exhaustion that occurs as the counselors' own wounds are continually revisited by their clients' life stories of chronic illness, disability, trauma, grief, and loss (Stebnicki, 1999, 2000, 2001, 2007, 2008, 2012). It is of paramount importance that professional counselors, counselor educators, clinical supervisors, and concerned others recognize this negative shift within the professional counselor's mind, body, and spirit that may signal an empathy fatigue experience. This chapter offers (a) a description of the empathy fatigue construct as it relates to other professional fatigue syndromes, (b) a recently developed tool (Global Assessment of Empathy Fatigue [GAEF]) that may be useful for screening and identifying professionals who may be experiencing empathy fatigue, and (c) resources for self-care of empathy fatigue and building resiliency.

Many counselors spend a tremendous amount of time and energy acting in compassionate and empathic ways, searching for the meaning of their clients' mind, body, and spirits that have been lost to trauma, incest, addictions, and other stressors that prompt questions concerning the meaning of their lives. As a consequence, professional counselors become affected by the same persistent or transient physical, emotional, and psychological symptoms as their clients. Thus, empathy fatigue is a type of counselor

*Permission granted by Springer Publishing Company to use Chapter 82, Stebnicki (2016), in from *The Professional Counselor's Desk Reference* (2nd ed.). © Springer Publishing Company.

impairment that affects the whole self: mind, body, and spirit. Identifying counselor impairment or fatigue syndromes requires the use of self-care practices to maintain competent and ethical practice in the counseling profession (Corey, Schneider Corey, Corey, & Callanan, 2015; Herlihy & Corey, 2015). As Corey and Corey (2016) suggest, helpers feel a great pressure being intimately connected with the welfare of their clients. This type of professional work-related stress has a psychological, physical, and behavioral cost, which may result in the symptoms of depression, anxiety, and emotional exhaustion. From the empathy fatigue perspective, there is a cost to one's mind, body, and spiritual growth.

## COMPARING EMPATHY FATIGUE WITH COUNSELOR IMPAIRMENTS

Similar observations and measurements of counselor impairment and fatigue syndromes have been noted in the nursing, psychology, counseling, and mental health literature. Compassion fatigue was first introduced in the nursing literature by Joinson (1992) and then expanded by Figley (1995, 2002), Pearlman and Saakvitne (1995), and Stamm (1995), as well as others later on in the psychology literature. Early in its development, compassion fatigue hypothesized that therapists who deal with survivors of extraordinary stressful and traumatic events are more prone to compassion fatigue or a secondary traumatic stress (STS) type of reaction as a result of feeling compassion and empathy toward others' pain and suffering. McCann and Pearlman (1989) refer to this experience as "vicarious traumatization" where the therapist becomes deeply emotionally affected by the client's traumatic stories. Consequently, the professional counselor experiences a special type of burnout (Maslach, 1982, 2003) where there is an organizational–environmental impact on the person who feels emotionally and physically exhausted, depleted, and has reached the point of depersonalization with his or her professional colleagues.

More recently as it relates to compassion fatigue, Stamm (2010) notes that over 500 papers, books, articles, and 130 dissertations have been written on this. Stamm has developed the Professional Quality of Life (ProQOL) Scale that is based on the foundations of the compassion fatigue construct. It is beyond the scope of this chapter to describe the ProQOL so readers should consult the resource list for a comprehensive discussion given the breadth of this work by Stamm.

### Empathy Fatigue as the Wounded Spirit

Clearly, the search for personal meaning in one's chronic illness, disability, or traumatic experience is an existential and spiritual pursuit (Stebnicki, 2006). Multiple client stories of extraordinary stressful and traumatic events, as well as exposure to clients with chronic illness and life-threatening disabilities, many times place the professional helper at risk for feeling helpless and hopeless. Many professional helpers search for spiritual and existential meaning within the context of their clients' pain and suffering. Such questions as *How could life and death, joy and suffering, love, self-acceptance, and healing exist all within the same day in the lives of my clients?* can be quite overwhelming and disorienting. So the question becomes: Who pays attention to, and takes care of, the wounded healer? Nouwen (1972) speaks to this type of counselor fatigue experience from his concept of the *wounded healer*. He suggests that paradoxically we withdraw into ourselves, thus creating a sacred space for no other person to enter. Miller (2003) suggests that from the wounded healer concept, as the counselor brings a compassionate spirit to the counseling relationship, the client's expectations of the counselor are that he or she does not have any psychological, emotional, or spiritual vulnerabilities. Thus, the counselor is seen as a role model for emotional and spiritual wellness by the client who feels wounded.

Spirituality is a natural part of being human (Assagioli, 1965; Jung, 1973; Worthington, 1988). In many cultures, one of the more significant and meaningful questions relate to where we came from before birth and where we will transcend at the time of our death (Pedersen, 2000), which is a deep spiritual and existential question. Accordingly, professional counselors have an ethical obligation to explore the spiritual identity of their clients' lives (Association of Spiritual, Ethical, and Religious Values in Counseling [ASERVIC], 2016; Pargament & Zinnbauer, 2000; Shafranske & Malony, 1996). Indeed, spirituality plays a prominent role in the lives of individuals from many different cultural and ethnic backgrounds. Spiritual connectedness is a cultural attribute and can be a form of social support that empowers individuals with chronic illnesses and disabilities to cope with their environment (Harley, Stebnicki, & Rollins, 2000). Thus, to work effectively with the client's spiritual identity and worldview, it has been suggested throughout the literature that counselor educators and supervisors need to intentionally prompt their supervisees to inquire about the client's spiritual health (Bishop, Avila-Juarbe, & Thumme, 2003; Cashwell & Young, 2004; Polanski, 2003; Stebnicki, 2006).

Overall, a major departure from the construct of empathy fatigue with other fatigue syndromes is the spiritual aspect. Facilitating empathic approaches in the counseling relationship requires that we help our clients unfold the layers of their stress, grief, loss, or traumatic experiences by searching through their emotional scrapbooks. The search for personal meaning and purpose of our client's pain and suffering may contribute to our own spiritual fatigue experience. If counselors are mindful of this experience and view this as an opportunity for nurturing personal growth and development, then they may create opportunities for resiliency so they can replenish their wounded spirits.

## A NEW LOOK AT COUNSELOR IMPAIRMENT AND FATIGUE SYNDROMES

One of the most troubling aspects of counselor impairment and fatigue syndromes is that counselor educators, supervisors, and professional counseling associations have been slow to prepare counselor supervisees for cultivating self-care approaches. We do a good job of preparing competent and ethical practitioners for diagnosing and treating a variety of mental health conditions and addressing other counseling-related issues. However, the roles and functions of professional counselors have expanded significantly in the past 10 years. Today, many counselors provide mental health and disaster relief services to those involved in a multitude of extraordinary stressful and traumatic events (e.g., hurricanes, fires, floods, school shootings, workplace violence, exposure to combat).

Consequently, providing mental health rescue to those at the epicenter of critical incidents profoundly affects the mind, body, and spirit of professional counselors.

Maintaining personal and professional wellness in one's career goes beyond acquiring continuing educational credits at conferences and workshops. Rather, some counselors require a transformative personal experience to continue in their chosen profession. There appears to be some promise for addressing issues in counselor impairment and fatigue syndromes that have drawn the interest of some state and national professional counseling associations. For example, the American Counseling Association (ACA) Taskforce on Counselor Wellness and Impairment was formed in 2003 to recognize the importance of self-care approaches to increase counselor wellness (ACA, 2014). The ACA website (www .counseling.org) provides a variety of stress and compassion fatigue self-reporting instruments for the identification and prevention of counselor impairment and fatigue syndromes. It also offers resources for building capacity for occupational and career wellness.

## EMPATHY: A NATURAL WAY OF BEING FOR PROFESSIONAL COUNSELORS

Throughout the history of the helping professions, the most fundamental approach to helping others has been rooted in compassion and empathy. In fact, empathy has a rich history of being at the core of most humanistic theoretical orientations within counselor education and training programs. Accordingly, possessing the skills of empathy is a prerequisite for becoming a competent helper and is a person-centered approach that practitioners can facilitate to increase interpersonal effectiveness and enhance client outcomes (Corey & Corey, 2016; Egan, 2010; Ivey, Bradford Ivey, & Zalaquett, 2010; Truax & Carkhuff, 1967). The richness of using the skills of basic- and advanced-level empathy can build a strong client–counselor relationship. If facilitated competently by the therapist, empathy can (a) help increase client self-awareness, (b) be a motivation for personal growth and change, and (c) cultivate new ways of thinking, feeling, and acting to achieve optimal levels of mind, body, and spiritual wellness.

Carl Rogers (1980) talked passionately about empathy and empathic listening as a "way of being" with a client. However, there is an emotional and physical cost to entering the private perceptual world of the client because the counselor may be a "sponge" for his or her client's emotional and physical pain. The conscious and unconscious absorption of the client's emotional, physical, spiritual, and existential issues is a natural artifact of helping others at intense levels of service. This is because many counselors are in "high touch" professions and are at the epicenter of their clients' life stories. Many client stories contain themes of extraordinary stressful and traumatic events, pain and suffering, and result in client transference and negative countertransference of toxic energy during the session. Accordingly, there is a shadow side to facilitating empathic approaches with clients during counseling interactions. If the experience of empathy fatigue is not recognized by self and others, then it can potentially lead to a deterioration of the counselor's resiliency or coping abilities.

Rogers (1980) appeared to have an understanding of counselor fatigue syndromes. He observed a significant need for therapists to rebalance their minds, bodies, and spirits after spending countless hours in psychotherapy sessions. As I have observed, counselors who work in a variety of professional practices experience professional fatigue. This includes professionals who work with clients who have experienced loss of a loved one (i.e., grief, divorce, extramarital affairs), trauma (combat, intimate partner sexual abuse, and violence), substance abuse (i.e., family, legal, career issues), career development issues (i.e., company downsizing, work-related job stress, career transitions), chronic health conditions (i.e., cancer, HIV/AIDS), and generalized anxiety and depression, as well as other general stress conditions.

This author hypothesizes that empathy fatigue may be different from other types of counselor impairment and fatigue syndromes. This is primarily because empathy fatigue (a) is viewed as a counselor impairment that can occur early on in one's career due to an interaction of variables that include, but are not limited to, personality traits, general coping resources, age and developmental related factors, opportunities to build resiliency, organizational and other environmental supports, and the interrelationship between the person's mind, body, and spiritual development; (b) many times goes unrecognized by the individual and the professional counseling setting or environment because of its subtle characteristics; (c) may be experienced as both an acute and cumulative type of emotional, physical, and spiritual stressor that does not follow a predictable linear path to total burnout or fatigue; (d) is a highly individualized experience for most individuals, because the counselor's perception toward the client's story and life events differs depending on the issues presented during session; and (e) is a dynamic construct where the search for personal meaning in one's chronic illness, disability, traumatic experience, pain, and suffering is an existential and spiritual pursuit (Stebnicki, 2006).

In view of this hypothesis, professional counselors who experience empathy fatigue appear to have a diminished capacity to listen and respond empathically to their clients' stories that contain various themes of acute and cumulative psychosocial stress, not necessarily stories of acute and posttraumatic stress. Client stories that have such themes as addictions, physical or sexual abuse, and psychological trauma can adversely affect the mind, body, and spirit of the counselor. Remembering emotions related to such painful or traumatic events and recreating an internal "emotional scrapbook" can be extremely painful and difficult for clients and counselors. This is especially relevant for new professional counselors who have not had the opportunity to cultivate self-care strategies for professional wellness.

Carl Jung appeared to have an understanding of counselor fatigue syndromes as he observed the need for therapists to rebalance their mind, body, and spirit after spending countless hours in psychotherapy sessions with their clients. Jung was inspired by the belief that humans are spiritual beings, not just biological, instinctual, or behavioral organisms. He explored manifestations of the soul and the process of transforming the mind, body, and spirit into a greater awareness of the self to increase one's purpose in life. In Jung's view, regaining psychic equilibrium, soul searching, and self-discovery appear to be paramount in maintaining one's therapeutic practice.

New studies on the mind–body connection report that the shared emotions and physiological arousal experienced between the client and the therapist can contribute to our knowledge of how empathic connections are developed during counseling sessions. For example, Marci, Ham, Moran, and Orr (2007) looked at 20 client–therapist pairs, with the client being treated for mood and anxiety disorders. The researchers specifically focused on the therapeutic relationships that were formed during psychotherapy sessions. They then took measures of the physiological reactions of both the client and the therapist and the client's perceived level of empathy as expressed by the therapist. They found that when high positive emotions and empathy were experienced by the client and therapist, then similar physiological responses were experienced as measured by electrical skin conductance recordings, heart rate, voice dynamics, and body movement.

It appears that a much stronger working alliance or social–emotional attachment is formed in therapy than once perceived (Barone, Hutchings, Kimmel, Traub, Cooper, & Marshal, 2005). Because an empathetic connection forms between the client and the therapist, there appears to be a potential for some degree of emotional and physical exhaustion experienced by intense, cumulative, and regular therapeutic interactions.

## Emotions and the Brain: The Neuroscience of Empathy Fatigue

In the study of emotions and the brain, it is hypothesized that there are discrete, basic, and universal emotions that persons react to on a mind, body, and spiritual dimension (Bar-On & Parker, 2000; Mayne & Bonanno, 2001). Advances in neuroimaging have provided scientific tools to measure the emotional and physiological experiences of empathic therapeutic interactions, showing a significant positive correlation between developing strong empathic ties through interactions and enhanced client/patient outcomes (Riess, 2010). Even though many individuals express universal emotions (e.g., anger, love, happiness, sadness) with varying levels of experience and intensity, Mayne and Ramsey (2001) indicate that this only constitutes a measure of personal experience and a self-report of emotional expression. From a purely dynamic physiological state, emotions involve different body systems and are measured much differently by neuroscientists than experimental psychologists. This is important to understand because our individual perception of critical events determines how our parasympathetic and sympathetic nervous systems are activated during times of an actual or anticipated stressful event. After prolonged periods of physiological stress such as seen by professionals who work with the traumatized, it is evident that chronic activation of the stress response has both a physiological and emotional cost. Consequently, professionals who work at such intense levels of service may experience anxiety and depressive disorders and may account for some aspects of the emotional and physical fatigue experienced by those who report counselor fatigue syndromes such as empathy fatigue.

Kabat-Zinn (1990; see Berger, 2006) indicates that empathy fatigue can be scientifically measured in the brain because there are specific neurological pathways to empathetic responses. The complexities of studying how emotions affect our mind, body, and spirit require studying such problems from a multidisciplinary perspective that includes the fields of psychology, neurology, immunology, and biology. The discipline of psychoneuroimmunolgy (PNI) has provided a model by which researchers can study emotions and the brain. The task of PNI researchers is a difficult one because as Sapolsky

(1998) suggests, our emotions, particularly the stress response, have their own unique physiological arousal patterns of magnitude, frequency, and intensity. This is so, in part, because people differ in how they turn on their stress mechanism and other emotional responses in the brain. As Sapolsky (1998) notes, if we are constantly trying to mobilize energy, we never have the opportunity to store it, so we can use this source of energy for calm and relaxed states of consciousness. Accordingly, there is a physical and emotional cost to persistent sympathetic arousal because of the heavy secretion of glucocorticoids released in the body that are markers for depression and anxiety disorders.

Brothers (1989) points to the amygdala-cortical pathway in the brain as part of the key neural circuitry that underlies the emotions associated with the empathy response. The amygdala appears to be the specific structure of the brain that orchestrates the most intense electrical activation when reading, interpreting, or trying to understand the emotions of others. Over time, the counselor's inability to express a healthy and facilitative emotional response (such as empathy) based on the client's expression of such feelings as stress, grief, or trauma appears to have a biopsychosocial–spiritual cost to the counselor. In other words, the chronic and cumulative activation of the emotional brain and habitual repression of emotions can compromise our immune system, which increases our resistance to infections, chronic illness, and diseases (Pert, Dreher, & Ruff, 2005; Sapolsky, 1998; Weil, 1995).

Even though we have no control over our autonomic nervous system, we do have some degree of control over our voluntary nervous system, such as is observed during a biofeedback session. Thus, becoming attuned to things we do have control over in life is central to the care we can provide for ourselves and our clients.

## RISK FACTORS IN EMPATHY FATIGUE

Stebnicki (2000) offers a functional risk factor assessment for empathy fatigue that may assist professional counselors, counselor educators, and supervisors to identify and recognize risk factors. The items in this particular functional assessment were developed from a meta-analysis of similar counselor impairments and fatigue conditions as noted in the literature (e.g., burnout, compassion fatigue, STS, depression, substance abuse, other mental health conditions). In the current development of an empathy fatigue measure, consideration will be given to content items that address the spiritual dimension. There is a constellation of areas to consider within the experience of empathy fatigue that includes, but is not limited to, the professional's:

1. *Current and preexisting personality traits and states:* type A personality traits, unrealistic or high expectations by the person, need for recognition, pattern of cynicism

2. *History of emotional or psychiatric problems:* underlying mental health issues or behaviors that may interfere with the counselor's competency, direct or indirect exposure to critical incidents, lethality issues or harm to self and others

3. *Maladaptive coping behaviors:* patterns of alcohol or substance abuse, increased use of tobacco, caffeine, food

4. *Age and experience-related factors:* younger professionals new to counseling versus older professionals' coping abilities, experience in working with different types of clients/consumers, experience in crisis response

5. *Organizational and system dynamics at the counselor's place of work:* organization or system is insensitive to or unappreciative of emotional needs of the counselor or the organization's or system's openness to trying new approaches

6. *Specific job duties of counselor in which the counselor is employed:* direct service versus supervisory, caseload size, work overly demanding, time-consuming

7. *Unique sociocultural attributes:* values, beliefs, cultural identity that may be different from that of the organization/employer

8. *Response to handling past critical and other stressful life events:* level of exposure to trauma or STS and the counselor's ability to cope, identification of any counselor isolation, detachment, or dissociative issues

9. *Level of support and resources:* individual, group, or family support, ability to seek out assistance

10. *Spirituality:* counselor questioning the meaning and purpose of life, occupation, spiritual and/or religious beliefs, anger toward God or religious affiliation, any spiritual emergencies

Generally, there are multiple risk factors in empathy fatigue that complicate one's competence and ethics, affect personal and professional relationships, and hinder one's capacity for personal coping and resiliency. Thus, consideration must be given to assessing empathy fatigue from a holistic perspective. Developing domains before scale items is essential in the scale development process. Other analysis and statistical procedures also assist the researcher in the design process. The following domains are suggested by which to measure the construct of empathy fatigue:

▶ *Individual traits:* current and preexisting personality traits, any history of emotional or psychiatric problems, maladaptive coping behaviors

▶ *Family:* level of support and resources, family history of poor coping abilities, lack of clear expectations and rules for occupation or career

▶ *Sociocultural:* worldview, personal cultural identity, choice of occupation, family and extended family members, coping resources, age, gender, race, ethnicity, disability

▶ *Developmental level:* experience level of the counselor: practicum, internship, postgraduate, or expert

▶ *Occupational setting:* organizational and system dynamics, setting where professional is employed, specific job duties, responsibilities, and position within the organization

▶ *Physical attributes:* medical–physical status, chronic illness, disability, health status, nutritional intakes, and lifestyle factors related to health

▶ *Cognitive behavioral:* dysfunctional thought patterns, ability to motivate oneself, flexibility in problem-solving tasks

▶ *Religious–spiritual:* connection to higher power, God, spirit helpers, patterns of religious practices in terms of rituals, ceremonies

## GLOBAL ASSESSMENT OF FUNCTIONING IN THE THEORETICAL MEASUREMENT OF EMPATHY FATIGUE

The GAEF rating scale is a theoretical measure of the holistic experience of empathy fatigue (see Table 19.1). The GAEF is categorized according to five different levels of functioning. Level V indicates the highest level and Level I the lowest level of the hypothetical construct of empathy fatigue. It is hypothesized that professional helpers may experience and project this felt sense of empathy fatigue in seven distinct content areas that are contained within each of the five levels: (a) cognitively, (b) behaviorally, (c) spiritually, (d) process/counseling skills, (e) emotionally, (f) physically, and (g) occupationally. Table 19.1 delineates each of these areas that may be observed by self and others in the professional helper's environment. The theoretical constructs involved in measuring this type of counselor impairment are currently being researched. As the GAEF is in its theoretical stage of development, the construct of empathy fatigue is differentiated theoretically from other counselor impairment and fatigue syndromes. There is no empirical evidence as of yet to report, however.

The intent and purpose of the GAEF in its early stage of development are to provide a means of viewing the overall level of functioning as the professional helper experiences empathy fatigue. The content contained within each of the five levels of functioning is based on a comprehensive review of the counselor impairment and fatigue literature in counseling, psychology, and mental health, as well as biopsychosocial research in the fields of nursing and medicine (see Stebnicki, 2008). The GAEF rating scale was also guided by the present author's clinical experiences.

Counselor impairments appear to involve a constellation of states, traits, behaviors, and other factors that encompass the person's experience of working with clients who have a diversity of issues ranging from daily hassles and life adjustment issues to extraordinary stressful and traumatic events. It is difficult to determine universal traits or states of counselor impairment because each professional experiences and perceives his or her client's general levels of stress differently. It is much like the difficulties in studying stressful life events. Overall, it is hypothesized that there are both conscious and unconscious factors that relate to the professional counselor's experience of stress and fatigue. Further, the frequency, intensity, level of intrusion, and avoidance of critical issues are considered to be both acute and cumulative in nature. Thus, some counselors may perceive more relevance of certain characteristics within each of the content areas in the GAEF than other areas. The theoretical continuum ranging from Level V (most impaired) to Level I (least impaired), it is hoped, can provide an anchor or benchmark for the optimal level of functioning for professional helpers within each of the content domains.

**TABLE 19.1 Global Assessment of Empathy Fatigue Rating Scale (GAEF)**

| | Level V | Level IV | Level III | Level II | Level I | |
|---|---|---|---|---|---|---|
| Cognitive | ▲ Diminished concentration<br>▲ Preoccupied<br>▲ Disorganized thoughts<br>▲ Detachment from client | ▲ Diminished concentration<br>▲ Preoccupied<br>▲ Slightly disorganized thoughts<br>▲ Detachment<br>▲ Possible irrational thinking | ▲ Exhibit some diminished concentration<br>▲ Somewhat preoccupied<br>▲ Thought organization loose<br>▲ Fair focus on therapeutic process<br>▲ Quiet attending of counselor to internal thoughts and feelings<br>▲ Having an "off day" | ▲ Slight problems in concentration<br>▲ Occasionally preoccupied<br>▲ Need to continually refocus<br>▲ Good focus on therapeutic process<br>▲ Some response to internal thoughts and feelings<br>▲ Thoughts of hopefulness<br>▲ Physical signs of being restless or impatient, but controls behavior<br>▲ Eye contact good<br>▲ Occasionally strained vocal quality and pace of speech | ▲ Slight problems in concentration and thought organization<br>▲ More preoccupied than usual<br>▲ Responding to internal thoughts and feelings more than usual, but therapeutic process good | |
| Behavioral | ▲ Impatience<br>▲ Irritability<br>▲ Aggression | ▲ Impatient<br>▲ Irritable<br>▲ Competitive | ▲ Exhibit signs of restlessness or impatience<br>▲ Slightly inattentive eye contact<br>▲ Slightly strained vocal tone and pace of speech | | ▲ Exhibit physical signs of restlessness or impatience, but controls behavior<br>▲ Eye contact good<br>▲ Vocal quality and pace of speech good, but sometimes strained | |
| | ▲ Cynical with the client<br>▲ Hypervigilance<br>▲ Poor eye contact<br>▲ Strained, erratic, slow, or fast-paced speech | ▲ Very cautious<br>▲ Eye contact fair<br>▲ Somewhat strained, erratic, slow, or fast-paced speech<br>▲ Somewhat cynical with clients | | | | |

| | | | | | |
|---|---|---|---|---|---|
| Spiritual | ▲ Detached from spiritual support<br>▲ Lack meaning and purpose in faith or spiritual beliefs<br>▲ Communication of these deficits | ▲ Lack some meaning and purpose with regard to faith or spiritual beliefs<br>▲ Some detachment of spiritual support<br>▲ Communication of lack of meaning and purpose spiritually | ▲ Confusion regarding meaning and purpose with regard to faith or spiritual beliefs<br>▲ Separation from spiritual support | ▲ Sense of awareness of refocusing on meaning and purpose with regard to faith or spiritual beliefs<br>▲ Attempts to remain connected spiritually<br>▲ Makes attempts to become reconnected to spiritual support | ▲ Sense of connectedness to faith restored after self-reassurance<br>▲ Attempts to become reconnected to spiritual support |
| Process skills | ▲ Lack of rapport with client<br>▲ Strained working alliance<br><br>▲ Nonexistent attending and listening<br>▲ No genuine empathetic responses<br>▲ Resistant<br>▲ Apprehensive<br>▲ Hypersensitive<br>▲ High degree of countertransference<br>▲ Lack of open-ended questioning<br>▲ Lack of solution-focused probes<br>▲ Diminished use of brainstorming techniques<br>▲ Basic information gathering sessions versus processing client story | ▲ Rapport difficult to establish<br>▲ No working alliance<br><br>▲ Poor attending and listening<br>▲ Gathers information in session versus processing client story<br>▲ Superficial empathic responses<br>▲ Some degree of countertransference<br>▲ Little use of open-ended questioning<br>▲ Little use of solution-focused probes<br>▲ Little use of brainstorming techniques with clients<br>▲ Somewhat resistant or apprehensive during session | ▲ Longer time to establish rapport<br>▲ Working alliance achieved more slowly<br><br>▲ Listening and attending to clients fair to good<br>▲ Empathetic responses more genuine<br>▲ Session involves gathering basic information<br>▲ Some missed opportunities in therapeutic interactions<br>▲ Responses have only basic empathy<br>▲ Somewhat resistant or apprehensive<br>▲ Little nonverbal interest during session<br>▲ Some degree of countertransference<br>▲ Little use of open-ended questioning | ▲ Working alliance takes longer to achieve but remains stable<br>▲ Empathic response more genuine, deeper, more frequent<br><br>▲ Session goes beyond data gathering<br>▲ Nonverbal incongruences in session<br>▲ Avoids dealing with countertransference<br>▲ Uses some open-ended questioning, solution-focused probes, or brainstorming techniques<br>▲ Rapport takes longer to establish, but eventually is good<br>▲ Working alliance takes longer to achieve<br>▲ Ongoing therapeutic work with client remains intact and stable | ▲ Rapport takes slightly longer to establish<br>▲ Working alliance takes somewhat longer to achieve, but work with client remains intact and stable<br><br>▲ Attending and listening are appropriate<br>▲ Integration of client content, experience, and affect better<br>▲ Few missed therapeutic opportunities<br>▲ Empathic responses somewhat deeper<br>▲ Somewhat hesitant to explore new areas of client support and resources<br>▲ Some nonverbal incongruences<br>▲ Increased interest in understanding countertransference |

(continued)

| | Level V | Level IV | Level III | Level II | Level I |
|---|---|---|---|---|---|
| | ▲ Misses opportunities to integrate client content, experience, and affect | ▲ Show little nonverbal interest during testing | ▲ Little use of solution-focused probes<br>▲ Little use of brainstorming techniques | ▲ Attending and listening is good | ▲ Open-ended questioning, solution-focused probes, and brainstorming techniques used |
| Emotional | ▲ Diminished affective state<br>▲ Moodiness<br>▲ Sadness<br>▲ Tearfulness<br>▲ Negative<br>▲ Pessimistic<br>▲ Clear high and low emotions<br>▲ Depleted<br>▲ Exhausted | ▲ Somewhat diminished affective state<br>▲ Moodiness<br>▲ Slight mood swings<br>▲ Moderate level of sadness<br>▲ Emotionally fatigued<br>▲ Exhausted<br>▲ Negative<br>▲ Pessimistic | ▲ Affective state fair<br>▲ Slight moodiness<br>▲ Dysthymic<br>▲ Appears emotionally tired<br>▲ Negative<br>▲ Pessimistic | ▲ Affective state good<br>▲ Sense of dysthymic mood<br>▲ Slightly emotionally tired<br>▲ Feeling negative or pessimistic | ▲ Affective state could be better<br>▲ Sense of a slightly "down" mood<br>▲ Somewhat emotionally tired<br>▲ Slightly negative<br>▲ Pessimistic, but initiates self-correction |
| Physical | ▲ Shallow breathing<br>▲ Sweating<br>▲ Fatigue<br>▲ Discomfort while sitting | ▲ Shallow breathing<br>▲ Slight sweating<br>▲ Fatigue<br>▲ Facial grimacing | ▲ Exhibit tiredness<br>▲ Sighs of frustration with breath<br>▲ Facial grimacing<br>▲ Lack of appetite | ▲ Exhibits slight tiredness but takes steps to avoid fatigue<br>▲ Occasional signs of frustration<br>▲ Uses internal dialogue to relax<br>▲ Some discomfort while sitting | ▲ Slight tiredness<br>▲ Takes steps to avoid fatigue<br>▲ Occasional sighs of frustration<br>▲ Uses internal dialogue to relax |

| | | | | |
|---|---|---|---|---|
| ▲ Dizziness<br>▲ Nausea<br>▲ Disturbance in visual acuity<br>▲ Facial grimace of pain<br>▲ Muscle tremors or twitches<br>▲ Severe headache | ▲ Feelings of wooziness<br>▲ Lack of appetite due to upset stomach<br>▲ Occasional muscle tremors or twitches<br>▲ Moderate degree of headache<br>▲ Disturbance in visual acuity | ▲ Occasional muscle twitches<br>▲ Slight sense of headache<br>▲ Dry eyes | ▲ Appetite and eating habits somewhat irregular<br>▲ Muscles slightly tense<br>▲ Needs constant reminder to rebalance physical wellness | ▲ Appetite and eating habits somewhat irregular<br>▲ Muscles feel slightly tense<br>▲ Constant reminder to rebalance wellness |
| **Occupational**<br>▲ Misses at least 1 day of work per week<br>▲ Cancels sessions<br>▲ Does not show up for sessions<br>▲ Avoids meetings<br>▲ Avoids colleagues at work<br>▲ Leaves work early every day<br>▲ Sick or cynical sense of humor<br>▲ Poor coping skills<br>▲ Shows little resiliency<br>▲ Difficulty separating professional and personal life | ▲ Misses 2 to 3 days of work per month<br>▲ Reschedules client appointments<br>▲ Avoids meetings<br>▲ Avoids colleagues at work<br>▲ Leaves work early on average<br>▲ Consistently cuts sessions short<br>▲ Exhibits cynical sense of humor<br>▲ Difficulties separating professional and personal life<br>▲ Struggles<br>▲ Exhibits decreased coping abilities and resiliency | ▲ Missing 2 days of work per month<br>▲ Some avoidance of starting session on time<br>▲ Hope that client "no shows"<br>▲ Cuts session shorter than usual<br>▲ Makes excuses to try and leave meetings and work early<br>▲ Superficial contact with colleagues at work<br>▲ Exhibits inappropriate sense of humor<br>▲ Some difficulties separating professional and personal life<br>▲ Some difficulties with coping abilities and resiliency | ▲ May feel the need to take 2 days off from work per month<br>▲ Has thoughts of client "no shows"<br>▲ Occasionally makes excuses for leaving meetings early<br>▲ Minimal contact with colleagues at work<br>▲ Has difficulties transitioning to social self<br>▲ Some difficulties separating professional and personal life<br>▲ Better coping abilities and resiliencies | ▲ May feel the need to take off 2 days of work per month<br>▲ Thoughts of client "no shows"<br>▲ Conducts sessions on time and for usual duration<br>▲ Will make excuses for leaving meetings early<br>▲ Contact with colleagues less than usual<br>▲ Exhibits usual sense of humor<br>▲ Difficulties transitioning to social self<br>▲ Some difficulties separating<br>▲ Better coping skills and resiliency |

## Use of Different Raters

The GAEF should be used to rate the professional helper's current level of functioning. Because individual behaviors, states, and traits are often dependent on the environment in which they are observed, observations should be documented based on multiple raters as listed in the following. A time sampling method should be used because the individual may differ in his or her experience of empathy fatigue with regard to events that take place at different times throughout the day (e.g., morning, afternoons, evenings, weekends, before client sessions, after client sessions, every other day). Persons considering rating themselves and/or others using the GAEF should be open to, and understand, the limitations and bias that are found in other subjective ratings of experiences such as mood, affect, personality, stress, attitude, motivation, level of satisfaction, and job burnout, as well as measures of spiritual well-being.

▶ *Self-ratings by the professional:* The individual himself or herself may use the GAEF as a self-report measure.

▶ *Ratings by the professional's colleagues:* The professional may request the involvement of his or her clinical supervisor, peer mentor, or another professional to rate his or her observations independently on the GAEF measure.

▶ *Ratings by clients/consumers:* Ratings may be carried out according to a well-designed scheme within the work environment that uses interrater agreement by the therapist's client/consumer and/or a triad of raters (i.e., client, therapist, and independent observer).

▶ *Ratings by independent observers outside the work environment:* The therapist may request ratings by close professional colleagues.

▶ *Ratings by another objective individual:* The professional may request ratings by others (i.e., personal therapists) who are closely committed to the professional's personal goals of self-care and personal growth.

As the rater(s) view the GAEF rating scale as shown in Table 19.1, they should rate the level of empathy fatigue experienced primarily within the past 2 weeks. Although the professional helper may not relate with all characteristics within each level, the therapist should choose the attributes that he or she identifies with more so than not. Also, the rater(s) may consider using the GAEF Levels (V, IV, III, II, and I) for each of the seven content areas and deriving a rating (i.e., Level V in Cognitive, Behavioral; Level III in Spiritual, Physical).

## CULTIVATING COUNSELOR RESILIENCY

A consistent finding in resiliency psychology research suggests that persons' attitudes and beliefs play a key role in the degree of resiliency that is exhibited or expressed. Resilient professionals almost always appear to possess a higher degree of internal locus of control, are inwardly directed and self-motivated, and thrive despite adverse conditions. Anecdotal evidence from professional helpers who have bounced back from adversity in their lives such as substance addiction, divorce, loss of a loved one, career transition, or traumatic stress have chosen to live in an optimal state of mental and physical well-being. They have incorporated the following principles, some of which are universal, in cultivating a resilient mind, body, and spirit:

*Making a Choice.* Professional helpers make a thinking, feeling, and behavioral choice on a daily basis when they must deal with client adversity. At the end of the day, counselors can choose to vent with their colleagues (and be a good listener for others) and not take home all their clients' stories of adversity. If they take on this stress (consciously or unconsciously) this may already be added to their own wounded soul. Thus, the alternative would be to choose more healthy thoughts and emotions. The act of choosing a healthier outlook basically is a choice to take responsibility for one's own thoughts and emotions. There will always be a professional responsibility of helping another person in a compassionate and empathic way. However, resilient professionals know how to manage client adversity throughout their work, home, social, and interpersonal lives. Thus, not moving forward into one's own program of personal wellness would be self-defeating. The alternative would inevitably be bleak by constantly ruminating over the client's adversity at the end of the day. Thus, making a choice to change one's stream of thoughts and emotions about a client's adversity can be very empowering for some therapists. Negative and destructive thought patterns must be replaced with a plan of personal self-care and wellness. This must be reinforced and supported by colleagues and others in the counselor's environment to be successful. Accordingly, professional counselors need to create opportunities to help cultivate personal wellness and self-care approaches.

*Positive Thinking.* The power of positive thinking is about believing in yourself, having faith in your abilities, and having a high level of confidence that you can effect a positive outcome with your clients. As counselors struggle with their own as well as their client's issues, it is easier for therapists to see the barriers and obstacles to living from a positive frame of reference. The counselor may have many negative recurring thoughts about the client's life in general. However, this can turn into a self-fulfilling prophecy. Professional counselors need to practice positive redirection in their thinking so that it can become a routine and intentional way of living.

*Taking Self-Responsibility.* Shifting blame to others does not provide an opportunity for the therapist to develop resiliency behaviors (e.g., "My clients drive me crazy sometimes by really pushing my buttons; if they think that they have problems, they should have seen the client from my previous session"). Metaphorically, "when you point a finger at someone else, there are four fingers pointing back at you." Taking responsibility is a challenge for many counselors even though we advocate the same with our clients. Many professionals were never taught how to do this. For example, some clients may be in denial of their son's or daughter's substance abuse behaviors and may be enabling the adolescent. The consequences of the adolescent's bad choices may be hindered by the therapist who has taken on all the emotional responsibility, or perhaps identifying with the adolescent's parent. Taking self-responsibility is a learned behavior that can generalize to other areas of the therapist's life. We all need to learn how to model self-responsibility and give up some control to the client. Allowing our clients to take safe risks and fail can be very therapeutic at times. It can build resiliency and promote healthy choices. Meanwhile, we may learn how our clients can live without our assistance. Overall, we should be internally responsible for our own thoughts, emotions, and actions and learn how to build resiliency traits.

*Self-Motivation.* Resilient individuals find their own unique style of internal motivation with school, work, home, social encounters, emotional considerations, and in other ways. Persons who have bounced back and pulled through adverse critical incidents demonstrate to others that they know how to achieve optimal and realistic control in their lives. These types of professional helpers tend to have an increased level of emotional, physical, and spiritual well-being. They are persistent with the tasks they take on and have an innate sense for knowing how to achieve their life goals. Many professionals have had the opportunity to observe healthy role models in their environment. They were fortunate to have a colleague, clinical supervisor, life coach, teacher, religious or spiritual leader, or others who have cared about them to help them overcome the more difficult challenges in their lives.

## CONCLUDING REMARKS

The experience of empathy fatigue is both similar and different from other types of counselor impairment or professional fatigue syndromes. Thus, it is hypothesized that the cumulative effects of multiple client sessions throughout the week may lead to a deterioration of the counselor's resiliency or coping abilities. Professional counselors who interact with clients who experience daily hassles and stressful life events may be at the same risk level as those professionals who assist those who are traumatized.

As the professional counselor engages in therapeutic interactions, this may predispose the counselor to experience an empathy fatigue reaction that ranges on a continuum of low to moderate to high. However, there are multiple risk factors that should be considered as identified in the GAEF. Consequently, the cumulative effects of multiple client stories can result in the depletion of the professional counselor's empathic energies, resulting in empathy fatigue. Developing a clearer understanding of the risk factors associated with empathy fatigue is pivotal in developing self-care strategies for the professional counselor.

## RESOURCES

American Counseling Association's (ACA) Taskforce on Counselor Wellness and Impairment: http://www.creating-joy.com/taskforce/tf_wellness_strategies.htm. The ACA is the largest professional counseling association in North America. This is a very comprehensive source for counselor self-care. There are multiple assessment and screening tools for professional counselors that include wellness, professional quality of life, traumatic stress, and a variety of other assessments.

Gift From Within: http://www.giftfromwithin.org. Gift From Within is an international not-for-profit organization for survivors of traumatic stress. This particular organization is dedicated to PTSD survivors and advocates multiple supports from family, friends, and peers. Educational materials, a list of retreats, workshops, and online support are offered.

Green Cross Foundation and Green Cross Academy of Traumatology: http://www.greencross.org. Green Cross is a professional organization of traumatologists founded by Dr. Charles Figley and colleagues who have developed the foundational research and educational materials related to compassion fatigue.

Mark Lerner Associates, Inc.: http://www.marklernerassociates.com. Dr. Lerner is a clinical psychologist and traumatic stress consultant with an international reputation in organizations and individuals who have experienced extraordinary stressful and traumatic events in their lives. Dr. Lerner offers consultations, workshops, and educational and training materials for individuals and organizations to thrive and survive after traumatic events.

Al Siebert Resiliency Center: http://resiliencycenter.com. Dr. Siebert (1934–2009) has been a resiliency researcher, trainer, and practitioner for well over 35 years. The Al Siebert Resiliency Center has over the years developed a culture of resiliency, as opposed to "managing one's stress," which is counter to the resiliency philosophy. The center has a plethora of resources and research articles on resiliency.

## RECOMMENDED BOOKS

Brennan, B. A. (1987). *Hands of light: A guide to healing through the human energy field.* New York, NY: Bantam Books.

Davis, M., Robbins Eshelman, E., & McKay, M. (1995). *The relaxation and stress reduction workbook* (4th ed.). Oakland, CA: New Harbinger.

Fanning, P. (1994). *Taking control of your life.* Oakland, CA: New Harbinger.

Figley, C. R. (2002). *Treating compassion fatigue.* New York, NY: Brunner-Routledge.

Fox, M., & Sheldrake, R. (1996). *The physics of angels: Exploring the realm where science and spirit meets.* San Francisco, CA: Harper San Francisco.

Goodwin, L. R. (2002). *The button therapy book: A practical psychological self-help book and holistic cognitive counseling manual for mental health professionals.* Victoria, BC, Canada: Trafford.

Hauck, R. (1994). *Angels: The mysterious messengers.* New York, NY: Ballantine.

Ingerman, S. (1991). *Soul retrieval: Mending the fragmented self.* San Francisco, CA: Harper San Francisco.

Kabat-Zinn, J. (1990). *Full catastrophe living: Using the wisdom of your body and mind to face stress, pain, and illness.* New York, NY: Dell Publishing.

Kabat-Zinn, J. (1994). *Wherever you go there you are: Mindfulness meditation in everyday life.* New York, NY: Hyperion.

LeShan, L. (1974). *How to meditate: A guide to self-discovery.* Boston, MA: Little, Brown.

Maslach, C. (2003). *Burnout: The cost of caring.* Cambridge, MA: Malor Books.

McKay, M., Davis, M., & Fanning, P. (1997). *Thoughts and feelings: Taking control of your moods and your life.* Oakland, CA: New Harbinger.

Mehl-Madrona, L. (1997). *Coyote medicine: Lessons from Native American healing.* New York, NY: Fireside/Simon & Schuster.

Merton, T. (1961). *New seeds of contemplation.* New York, NY: New Directions.

Mitchell, K. K. (1994). *Reiki: A torch in daylight.* St. Charles, IL: Mind Rivers Publications.

Monaghan, P., & Diereck, E. G. (1999). *Meditation: The complete guide.* Navato, CA: New World Library.

Moodly, R., & West, W. (2005). *Integrating traditional healing practices into counseling and psychotherapy.* Thousand Oaks, CA: Sage Publications.

Myers, J. E., & Sweeney, T. J. (2005). *Counseling for wellness: Theory, research, and practice.* Alexandria, VA: American Counseling Association.

Schaper, D., & Camp, C. A. (2004). *Labyrinths from the outside in: Walking to spiritual insight: A beginner's guide.* Woodstock, VT: Skylight Paths.

Seaward, B. L. (1997). *Stand like mountain flow like water.* Deerfield Beach, FL: Health Communications.

Seaward, B. L. (2006). *Essentials of managing stress.* Sudbury, MA: Jones & Bartlett.

Siebert, A. (2005). *The resiliency advantage: Master change, thrive under pressure, bounce back from setbacks.* San Francisco, CA: Berrett-Koehler Publishers.

Weiss, L. (2004). *Therapist's guide to self-care.* New York, NY: Brunner-Routledge.

## REFERENCES

American Counseling Association. (2014). ACA Taskforce on counselor wellness and impairment. Retrieved from http://www.creating-joy.com/taskforce/tf_wellness_strategies.htm

Assagioli, R. (1965). *Psychosynthesis.* New York, NY: Viking Press.

Association for Spiritual, Ethical, and Religious Values in Counseling. (2016). Spiritual competencies. Retrieved from http://www.aservic.org/resources/spiritual-competencies

Bar-On, R., & Parker, J. D. (2000). *The handbook of emotional intelligence: Theory, development, assessment, and application at home, school, and in the workplace.* San Francisco, CA: Jossey-Bass.

Barone, D. F., Hutchings, P. S., Kimmel, H. J., Traub, H. L., Cooper, J. T., & Marshal, C. M. (2005). Increasing empathetic accuracy through practice and feedback in a clinical interviewing course. *Journal of Social and Clinical Psychology, 24*(2), 156–171.

Berger, R. M. (2006). Prayer: It does a body good. *Sojourners Magazine, 35*(2), 17.

Bishop, D. R., Avila-Juarbe, E., & Thumme, B. (2003). Recognizing spirituality as an important factor in counselor supervision. *Counseling and Values, 48*(1), 34–46.

Brothers, L. (1989). A biological perspective on empathy. *American Journal of Psychiatry, 146*(1), 1–16.

Cashwell, C. S., & Young, J. S. (2004). Spirituality in counselor training: A content analysis of syllabi from introductory spirituality courses. *Counseling and Values, 48*(2), 96–109.

Corey, G., Schneider Corey, M., Corey, C., & Callanan, P. (2015). *Issues and ethics in the helping professions* (9th ed.). Stamford, CT: Brooks/Cole Cengage Learning.

Corey, M. S., & Corey, G. (2016). *Becoming a helper* (7th ed.). Boston, MA: Cengage.

Egan, G. (2010). *The skilled helper: A problem-management approach to helping* (9th ed.). Pacific Grove, CA: Brooks/Cole.

Figley, C. R. (1995). *Compassion fatigue: Coping with secondary traumatic stress disorder in those who treat the traumatized.* Bristol, PA: Brunner/Mazel.

Figley, C. R. (2002). Psychotherapist chronic lack of self care. *Journal of Clinical Psychology, 58,* 1433–1441.

Harley, D. A., Stebnicki, M. A., & Rollins, C. W. (2000). Applying empowerment evaluation as a tool for self-improvement and community development with culturally diverse populations. *Journal of Community Development Society, 31*(2), 348–364.

Herlihy, B., & Corey, G. (2015). *Boundary issues in counseling: Multiple roles and responsibilities.* Alexandria, VA: American Counseling Association.

Ivey, A. E., Bradford Ivey, M., & Zalaquett, C. P. (2010). *Intentional interviewing and counseling: Facilitating client development in a multicultural society* (7th ed.). Pacific Grove, CA: Brooks/Cole.

Joinson, C. (1992). Coping with compassion fatigue. *Nursing, 22*(4), 116–122.

Jung, C. G. (1973). Psychology and religion: East and west. In W. McGuire & R. F. C. Hull (Eds. & Trans.), *The collected works of C. G. Jung* (Vol. 11, pp. 5–105). Princeton, NJ: Princeton University Press. (Original work published 1937.)

Kabat-Zinn, J. (1990). *Full catastrophe living: Using the wisdom of your body and mind to face stress, pain, and illness.* New York, NY: Dell Publishing.

Marci, C., Ham, J., Moran, E., & Orr, S. (2007). Physiologic correlates of perceived therapist empathy and social-emotional process during psychotherapy. *Journal of Nervous and Mental Disorders, 195*, 103–111.

Maslach, C. (1982). *The burnout: The cost of caring.* Englewood Cliffs, NJ: Prentice-Hall.

Maslach, C. (2003). *Burnout: The cost of caring.* Cambridge, MA: Malor Books.

Mayne, T. J., & Bonanno, G. A. (2001). *Emotions: Current issues and future directions.* New York, NY: Guilford Press.

Mayne, T. J., & Ramsey, J. (2001). The structure of emotion: A nonlinear dynamic systems approach. In T. J. Mayne & G. A. Bonanno (Eds.), *Emotions: Current issues and future directions* (pp. 1–37). New York, NY: Guilford Press.

McCann, L., & Pearlman, L. A. (1989). Vicarious traumatization: A framework for understanding the psychological effects of working with victims. *Journal of Traumatic Stress, 3*(1), 131–149.

Miller, G. (2003). *Incorporating spirituality in counseling and psychotherapy: Theory and technique.* Hoboken, NJ: Wiley.

Nouwen, H. J. M. (1972). *The wounded healer.* New York, NY: An Image Book/Doubleday.

Pargament, K. L., & Zinnbauer, B. J. (2000). Working with the sacred: Four approaches to religious and spiritual issues in counseling. *Journal of Counseling & Development, 78*, 162–171.

Pearlman, L. A., & Saakvitne, K. W. (1995). *Trauma and the therapist: Self-care issues for clinicians, researchers, and educators.* Lutherville, MD: Sidran Press.

Pedersen, P. (2000). *A handbook for developing multicultural awareness* (3rd ed.). Alexandria, VA: American Counseling Association.

Pert, C. B., Dreher, H. E., & Ruff, M. R. (2005). The psychosomatic network: Foundations of mind-body medicine. In M. Schlitz, T. Amorok, & M. Micozzi (Eds.), *Consciousness and healing: Integral approaches to mind-body medicine* (pp. 61–78). St. Louis, MO: Elsevier, Churchill, & Livingstone.

Polanski, P. J. (2003). Spirituality and supervision. *Counseling and Values, 47*(2), 131–141.

Riess, H. (2010). Empathy in medicine: A neurobiological perspective. *Journal of the American Medical Association, 304*(14), 1604–1605.

Rogers, C. R. (1980). *A way of being.* Boston, MA: Houghton Mifflin.

Sapolsky, R. M. (1998). *Why zebras don't get ulcers: An updated guide to stress, stress-related diseases, and coping.* New York, NY: W. H. Freeman.

Shafranske, E. P., & Malony, H. N. (1996). Religion and the clinical practice of psychology: The case for inclusion. In E. P. Shafranske (Ed.), *Religion and the clinical practice of psychology* (pp. 561–586). Washington, DC: American Psychological Association.

Stamm, B. H. (1995). *Compassion fatigue: Coping with secondary traumatic stress disorder in those who treat the traumatized.* New York, NY: Brunner-Routledge.

Stamm, B. H. (2010). *The concise ProQOL manual.* Retrieved from http://www.proqol.org/uploads/ProQOL_Concise_2ndEd_12-2010.pdf

Stebnicki, M. A. (1999, April). *Grief reactions among rehabilitation professionals: Dealing effectively with empathy fatigue.* Presentation made at the NRCA/ARCA Alliance Annual Training Conference, Dallas, TX.

Stebnicki, M. A. (2000). Stress and grief reactions among rehabilitation professionals: Dealing effectively with empathy fatigue. *Journal of Rehabilitation, 6*(1), 23–29.

Stebnicki, M. A. (2001). Psychosocial response to extraordinary stressful and traumatic life events: Principles and practices for rehabilitation counselors. *New Directions in Rehabilitation, 12*(6), 57–71.

Stebnicki, M. A. (2006). Integrating spirituality in rehabilitation counselor supervision. *Rehabilitation Education, 20*(2), 137–159.

Stebnicki, M. A. (2007). Empathy fatigue: Healing the mind, body, and spirit of professional counselors. *Journal of Psychiatric Rehabilitation, 10*(4), 317–338.

Stebnicki, M. A. (2008). *Empathy fatigue: Healing the mind, body, and spirit of professional counselors.* New York, NY: Springer Publishing.

Stebnicki, M. A. (2012). Psychosocial impact of empathy fatigue on professional helpers. In I. Marini & M. A. Stebnicki (Eds.), *The professional counselor's desk reference* (pp. 423–432). New York, NY: Springer Publishing.

Stebnicki, M. A. (2016). From empathy fatigue to empathy resiliency. In I. Marini & M. A. Stebnicki (Eds.), *The professional counselor's desk reference* (2nd ed., pp. 533–545). New York, NY: Springer Publishing.

TaFoya, T., & Kouris, N. (2003). Dancing the circle: Native American concepts of healing. In S. G. Mijares (Ed.), *Modern psychology and ancient wisdom: Psychological healing practices from the world's religious traditions* (pp. 125–146). New York, NY: Haworth Integrative Healing Press.

Truax, C. B., & Carkhuff, R. R. (1967). *Towards effective counseling and psychotherapy.* Chicago, IL: Aldine.

Weil, A. (1995). *Spontaneous healing.* New York, NY: Ballantine.

Worthington, E. L. (1988). Understanding the values of religious clients: A model and its application to counseling. *Journal of Counseling Psychology, 35*(2), 166–174. http://dx.doi.org/10.1037/0022-0167.35.2.166

# CHAPTER 20

# The Personal Growth Program to Heal Trauma (PGP-HT)

During my master's and doctoral programs, I had the opportunity to be mentored by one of the most skillful, compassionate, empathic, and insightful persons I have ever encountered in the counseling field: Dr. Harry Allen, Professor Emeritus-Posthumous, Southern Illinois University Carbondale. Dr. Allen, who preferred to be called "Harry," was not only a highly creative and enlightened counselor educator and productive researcher, but he also had a reputation among his peers as an extraordinary practitioner; a shaman of sorts. Harry's lineage grew deep. He earned a master's degree of divinity at Duke University, a PhD in counseling psychology from the University of Arkansas, and I believe he stated that he had specialized training with Dr. Carl Rogers.

Harry developed a graduate-level foundational counseling course that he called the *Empathy Lab*. In today's counselor education programs, this course would be titled "prepracticum"; if not conducted by a skilled and competent practitioner, the experience would end up being more counseling lectures (e.g., ethical dilemmas, counseling disclosure statements, suicide assessment, treatment planning) than actual practice. As a matter of practicality, the Empathy Lab prepared students regarding how to respond to real client issues during their practicum and internship experience.

Harry would begin the first class of the semester by telling students, "There are only three things that I want you to gain from this course: show up; pay attention; and be open to the outcomes." After Harry made this statement, there was silence in our small group of six to eight students. From what I remembered, there was little explanation beyond this mantra. Being the first class of the semester, it was respectful to sit and listen, rather than stating my needs for the course and what it takes to get an "A." As the semester rolled along I became enlightened as to what Harry meant by these three simple rules or learning objectives to show up, pay attention, and be open to the outcomes.

To truly understand Harry's mission, vision, and purpose for the Empathy Lab required participation in various experiential activities throughout the semester. The Empathy Lab, as I experienced it, facilitated my own interpersonal awareness of self and others; it cultivated an increased understanding of my own emotional and interpersonal

IQ and how I experienced my clients' thoughts and feelings, moment to moment. The Lab also provided me with the opportunity to acquire the foundations of the helping profession that included responding to others with a high level of empathy and compassion, establishing a genuine and trusting relationship with others, and strategies that helped build a working alliance with my clients. This was accomplished through video-taped client–counselor role-plays, one-on-one feedback sessions with Harry, and other relationship building person-centered activities.

Mostly, I had the opportunity to learn from a highly intuitive person who could empower others to nourish their spirit for serving others in the world compassionately and empathically. It was also an opportunity to learn how to grow personally and professionally in the helping profession. Indeed, the Empathy Lab was something that one would need to experience firsthand to gain the full range of lessons. It also became my passion as I transitioned into academia teaching in counselor education programs for more than 20 years.

Through these experiences were born the principles of the three-step program I call the Personal Growth Program (PGP). Originally designed as a self-care practice to heal empathy fatigue, it has been adapted and redesigned as a resiliency approach to heal trauma. The acronym I have chosen to represent this approach is PGP-HT

## PERSONAL GROWTH PROGRAM TO HEAL TRAUMA

### Introduction to PGP-HT

The PGP-HT is a dynamic, interactive, and solution-focused approach for exploring posttraumatic growth and resiliency. Mostly, it provides an opportunity for early identification, assessment, and recommended interventions to deal with a range of issues affecting the mind, body, and spirit of trauma survivors. This approach is based on my own personal growth experiences, clinical experiences in rehabilitation counseling and mental health, and particularly treating others who have acquired posttraumatic stress and co-occurring conditions. Also integrated in the PGP-HT are 30 years of teaching and research experiences that I would describe as holistic in nature. The theories, models, and approaches were drawn from a range of humanistic, cognitive behavioral, mindfulness-stress reduction, and culturally indigenous healing methods as I have learned in my Level I, II, and III Reiki Master training, as well as my beginning- and intermediate-level shaman training I began through the California-based Michael Harner's Foundation for Shamanic Studies (Harner, 2016). Essentially, the PGP-HT provides a model for helping others to (a) show up and receive help from professionals and other natural supports; (b) pay attention to their mind, body, and spirit with the intention to heal their trauma; and (c) be open to the outcomes with the journey they began.

### Benefits of PGP-HT

Persons who have extraordinary stressful and traumatic experiences require the highest level of attention, compassion, and empathy through a skilled and competent mental health professional. It is critical as professionals that we understand we are just a conduit to facilitating healing resources, which may or may not include approaches in traditional mental health settings. Attuned mental health professionals understand their clients' cultural significance, personality traits/states, behaviors, thoughts, feelings, and experiences in life, and know how to draw in other resources. This may include activities such as expressive arts, animal-assisted therapy, mindfulness meditation, yoga, tai chi, acupuncture, and many other approaches unique to the client's values and beliefs.

Accordingly, the PGP-HT challenges individuals to *show up* to begin their journey of healing trauma; *pay attention* to all traditional, complementary, and alternative options that are available for healing trauma; and *be open to the outcomes*, knowing that being flexible and trying out new things are key in resiliency and posttraumatic growth. The PGP-HT requires one to make a commitment to self and others in an intentional way, to ask for help from other trusted and natural supports, and to be in a journey of self-care practices that can be carried on throughout one's daily routines.

One of the unique features of the PGP-HT is that it employs both a group and individual approach. It is recognized that the individual may have preferences for either/or and that personal change varies with the individual's level of motivation. Thus, a stage-change approach is used with the PGP-HT to deal with problems and opportunities that relate to mental and physical symptoms experienced as a result of being at the epicenter of trauma. Basically, the PGP-HT invites the person to change something in his or her life (e.g., way of thinking, feeling, perceiving others, work behaviors, physical symptoms). This is very similar to the therapeutic stages of change that individuals go through as they transition to increased levels of wellness. The PGP-HT encourages the person to chart these experiences with the use of a journal or diary. The benefits are useful in recording and processing feelings, thoughts, and experiences.

## Preliminary Issues of Showing Up

For some survivors of trauma, there may be several hours or days that pass before they have any intensive interactions with mental health professionals. Thus, establishing rapport is a critical first step in realizing that survivors may not be ready for a structured system of support. Rather, the survivor may heal better with his or her family, friends, coworkers, and other natural supports such as religious and spiritual practices. Thus, the concept of *readiness* is important to understand before the trauma survivor is ready to *show up*. This may take months for some, depending on the severity of mental and physical injury that occurred as a result of their traumatic experiences.

Skilled and competent mental health professionals complete preliminary assessments and mental health screenings with their clients. Given the nature of extraordinary stressful and traumatic events, it is quite natural for survivors to isolate themselves from family, friends, and coworkers and detach socially. Thus, there is a balance between allowing the person to process his or her trauma and intervening as a professional. The discovery of client readiness is ongoing. It may change from day to day. However, mental health professionals should be available to assess the degree of stress, depression, anxiety, posttraumatic stress, poor coping skills such as substance use, and any level of suicide ideation. Monitoring any medical, physical, or chronic health conditions is also critical and referrals need to be made to the appropriate health care providers.

Overall, the survivor's vulnerability can be reduced by cultivating a program of self-care that may lead to opportunities for increased personal awareness, growth, and hope for the individual's future optimal wellness. However, first the individual must *show up*. This can be introduced to the trauma survivor as follows.

## STEP 1: SHOW UP AND BE PRESENT

Showing up is the first step in any self-care structured program. Since you are reading *Disaster Mental Health Counseling* or have introduced the PGP-HT to clients, coworkers, or others, you have made a choice to show up. So welcome! You have taken a significant step thus far. The primary emphasis in Step 1 is for you to be physically, mentally, cognitively, and spiritually present in the here and now. If you feel that you are not ready currently, that is okay. Many individuals who felt they were not ready to begin their healing journey were in the exact same spot as you. For now, invite yourself to be open, honest, flexible, and begin to conceptualize how you might deal more effectively or creatively with some specific issues related to your experiences. It may or may not be related to your symptoms of posttraumatic stress. It may relate to a goal you have to decrease or stop smoking cigarettes or feel less stressed, depressed, or something else in life. These issues may concern your sense of mental, physical, or spiritual depletion or exhaustion. You may be an individual just beginning a career, marriage, living in a new geographic location, or may be anticipating some changes in your future. Showing up in Step 1 may challenge you to be mindful of all the issues that may hinder your ability to move forward. Please do not place a value on any of these issues in terms of I "shoulda-coulda-woulda." There are not "good and bad" emotions; rather, they are all just emotions. We feel because we are human.

To begin the process with the PGP-HT, pay attention and be mindful of the things you want to change in your life. Find a quiet place in your home, in an outdoor environment, or go on a retreat and invite yourself to explore the following questions:

▶ What do I currently feel emotionally, physically, spiritually, career-wise, educationally, academically, and in my relationships with others?

▶ Which areas of my life do I want to grow—what do I want to transform?

▶ What can I do to go about changing or growing in specific life areas?

▶ What are some things that I need to achieve my goals?

▶ How will I know when I have arrived and have met what I set out to accomplish?

In this first step, please be open to the idea that you can choose a more conscious and intentional way of living and being mindful in the moment with yourself and others. You may have already developed a program of self-care; however, being creative and incorporating other activities may inspire your mind, body, and spirit in other ways.

## STEP 2: PAYING ATTENTION AND BEING MINDFUL

Paying attention and being mindful actually involves more than working on a cognitive level of awareness and understanding. This requires a shift in your level of consciousness by becoming aware of your feelings, emotions, and mental and physical wellness. Paying attention to deeper levels of consciousness through activities such as meditation, focusing, quieting the mind, and expressive arts can help you cultivate a felt sense of meaning and purpose concerning your life. It has the potential to open the door to nonordinary states of consciousness or deeper contemplation, which can assist you in accessing your intuitive sense (or gut feelings) of a higher power that can lead you in your plan of self-care.

You do not have to be a spiritual person to benefit from quieting your mind, body, and soul, or relaxing your spirit. There are so many distractions throughout the day that quieting your mind, body, and spirit should become as natural as exercising, eating, sleeping, or breathing. If you are already engaged in a program of wellness, personal growth, or spiritual or religious ritual, then you are nurturing your body. To nurture your mind requires that you begin paying attention to the different levels of consciousness but at a much deeper level than ever before. You also may want to identify your unused opportunities and resources by starting with a variety of structured or nonstructured self-guided activities.

The primary emphasis in Stage 2 is for you to communicate your plan of action to self and others in your environment. To begin this process, it will be helpful to keep a daily journal or diary. The journal entries may be a combination of words, symbols, sentences, drawings/sketches, or other forms of expression. Documenting your thoughts, feelings, emotions, cognitions, and experiences allows you to analyze the different levels of your consciousness. After you have written down any thoughts, emotions, or experiences, you should interpret, translate, and find meaning in your journal entries.

You may want to seek out another person or a group of peers to discuss and share your personal journal entries. For some individuals, writing down their life's mission and purpose or developing a vision statement can help bring some meaning and purpose to their healing. Some may pose a question in their journals. Others may state a plan of self-care that has a specific measurable goal that supports one's personal growth. Since this is your personal journey, it is your decision on how to disclose your vision, goals, and plans for change.

If you are not the type of person who approaches life with specific behavioral objectives and lives "one-day-at-a-time," this is okay too. Each person finds his or her own way of paying attention and being mindful by proposing a plan of self-care. At a minimum, you should begin learning how to pay attention, living life more consciously, and being more aware of your thoughts, feelings, and behaviors.

For now, clear a space in your life and begin to visualize how you want to feel emotionally, physically, spiritually, and in other ways. Be creative in your solutions to finding new ways to approach old problems. There is no "right way" or "wrong way." There are not "good feelings" or "bad feelings." Having conscious and/or unconscious rules set up only serves to restrict your creativity. It draws boundary lines around your ideas, thoughts, feelings, or creative expression of healing from trauma.

## STEP 3: BE OPEN TO THE OUTCOMES AND EXPERIENCES

In this step you will want to review your PGP-HT journal and search for any significant themes or information that you may have overlooked. Review your journal notes and try to read between the lines. Search beyond the literal meaning of what you have written. Review your notes for any daily progress, creative ideas, or successes you have documented. Explore your journal entries for any challenges or obstacles that you may have encountered on your wellness journey. Remember that in most situations outside of the uncontrollable (e.g., weather conditions, chronic health conditions, disability, or socio-economic status) we create most of our own obstacles.

There is an old Hindu story of the monkey and the coconut, also told as a "South American Indian Tribe" story by Pirsig (1976). A group of hunters wanted to capture a monkey, so they tied a coconut to a tree, drilled two small holes on each side of the coconut, and then planted/baited the coconut with a banana. They waited for hours and then finally a monkey approached. The monkey slipped his hands through the two small openings on each side of the coconut and grabbed the banana with both hands. The monkey could not pull the banana out of the coconut because his hands were in a fist. Quickly, the monkey was caught. Had the monkey not made a fist and could let go of the banana, he could have easily freed his hands from the coconut. However, the desire to hold tight and try and pull the banana from the coconut was much stronger than his will to let go. Basically, the monkey was so consumed with holding on so tight to something (metaphorically) that may have been an object of desire, high-risk thrill-seeking activity, or an addiction that the monkey forgot how to free himself; how to let go. Thus, the hunters caught their monkey.

It is essential that we: (a) are aware of things that can trap us, (b) know how to get unstuck once we are in the midst of things that can harm us, and (c) learn how to let go. Despite what animal researchers have shown us, our critical thinking and problem-solving skills are much more sophisticated than those of the monkey. However, sometimes we get trapped like the monkey in the Hindu parable. So we must be open to the outcomes by conducting an open and honest assessment of our self-care and PGP-HT progress. It is essential that we explore how we can let go and grasp the things in life that can nurture and support our mind, body, and spirit. Expanding our list of options, resources, and natural environmental supports help us become unstuck.

## ASSESSING PERSONAL GROWTH

There are many tools for assessing personal growth. It is based on what you might be measuring (e.g., improvement in mood and affect, smoking cessation, weight loss program, decreased negative thoughts). However, in reality, you and others around you may be the most important tool for measuring change. If you made an attempt to get through the PGP-HT three-step program you already have shown some level of commitment and motivation to change something in your life and to begin a program of self-care. Holistically, this may look like you have taken care of your body (e.g., an exercise program, nutritional intake, weight loss), taken care of your mind (e.g., reading a self-care book, thinking positive thoughts), or caring for your spirit (e.g., attending a church service, going to a yoga class, or participating in a meditation group). You should not be satisfied with just a traditional behavioral health plan (e.g., stress reduction activities, exercise, nutrition, dieting) as a self-care approach. This may be a great start for some. However, it is important to be mindful that optimal functioning requires feeling whole and back to balance in our mind, body, and spirit.

Making the necessary changes in your life sometimes takes a few weeks or months just to get started. Many mental health researchers and clinicians emphasize that individual change and personal growth do not occur spontaneously. There are a large number of personal testimonials in books, articles, and online that discuss significant life changes others have made for the survival of their mental, physical, and spiritual well-being. Further, there are qualitative studies in peer-reviewed journals that report spontaneous remission from a chronic medical, physical, or mental health condition. In many of these studies, the person provides details about a profound transformation he or she experienced. Others provide testimonials about the wellness and lifestyle changes they have achieved.

The PGP-HT does not propose that you attempt a rapid journey into mental, physical, or spiritual health. This would be unnatural for most. You are smarter than the monkey in the Hindu parable. Some individuals may want to consider the PGP-HT as an opportunity to begin the experience of extraordinary personal growth and/or transformation. Such a rehabilitation of the mind, body, and spirit typically occurs over time. It is essential that we are mindful of the "baby steps" to wellness that we can take. At a minimum, it is essential that you empower yourself by taking responsibility to seek out multiple resources and support systems that will assist you in accomplishing your goals or vision for personal change and growth.

Whichever stage of personal growth and development that you experience (i.e., Steps 1, 2, or 3), it is helpful to go back and review the principles of resiliency. As the resiliency literature suggests, every negative action, feeling, and thought has a cost to your mind–body–spirit. Thus, a resilient mind, body, and spirit are essential to your well-being, especially for those closest to the epicenter of disaster and trauma. The following questions are offered as a way to cultivate a deeper meaning and purpose in your life for resiliency.

## Questions That Cultivate a Deeper Meaning and Purpose

Healing trauma requires much more than reading a self-help book or attending a counseling session. Some of the most prolific spiritual leaders of our time strongly believe that transformation of the mind, body, and spirit happens when we create a place in our consciousness that takes us to a much deeper level than ever before. Access to the human spirit happens from a meditative or nonordinary state of consciousness, not from ordinary everyday states of consciousness.

The following existential and spiritual questions may be helpful to begin cultivating your program of self-care. Some of these questions have been developed through personal interviews (see Elliott, 1996) from some of the world's greatest spiritual healers (i.e., Mother Teresa, Norman Vincent Peale, Dalai Lama, Ram Dass, Rabbi Zalman Schachter-Shalomi). Thus, listening and paying attention to your inner voice experiences by asking the following questions may bring a higher level of wisdom and insight to begin your journey into wholeness.

*Ask yourself the following questions using the deeper reaches of all five senses:*

1. On what main beliefs, truths, or values do I base my life?
2. Do I believe in a divine source of power, Great Spirit, or Supreme Being who has the ultimate compassion for my life and its purpose? How do I experience this spirit entity?
3. How would I characterize or describe the ultimate purpose of my life?
4. What is the highest ideal that a person can reach in his or her life?
5. How have I achieved or attained a goal that I really desired? What was the process I went through to achieve this goal for myself?
6. What has been or what is the greatest obstacle to obtaining what I want in my life?
7. Do I see myself achieving the ultimate happiness or harmony in life? If not, what are some things that may be an obstacle to me?
8. What is the meaning or purpose to my life at this moment?
9. If I could change anything about my life, what would I want to change?
10. What advice has a family member, close friend, mentor, consultant, or spiritual leader given me in regard to my particular life issues? Has any of this been valid?
11. If I could meet anyone throughout history, who would I want to meet? What would I want to know or ask this person?
12. What was the most significant thing or event (positive or negative) that ever happened in my life? How did this affect me and what lessons did it teach me?
13. Some people believe that certain things interfere with reaching personal growth. What things have I noticed in my life that have hindered my abilities to achieve?
14. If I only had a few days left on the Earth before I passed on to some other dimension, what advice would I have for my friends, family, children, or others?
15. If I only had a few days left on the Earth before I passed on to some other dimension, what would I want others to know or say about me when I am gone?

Now that you have had an opportunity to review these 15 questions, you might notice how difficult they are to answer in a direct or concrete way. Some are deeper questions that require thoughts, feelings, cognitions, insights, and reflections that may challenge you. Thus, there is no right or wrong responses to the questions given previously. In fact, you may have already asked yourself these questions as you go through the PGP-HT model. Despite the uncertainty that exists as we contemplate the nature of these 15 questions, it is critical that we probe the deeper reaches of our mind, body, and spirit. This may require a weekend meditation retreat or finding a natural environment in which to write in a journal. A journey of inner healing requires that we come out of the darkness and into the light to face the fear of changing something in our life.

## Solution-Focused Questions: Getting to the Core of the Problem Issue

Highly skilled professionals know the importance of implementing the right strategies to facilitate client change. After professional helpers listen to their clients' story and assess their motivation for change, they then may match specific counseling theories and techniques that assist individuals in putting their plans into action. Before this process begins, however, it is essential to have a direction that leads to successful coping or problem-solving strategies. The following solution-focused questions are offered as a way to point yourself in a specific direction. These probes may provide you with a clearer understanding of what you would like to change.

- ► What is it that I would like to change?
- ► Given my present situation, what changes in my life make sense?
- ► If I made these changes, what would I be doing differently in my life right now?
- ► What would these changes look like?
- ► What particular behaviors, thoughts, emotions, and experiences would I be feeling or doing differently?
- ► What would I be doing differently that I am not doing currently?
- ► What resources have I thought about that would help support my goals/vision?
- ► If I no longer had these issues, what would others notice different about me?

## STAGES OF CHANGE IN PERSONAL GROWTH

The following model presented is based on stages of change theory. Prochaska and DiClemente (1982) and Prochaska, DiClemente, and Norcross (1992), as well as their other colleagues, developed the foundational research in this area, which explains how individuals progress through five different stages of change to transform their pattern of simple and complex behaviors. The model offered here is to assess, predict, and monitor activities that relate to one's self-care, which will assist in moving an individual beyond trauma victim to trauma survivor. It follows the five stages that were originally proposed in the foundational research: precontemplation, contemplation, preparation, action, and maintenance.

The intent of this proposed model is to predict patterns of negative or unwanted thoughts, behaviors, emotions, cognitions, and personality states or traits that may be observable by self and others. The purpose of integrating the PGP-HT with a stage change model is for you to assess and predict some of the challenges of self-defeating and unwanted behaviors, thoughts, or experiences that may hinder your ability to achieve optimal wellness of your mind, body, and spirit and heal your trauma. This particular stage change model makes the assumption that you want to heal your mind, body, and spirit and that you feel stuck, vulnerable, and are trapped like the monkey in the Hindu parable. To guide you through the stages of change, I have offered four specific areas of evaluation that are typically associated with each stage: (a) issues, (b) typical feelings experienced, and (c) self-assessment questions associated with each stage. The last area relates to suggested *interventions* that may be helpful for you in this process of change.

## Precontemplation

▶ *Issues in this stage:* In this stage, you are typically not interested in changing certain behaviors, thoughts, feelings, and emotions. You are likely in denial that you have any significant problems related to your traumatic experience. Basically, you are not motivated to act at this time. Cognitively, you may feel somewhat disorganized and detached from your friends, family, coworkers, or socially because you are too preoccupied with the internal dialogue or interplay between your mind, body, and spirit, all of which are in disharmony. There may be a sense of mental, emotional, physical, or spiritual exhaustion where you feel vulnerable or not securely attached to family, friends, relationships, or your job. You may also feel a sense of mental, emotional, social, physical, spiritual, and/or occupational depletion. Your career and day-to-day routine may feel meaningless. You may have a sense that "I need to suck it up."

▶ *Typical feelings experienced at this stage:* In this stage, you may feel that there are no possibilities for natural supports or a system that can provide a foundation to nourish your mind, body, and spirit. You may exhibit a pattern of negative thinking that may create problems for self and others around you. You would like to see others change, rather than you changing something about yourself. You may be coerced or forced into change because of poor coping abilities and choices you have made prior to your traumatic experiences (e.g., driving under the influence [DUI], divorce, chronic mental and/or physical illness). This may lead to further resistance and defensiveness.

▶ *Self-assessment:* Ask yourself: Do I become defensive or resistive when discussing certain aspects of my mind, body, or spirit with others? Do I tend to avoid relevant and important information about the health and wellness of my mind, body, and spirit? Do I avoid taking responsibility for trying to harmonize or rebalance my mind, body, and spirit? Do I intend to do something about these issues in the next few days, weeks, or months? When can I anticipate that I will make a commitment to change?

▶ *Interventions:* Share and communicate your concerns related to how out of balance your mind, body, or spirit is. Discuss these concerns with someone close to you or that you perceive can help guide you through this process. Try and understand your reason for wanting to avoid change or resist personal growth. Ask yourself the solution-focused probes listed previously such as: "How would things be different if I. . . ." Make some attempt to gain a small commitment toward personal change or growth.

## Contemplation

▶ *Issues in this stage:* In this stage, you may struggle to understand why your life is so out of balance. Stress and anxiety may be at its peak because you are experiencing the need for change. You begin to understand that change and growth require some kind of commitment. You may have to give up some type of self-destructive lifestyle habit, negative thoughts, self-defeating emotions, or some other negative behavioral or personality patterns.

▶ *Typical feelings experienced at this stage:* In this stage you may be premature in your actions to change or have a fear of failing. Be cautious because many individuals search for the perfect solution to their problems and attempt to make changes that are not natural to them. Many change a self-destructive lifestyle habit (e.g., quit smoking, stop drinking, decrease poor nutritional habits). However, these changes may be superficial for you because it requires that your mind, body, and spirit work in concert to achieve an optimal level of well-being.

▶ *Self-assessment:* Ask yourself: Am I willing to discuss this with someone else without blaming others? Am I interested in being educated or increasing my insight and awareness about my particular issues? Am I intending to take action on this? Does this problem behavior, thought pattern, or dysfunctional coping ability serve some higher purpose in my life?

▶ *Interventions:* Become aware and conscious of issues by balancing your mind, body, and spirit. Attempt change through breathing awareness, relaxation, meditation, or a visualization program of self-care. Notice how this impacts your life (i.e., job, relationship with others, lifestyle habits). What things must realistically be approached first? Identify some triggers, responses, or obstacles that could hinder your ability to change and rebalance your mind, body, and spirit.

## Preparation: Building a Foundation for Success

▶ *Issues in this stage:* If you are truly in this stage, you will make a commitment by taking action in the very near future. You will recognize this by developing a plan of action or a clearer vision of the purpose and meaning of doing the work that is essential in healing traumatic experiences and other co-occurring symptoms you may be experiencing. If you are truly in this stage, you are actively beginning a path to make the necessary changes and initial first steps into taking action.

▶ *Typical feelings experienced at this stage*: You may make a premature leap into change. This may be due to a vague plan of action. You may feel that you are being "pushed" into personal change or growth because your traumatic experiences are so intense that this will open up a "can of worms." Your thinking may be such that by confronting and challenging yourself you could potentially affect your job, marriage, or mental, physical, or spiritual health. You may feel some degree of balance already but it is not worth the risk of working on traumatic experiences at this point. It may be that you are not ready to make difficult life decisions and transitions. Another problem at this stage is that you do not have an environment this time that could support change. You may also lack the resources that do not support your change or growth.

▶ *Self-assessment:* Ask yourself: Am I only making excuses not to change or achieve personal growth? Are there some real issues that I cannot control (e.g., brain chemistry, hormones) when it comes to rebalancing my mind, body, and spirit? If I do change something in my life, have I considered the consequences of this change? What would I be giving up? What challenges would possibly lie ahead for me? Do the "positives" of change clearly outweigh the "negatives"? Am I focusing on the future benefits of change? Have I developed some specific ideas about how to change my behaviors, thoughts, or feelings?

▶ *Interventions:* Not having the support and resources to make changes in your life are in fact real issues. However, you have some resiliency traits because you have already done some of the hard work that got you to this point. Thus, it is worth going over your journal entries, reviewing resiliency traits, and looking at other creative solutions that have helped you to this point.

You may also want to increase your commitment to act by making a "public" commitment or asking others for help and support. Document a plan that has specific goals/objectives, meaning, and purpose for your mind, body, and spirit. State a clearer vision with specific start and completion times. Prepare your environment so it can support personal change and growth. Take responsibility and hold yourself accountable.

## Action: Attempting Change

▶ *Issues in this stage:* In this stage, you will clearly recognize that you are making an honest attempt to change your behaviors, thoughts, emotional reactions, maladaptive (codependent) behaviors, and your environment. The ultimate purpose is to achieve optimal wellness and much better self-control over your mind, body, and spirit. Other persons and supports that are in your environment should also notice these changes. You may be reluctant to ask for help. Most persons require assistance from a supportive network of family, friends, or professionals. If in fact you are in the *action* stage of change, you will not be shy about asking for help from others.

▶ *Typical feelings experienced at this stage:* You may feel hopeful. The chances of resisting or terminating your PGP-HT are less risky because you have prepared yourself much better in this stage. Thoughts of failure may be sporadic but one's confidence abounds because you have transitioned through the previous intense feelings and have made some sense and meaning of your thoughts, emotions, and experiences. At the present time, the worry and anxiety you may have about making personal change and growth may not be a dominant feature of your mind, body, and spirit because you have already taken action. You may become less impatient or frustrated because you have witnessed small changes or progress. You may feel less overwhelmed with making change. A small step backward is viewed as a "slip" rather than a "full-blown relapse." You have more good days than bad while at work, during therapeutic interactions with others, and in social, family, or interpersonal relationships. Any "slip" you experience does not become interpreted as a complete failure or disaster. Basically, giving up is not a consideration because of the level of success you have achieved. A very supportive environment is also responsible for your success at this stage.

▶ *Self-assessment:* Ask yourself: Am I continuing to actively pursue personal change and growth in my behaviors, thoughts, emotions, environment, mind, body, and spirit? Am I using my plan, supports, and other resources to my advantage? Am I empowered to neutralize or counteract any doubts or issues with my well-designed plan? What incentives am I using to sustain or reinforce my personal change or growth? Does my plan actually feel like it is working? Do I feel better emotionally? Physically? Spiritually? Cognitively? Does my life have more meaning and purpose? Do I feel somewhat more in balance with my mind, body, and spirit?

▶ *Interventions:* Use a variety of settings or environments to structure your interventions. Try to avoid or minimize your exposure to negative elements, people, or places in your life, knowing full well that you are the person empowered to control and maintain a balance of your mind, body, and spirit. Design your plan so that you can identify and interrupt the negative thoughts or chain of events that may be environmental, cognitive, behavioral, social, emotional, physiological, spiritual, or occupational. Have a deeper awareness of things you can control in your life and things that you cannot.

## Daily Maintenance and Preserving What Works

▶ *Issues in this stage:* In this stage, you make an honest and genuine attempt to sustain long-term personal change, growth, and commitment to your PGP-HT, which has enhanced your overall physical, mental, and spiritual well-being.

▶ *Typical feelings experienced at this stage:* It is typical that there may be protective factors or strategies that worked well for you at one point in time. Recognize that this may not be working currently. Progress or advancement within the PGP-HT may be viewed as a success by self and others. Be mindful that sometimes you may rationalize, celebrate, or reward yourself prematurely. This could cause a "slip" or backslide. Thus, be aware that achieving mind, body, and spiritual wellness is not an end goal. Rather, maintaining a balance in your life is an ongoing process.

▶ *Self-assessment:* Ask yourself: Do I know how to cope with high-risk situations in my PGP-HT? Is my mind, body, and spirit aware enough to know what to do if I have a slip or relapse? What elements of my plan do I need to modify or adjust to fit with my changing life needs? Am I continually being open and flexible to other possibilities and outcomes? Am I being creative enough to have a good level of self-fulfillment?

▶ *Interventions:* Be open to the idea that there is no one correct way of doing things. Try and view any slips or relapses as a lesson to be learned. Understand that your goals and objectives may include a long journey where staying focused and in balance is a major accomplishment. It may be helpful for the person to return to "baby steps" again. Most of all, your plan of action must change as you grow and develop.

## ADDITIONAL STRATEGIES FOR ACCOMPLISHING YOUR PGP-HT

### Brainstorming

Brainstorming is a technique that psychologist Gerald Egan (2014) uses to help persons move beyond problem solving and thoughts that are overly constricted or narrow. It is a tool to help persons develop both opportunities and possibilities for a better future. A good brainstorming session should empower you with the resources to take control of your life, anticipate any obstacles, and plan for a more functional and healthy future.

Egan has several prescripts before facilitating a brainstorming session. These include: (a) suspending your own bias and judgment about how the world functions, (b) encouraging quantity of ideas no matter how "wild" they may seem to be, (c) coming up with as many possibilities as imaginable, then dealing with the quality or realistic aspects of the solution later on, and (d) using one idea to stimulate others by combining one solution with another, which ultimately creates new ideas. Be mindful that brainstorming is an ongoing process because as you develop as a person, you will try out new behaviors, see what works, and hopefully make adjustments in your plans. Egan suggests that during brainstorming sessions, you should form probes that are based on the following solution-focused questions:

▶ *How:* How can I get to where I would like to go and how many different ways are there to accomplish what I want to accomplish?

▶ *Who:* Who can help me achieve my goals and who can serve as a resource for me to accomplish these goals?

▶ *What:* What resources, both internal and external, can help me accomplish my goals?

▶ *Where:* Where are the places that can help me achieve my goals?

▶ *When:* When are the times (what kind of timing) that can help me achieve my goals?

One way of cultivating a program of self-care is to invent a better future for yourself. You may want to challenge the insight and awareness that you have already gained by asking yourself the following solution-focused questions. Notice that these questions are all future-oriented. This will assist you in the action and planning stage.

▶ What would this problem situation look like if I were to manage it better?

▶ What changes in my present situation/life would make sense?

▶ What would I be doing differently with my problem situation if I made the changes that I would like to make?

▶ What things have I thought about that would make life better for me right now?

▶ What things/feelings in my life would I like to eliminate right now?

▶ If I eliminated certain things in my life, what would that feel like?

▶ When do I plan on making these changes?

## Discovering Multiple Resources

A good brainstorming session should bring about some positive changes in your life. One essential component to the PGP-HT is making sure that you have access to multiple resources to begin or maintain your overall program of self-care. There are multiple persons and life areas to draw upon. Here are a few suggested resources:

▶ *Individuals:* Trauma survivors who are successful in reaching optimal mental, physical, and spiritual well-being seek help from qualified health care professionals for medically related problems. Others seek out professional counselors, spiritual leaders, folk healers, or a family member for counseling and advice. There may be complementary and alternative health care practitioners that may be of value to you, such as acupuncturists, massage therapists, or yoga or tai chi classes. It is critical that you cultivate healing partnerships with others.

▶ *Role models:* Trauma survivors who are successful in reaching optimal mental, physical, and spiritual well-being seek out persons who have been successful in healing others. Search for others that have the wisdom, knowledge, advice, and counsel you seek. Think about those persons in your environment who have been through what you have been through emotionally, physically, medically, spiritually, and occupationally and talk with them.

▶ *Communities/groups:* Trauma survivors who are successful in reaching optimal mental, physical, and spiritual well-being seek out communities and groups that are therapeutic and supportive. Create your own support group. There are also a number of legitimate online support groups and chat rooms.

▶ *Eco-environment:* Trauma survivors who are successful in reaching optimal mental, physical, and spiritual well-being seek out geographic locations (e.g., mountains, rivers, lakes, oceans) that can help you connect with the Earth or natural environment.

▶ *Technology:* Trauma survivors who are successful in reaching optimal mental, physical, and spiritual well-being seek out assistive devices or other technology that will empower your independence, knowledge, and wisdom.

▶ *Organizations:* Trauma survivors who are successful in reaching optimal mental, physical, and spiritual well-being seek out associations and organizations that adhere to your philosophy and ideology about what you have experienced. Many of these organizations have networking, video education, and training opportunities at a distance. There are also face-to-face or online discussion groups and other activities that can help you achieve your goals.

▶ *Model programs:* Trauma survivors who are successful in reaching optimal mental, physical, and spiritual well-being seek out specific model programs that can assist you in achieving your goals. Some universities and teaching hospitals have opportunities to become involved in a study group for a variety of things including stress reduction, nutrition, weight loss, exercise, smoking and alcohol cessations, and many other wellness and lifestyle enhancement programs.

## Optimizing Your Mind, Body, and Spiritual Health

Optimizing your PGP-HT may require that you make a commitment in writing to begin your journey along the path of wellness. Be open to the idea that your PGP-HT may be a long-term building project and there may be specific issues that challenge your ability to achieve personal growth and development. Dr. Andrew Weil (1995) in his book *Spontaneous Healing* proposes that there are specific areas in a person's life that create obstacles to health, healing, and wellness. Many of the areas listed next are things that we have direct control over. Weil has met with healers throughout the world to try and discover what things can optimize our natural healing system. Interestingly, he suggests that illness is not caused purely by a deterioration of our physical wellness. Rather, our mind, body, and spirit interact to affect our overall healing and well-being. This belief characterizes a non-Western medical and mental health system of health care. The fact is that there is some degree of control we have in our lives. This takes responsibility, motivation, persistence, and support from others to achieve an optimal level of wellness. Weil is indeed an advocate of taking responsibility for our overall health and healing. Weil proposes that the following areas can help us achieve an optimal level of functioning.

### Weil's Proposal to Optimize the Mind, Body, and Spirit

*Lack of energy:* Energy supplied by our metabolism (the conversion of food to chemical energy) is essential for health and healing. An adequate nutritional intake, good digestion, and proper breathing are all within our control to effect energy. Overwork, overexertion, not getting enough rest and sleep, and other things we may be addicted to (too much alcohol, caffeine, and cigarettes) can all pull energy away from our physical being. Ultimately, a healthy mind is sacrificed because of poor concentration, focus, and other attention deficits that cause a drop in performance.

*Poor circulation:* Our natural healing system depends on the circulation of blood through our body to bring nutrients to our body system and organs. Circulation can be enhanced by following a healthy diet, not smoking, and getting enough exercise.

*Restricted breathing:* Restricted breathing can reduce circulation, metabolism, and interfere with the natural healing system in many other ways. The brain and nervous system especially require taking a good cleansing breath.

*Impaired defenses:* Natural healing is unlikely to occur if the body's defenses are weak. Decreased immunity happens when we have acquired: (a) persistent or overwhelming infections, (b) toxic forms of matter and energy that have entered our immune system, and (c) multiple stressors due to various mental health conditions. We can protect our immune system through good mental and physical health practices.

*Toxins:* Toxic overload is much more common than you think. We take in toxins through the food we eat, water we drink, air we breathe, use of pharmaceutical products, and unhealthy thoughts, feelings, and emotions. Toxic overload may be a significant cause of allergies, cancers, autoimmune diseases, and a variety of other chronic health conditions. Being educated about the various toxins we are exposed to on a daily basis is essential for good health.

*Age:* The myth that everyone who grows old will have lower immunity and become sick and diseased is not necessarily true. There are many cultures of the world that grow into extremely healthy individuals at an older age. The number one risk factor associated with age may be the American lifestyle.

*Obstruction of the mind:* Our thoughts and feelings have a major impact on our physical health. Persons who have acquired mental health conditions (e.g., depression, anxiety, substance abuse, stress-related disorders) become physically ill at much higher rates than individuals who are mentally and spiritually healthy. Thus, it is critical to maintain good mental health.

*Spiritual problems:* Many other world cultures believe that a harmony must exist between the mind, body, and spirit. Thus, increasing one's spiritual life is a protective factor. It is essential to maintain a balance of the mind, body, and spirit.

## Developing Goals and Opportunities for Personal Growth

There are three kinds of people in this world: (a) *list people*—those who write out "to-do" lists that need concrete and structured plans to live by; (b) *nonlist people*—those who do little preparation ahead of time, but when the time is right, they can get down to business and achieve at an optimal level of functioning; and (c) *combo people*—persons who combine both structured and nonstructured ways of living, depending on the situation and setting.

Developing concrete goals and objectives may not be a priority for you. It may work for others but not for you. Just the thought of structuring your day with a "to-do list" may really turn off your mind, body, and spirit. Regardless of your style of making commitment, you may benefit from reviewing the following examples of goal-oriented opportunities that some others have committed to and have achieved in optimizing their minds, bodies, and spirits.

I make an important distinction between *problem issues* and *goal-oriented opportunities*. If you are always dealing with a problem situation or issue, then you tend to be focused on things you are trying to avoid, reduce, or decrease in your life. However, if you can reframe your "problems" into goal-oriented opportunities, then your focus will be on things you can increase, draw closer to, and feel motivated by in your life. So, take this opportunity to review some sample goal-oriented opportunities listed next.

## Examples

► Identify the goal-oriented opportunity from your list (or nonlist) of things you want to change.

*Example:* I do not feel focused in life because I cannot concentrate. I feel overly anxious at times and can never seem to break away from my emotional stress.

► Turn the problem issue into a specific goal-oriented opportunity by stating the issue as something that needs to be done differently.

*Example:* I need to begin a program of stress reduction, perhaps using mindfulness meditation approaches. I would also like to begin journaling and then analyzing what I have written.

► For each goal-oriented opportunity, create a short-term objective that is measurable.

*Example:* You may want to state your short-term objectives in terms of:

- Frequency (e.g., I will meditate using a guided meditation/relaxation tape for 15 minutes a session, twice per day—once in the morning and once in the afternoon)

- Intensity (e.g., I will rate myself after each meditation session and during client sessions using my own Peace–Compassion scale that ranges from 1 to 10)

- Duration (e.g., I will use a guided meditation approach every day for 2 weeks with the anticipation that my stress levels will decrease during my client sessions)

- Amount (e.g., I will monitor the scores on my self-rating scale of Peace–Compassion and try to decrease my stress level by 10% each day)

► List out multiple support systems and resources to help achieve your goal-oriented opportunities.

*Example:* I will alternate using three different guided meditation tapes. I will spend a portion of my lunch break in meditation. I will ask my spouse for some quiet time so that I can focus on my self-care. I will review my journal entries daily so I can bring some meaning to this experience.

► Observe indicators of improvement—Make sure to include items that are measurable along with feelings, thoughts, behaviors, and experiences.

*Example:* My Peace–Compassion scale ratings have decreased from an "8" at work to a "5" this week. I appear to feel less distracted and more focused during client sessions. I also have an increased sense of compassion and empathy for the people I serve. Reading my journal entries helped me clarify why I chose this profession.

► List a plan of action for maintaining your goal-oriented opportunities by specifying multiple resources and opportunities.

*Example:* Buy new meditation tapes that have a variety of visualization and contemplative meditation experiences. Start a meditation group with my close friends or colleagues. Search for a yoga or tai chi instructor.

## WORKING WITH PERSONAL GROWTH IN GROUP WORK

### Purpose of Group Work

The purpose of facilitating or being a member of a process group is to cultivate a caring community of like-minded individuals who are having difficulties dealing with issues related to disaster and posttraumatic stress. Individuals function most of their lives within group settings (e.g., at work, home, community, church). There may be little opportunity for trauma survivors to be involved in a process group. Theefore, a process group may have to be formed in your community. You can ask your therapist or search the Internet for a support group in your town. It can be very beneficial and assist in building long-term relationships. The primary purpose of a process group is to: (a) provide a safe, secure, and confidential environment for the release of emotions in front of others who have the same or similar feelings, reactions, and experiences of trauma or disaster; (b) provide a support system of accountability where others can identify individuals within the group that may require more intensive help or special attention; (c) provide a resource for recommitment to personal growth opportunities; (d) share information, resources, and other supports with group members to assist one another in building coping and resiliency; and (e) cultivate seeds of hope by building a caring community of others that may be dealing with many of the same issues of trauma and disaster recovery.

### Choosing a Group Facilitator

It is strongly suggested during the first process group meeting that group participants select a facilitator or leader. In some cases, groups may choose a cofacilitator. Sometimes it is healthy for a group to rotate group facilitators. This can be arranged so each week a different person can be prepared to lead the group or group activity. Regardless of what your group chooses, the primary task of the group facilitator is to: (a) lead, present, or facilitate guided activities for the week; (b) take responsibility for keeping the group structure and rules intact; (c) ensure that the group as a whole is moving in a solution-focused oriented direction; and (d) model a cohesive environment that enhances positive interactions for the purpose of reducing empathy fatigue and increasing positive support and resources outside the group.

### Basic Protocol

Consider forming peer groups of approximately six to eight participants who all have similar experiences related to trauma and co-occurring conditions. It is important to meet on a regular basis and decide a beginning and ending point as well as how frequently you will meet. Group participants should choose a facilitator or be in agreement who the facilitator will be on a week-by-week basis. The facilitator should: (a) make sure that all participants introduce themselves or check in with the group; (b) discuss group rules, attendance, goals, issues of confidentiality, and the overall group process; (c) obtain consensus from the group regarding what issues will be dealt with and what is to be accomplished within each session; and (d) focus on positive coping strategies, attitudinal healing, and wellness among the group participants, with the goal of reducing posttrau-matic stressor and co-occurring conditions.

## Group Rules and Guidelines

1. *Maintain confidentiality:* This is absolutely critical in developing trust among other group participants. Building a working alliance is essential for disclosure and trust. Talking outside the group regarding others' personal issues is considered unethical and violates the person's privacy. Persons who violate such rules should not be asked back unless there is a consensus among group participants other-wise.

2. *Be an active listener:* Every group participant has something important to say. Even though there may be other group members who dominate the group, it is essential to listen carefully to what others have to communicate. Listening with compassion and empathy demonstrates respect for others in the group and will help you understand their point of view on a particular issue. There are other members who also want to express their thoughts and opinions. We forget this group etiquette sometimes. Be open to the idea that we may learn something from other group members although we do not always have to accept their worldview on certain issues.

3. *Express your own ideas:* You have something important to say also. Sharing your thoughts, feelings, and experiences with the group on a particular topic makes a contribution and may stimulate other creative ideas.

4. *Communicate honestly, concretely, and openly:* Giving positive feedback to other group participants is important. You can accomplish this by being genuine and communicating openly and honestly with others. As a group participant, you can expect to receive from the group what you are willing to contribute. How you respond to others also affects how they respond to you.

5. *Problem solve as a team:* Problems are best solved when working together coopera-tively with others. When conflict or problems arise, think of creative alternatives and options for resolution to keep the group moving in a positive direction.

## Suggested Group Protocol: A Three-Phase Approach

Since some individuals in your process group may have had other experiences leading a peer-process group, too many leaders can be toxic to the group process. If each partici-pant takes responsibility as a group facilitator, then each is empowered with the same responsibility for a healthy process group environment. In the following, I have offered a three-phase group structure to help initiate specific activities. This protocol also serves as a way to monitor the progress of your process group. Be mindful that the three-phase protocol is flexible and should be designed for your particular agency, organization, and interests. Each phase varies depending on the participants in your group. Some groups may take several sessions to complete one particular phase, while others may take longer in other phases.

## Phase 1: Opening and Emotional Check-In

1. Assuming that all the group rules and structure have been fully determined and discussed, the group facilitator should provide an opportunity for each participant to give a check-in. The group check-in process should allow individuals 4 to 5 minutes each to disclose a particular issue, emotion, or experience that they are struggling with as it relates to their experience of extraordinary stressful or traumatic events. The purpose of the check-in is to allow all group members to become aware of how each participant is currently functioning and what issues each individual plans to work on during the process group. Members should be encouraged to begin their check-in statements using feeling words and good "I" statements so they can take ownership with their current mind, body, or spiritual wellness.

2. After all members have checked in, the group facilitator can begin the group process by asking participants what issues they would like to deal with first, second, third, and so forth. There should be group consensus on what issues need to be addressed within the average 90-minute group session.

3. Participants are encouraged to initiate the PGP-HT, as described earlier in this chapter. Individuals may use this opportunity to share and discuss the obstacles or struggles they may be experiencing with their personal growth.

## Phase 2: Working Phase—Mapping Your Path

1. The goal of this phase is to further build a trusting and working alliance within the group so that each person feels comfortable enough to disclose personal issues. Groups that work well together in this phase have a high level of trust and provide support for one another, even through difficult emotional periods.

2. The group facilitator should allow members to vent. However, the goals of this phase must be solution focused on developing a more effective and functional personal and professional life. Group participants should assist others within the group to look for any obstacles that may be in the way for achieving a more effective personal and professional quality of life. The most important aspect of this phase is insight, awareness, and being able to look at one's unused talents and opportunities.

3. Participants are encouraged to discuss the "Self-Assessment" questions as delineated in the PGP-HT as a means for looking at individual growth and change.

## Phase 3: Choosing a Path—Getting Group Closure

1. A primary reason that we do not meet our own expectations in life is that we fail to take responsibility and follow-through on the plans we have made. The PGP-HT was developed as a way to try and initiate a plan of action and take responsibility for your own personal and professional wellness. The final phase of your process group or last several sessions is to choose a path and cultivate those resources that can support you in accomplishing your goals. Remember that there are many different paths you can take to get you to where you are going in life. It may not necessarily include the PGP-HT model.

2. Suggested guided activities:

   Individuals may want to create *goal-oriented opportunities* as developed by the PGP model, or verbally make a commitment to others in the group. This may begin by listing resources in your environment that have the potential for making a significant impact in your life (e.g., teacher, mentor, minister/spiritual person, family, friends, a particular professional helper or provider of services). Participants may want to continue to network with others in the group after termination of the process group. It may be helpful to share specific resources, contacts, or other activities that have helped you accomplish your *goal-oriented opportunities* as you have documented in your PGP-HT. After you have fully addressed an issue and have gotten closure, choose another item that you may have rank ordered and begin working on this.

3. Group closure is an important aspect of Phase 3. Some groups may have reached their goals after several sessions together, while others may stay together for several months. Regardless of how many sessions your group has spent together, the facilitator should allow each person to make some final comments regarding the group process or about someone else in the group. The facilitator may challenge group members with solution-focused questions such as: *If we came in contact with you a few weeks or months from now, what would we see different about you (e.g., emotionally, physically, cognitively, spiritually)?*

## CONCLUDING REMARKS

The PGP-HT is a dynamic, interactive, and solution-focused approach for exploring posttraumatic growth and resiliency. Mostly, it provides an opportunity for early identification, assessment, and recommended interventions for dealing with a range of issues affecting the mind, body, and spirit of trauma survivors.

Personal growth and development are essential to maintain wellness of the mind, body, and spirit. The PGP-HT is adaptive, flexible, organized, and has intentions to offer guidelines to disaster mental health counselors as a structured approach for cultivating resiliency for healing trauma. It also has the potential for healing empathy fatigue and other professional fatigue syndromes that draw energy away from one's mind, body, and spirit. Overall, the journey to heal from disaster or trauma should begin with leaving "no stone unturned."

## REFERENCES

Egan, G. (2014). *The skilled helper: A problem-management and opportunity-development approach to helping* (10th ed.). Belmont, CA: Brooks/Cole.

Elliott, W. (1996). *Tying rocks to clouds: Meetings and conversations with wise and spiritual people.* New York, NY: Image Books/Double Day.

Harner, M. (2016). The foundation for shamanic studies. Retrieved from https://www.shamanism.org

Pirsig, R. M. (1976). *Zen and the art of motorcycle maintenance.* New York, NY: Bantam Books.

Prochaska, J. O., & DiClemente, C. C. (1982). Trans-theoretical therapy: Toward a more integrative model of change. *Psychotherapy: Theory, Research and Practice, 19*, 276–288. http://dx.doi.org/10.1037/h0088437

Prochaska, J. O., DiClemente, C. C., & Norcross, J. C. (1992). In search of how people change. *American Psychologist, 47*, 1102–1104.

Weil, A. (1995). *Spontaneous healing.* New York, NY: Ballantine.

# INDEX

Printed in the USA
CPSIA information can be obtained
at www.ICGtesting.com
CBHW051226210124
PP14819300001B/6